Sexy Hormones

Unlocking the Secrets to Vitality

Lorna R. Vanderhaeghe M.S.
and
Dr. Alvin Pettle M.D.

Fitzhenry & Whiteside

Sexy Hormones: Unlocking the Secrets to Vitality
Copyright © 2007 Lorna R. Vanderhaeghe M.S. and Alvin Pettle, M.D.

Fitzhenry and Whiteside Limited
195 Allstate Parkway, Markham, Ontario L3R 4T8
In the United States:
311 Washington Street, Brighton, Massachusetts 02135
www.fitzhenry.ca   godwit@fitzhenry.ca

Fitzhenry & Whiteside acknowledges with thanks the Canada Council for the Arts, and the Ontario Arts Council for their support of our publishing program. We acknowledge the financial support of the Government of Canada through the Book Publishing Industry Development Program (BPIDP) for our publishing activities.

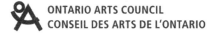

Library and Archives Canada Cataloguing in Publication
Vanderhaeghe, Lorna R.
Sexy hormones : unlocking the secrets to vitality / Lorna R.
Vanderhaeghe & Alvin Pettle.
Includes bibliographical references and index.
ISBN 978-1-55455-015-9
1. Middle-aged women—Sexual behavior. 2. Menopause.
3. Hormones, Sex. I. Pettle, Alvin, 1945- II. Title.
RG121.V35 2007   613.9'54   C2006-904452-X
United States Cataloguing-in-Publication Data
Vanderhaeghe, Lorna R.
Sexy hormones : unlocking the secrets to vitality / Lorna R. Vanderhaeghe ; Alvin Pettle.
[256] p. : cm.
Summary: A complete guide to realizing sexual potential through hormones.
ISBN-13: 978-155455-015-9 (pbk.)
1. Hormones, Sex. I. Pettle, Alvin. II. Title.
613.954 dc22   RG121.V3634 2007

Permission granted by ZRT Laboratory http://www.zrtlab.com for illustration on page 4.

All drawings on pages 186 – 197 are from Lorna Vanderhaeghe, The Body Sense Natural Diet: Six Weeks to a Slimmer, Healthier You, courtesy John Wiley & Sons Canada, Ltd.
NOTE: If you are taking prescription medications consult your physician before applying the recommendations in the book. If you are taking Coumadin or Warfarin you should not change your diet, add any new drugs either over-the-counter or prescription or add any new supplements without consulting your physician.

DISCLAIMER: This publication contains the opinions and ideas of its authors and is designed to provide useful advice in regard to the subject matter covered. The authors and publisher are not engaged in rendering medical, therapeutic, or other professional services in this publication. This publication is not intended to provide a basis for action in particular circumstances without consideration by a competent professional. The authors and publisher expressly disclaim any responsibility for any liability, loss, or risk, personal or otherwise, which is incurred as a consequence, directly or indirectly, of the use and application of any of the contents of this book.

Cover design by Kerry Plumley
Interior design by Karen Thomas, Intuitive Design International Ltd.
Illustrations by Michael Petherick
Printed and bound in Canada

1 3 5 7 9 10 8 6 4 2

Contents

Prologue

AN ANCIENT ADAGE from Chinese medicine states, "A doctor would rather treat 10 men than one woman." In a way, this validates what women have always known—that they are indeed intricate creatures. At the heart of a woman's complexity are her hormones, their ebb and flow influencing all aspects of physical, emotional and mental wellness. Sexy hormones are sex hormones including, but not limited too, estrogen, testosterone, DHEA and progesterone. When a woman's hormones are in balance, she feels fabulous, has energy and is vital. She is also far less likely to experience symptoms through her fertile years and during the transition through menopause. Unfortunately, all it takes is one alteration to this perfectly orchestrated process for hormone havoc to ensue.

Understanding the ebb and flow of female sex hormones means untangling a complex feedback loop between the brain, ovaries and adrenal glands. Correcting an imbalance in hormones is complicated by the fact that not only does the body produce hormones but the environment is loaded with hormone mimickers that are adding to the overall hormonal confusion.

In the last five years women have finally been told that commonly prescribed synthetic hormones may come with enormous health implications. In 2002 the Women's Health Initiative Estrogen and Progestin Study (WHI) was halted due to serious safety concerns. For over five decades women used estrogen and progestin to treat menopause symptoms and to prevent heart disease, Alzheimer's, bone loss and more. The WHI study found that women taking a combination of synthetic estrogen and progestin had a 26 percent increase in invasive breast cancer, a 29 percent increase in heart attacks, double the risk of dementia, double the risk of blood clots and a 41 percent increase in stroke. It also found that breasts became so dense breast cancer could not be read on a mammogram, and asthma and hearing loss were also increased. An extension of this study using estrogen only was halted less than a year later because of an increased risk of stroke and dementia. Millions of women threw their hormones in the garbage and many doctors stopped prescribing them altogether. The results left many women suffering severe menopause symptoms and fearing that maybe all those years of taking hormones potentially increased the risk of those conditions they were trying to prevent. Since the decline in synthetic hormone use, the United States recorded in 2003 the largest single yearly decline in the incidence of estrogen-receptor positive breast cancer for woman aged 50 to 69.

Physicians and women alike are learning that the love affair with estrogen, in particular, can be a very dangerous liaison. Dr. Jerilynn Prior, reknowned professor of endocrinology at the University of British Columbia's Center for Menstrual Cycle and Ovulation Research, has found many of her patients are experiencing what she calls "estrogen's storm." Estrogen dominance or too much estrogen put women at greater risk of developing breast cancer, uterine fibroids, endometriosis, no sex drive, ovarian cysts and much more.

Estrogen is responsible for the soft curve of a woman's body and fertility. A natural rise in estrogen every month in a reproductive-aged woman is designed to get her uterus ready for pregnancy. Every woman is unique regarding "how much" estrogen is needed. However, estrogens found in the environment, in such common products as cosmetics, plastics, water, dairy products, red meat, chicken and pesticides, to name but a few, create chronically high out-of-balance hormones that lead to "estrogen dominance." Dr. John Lee, M.D. pioneer of natural progesterone therapy coined this term. Before his death Lee worked tirelessly to convince the medical establishment that too much estrogen—not a deficiency in estrogen—was the root cause of most women's hormonal problems.

Dr. Prior has continued his work and today estrogen dominance remains contentious. And it should not considering we are being bombarded by estrogens and other hormones on a daily basis. Synthetic estrogens found in birth control pills, fertility drugs, and other hormone therapies are major sources of estrogen that contribute to estrogen overload. Women are fooled into believing the birth control pill is safe because it is "low dose." Low dose means lower than previous years but the pill contains many times a woman's natural level of estrogen. The birth control pill launched in the 1960s to provide women with sexual freedom and liberation from unwanted pregnancies is known to increase the risk of breast cancer, promote endometrial and fibroid tissue growth and halt testosterone's libido enhancing effects. New research found in the pages of this book shows that women may have traded the freedom to have sex without worry of pregnancy for a reduction or elimination of sex drive. What's worse the pill is being prescribed for acne, endometriosis, heavy periods and uterine fibroids—yet no research has been done on using the pill for these conditions. We believe that future research on the pill's safety will confirm what we have learned about estrogen and progestin used for menopausal concerns—that the pill is contributing to hormone diseases in women.

Food is also a contributor to hormone havoc. Two watch dog groups the Toronto-based Environmental Defence and the U.S. Environmental Working Group, state a large percentage of our exposure to dangerous hormone-mimickers comes from our diet, especially fish, meats, chicken, dairy products and pesticide-laden fruits and vegetables. The Sexy Hormone Diet in Chapters 6 and 7 teaches you which foods balance or disrupt hormones and which foods rev up sex drive.

Hormone-mimicking foods have added to the obesity epidemic. Too much fat on the body adds to hormone hell because fat cells, through an enzyme, convert testosterone into estrogens. The more fat cells you have the higher your total estrogen. Excess insulin or insulin resistance, common in the overweight, also causes estrogen dominance. As insulin levels spike, estrogen is secreted in higher amounts. And cortisol, our stress hormone, promotes estrogen dominance and more weight gain creating a viscous cycle of more fat cells that become even fatter and produce even more estrogen.

Sexy Hormones delves deep into these issues weeding out the hype from the research. And there is a lot of hype. You will learn that hormones are powerful messengers that direct and control every function in the body from heart rate to orgasms.

We called this book *Sexy Hormones* because all sex hormones contribute to the vibrancy of your health, stamina and vitality. We wanted to clear up the confusion on how to use hormones safely to treat female conditions. Suzanne Somers made a valiant attempt to bring bioidentical hormone therapy to the masses in her book the *Sexy Years*. Unfortunately, the medical profession attacked her and the media was more than happy to cover the story. In this book bioidentical hormone therapies are discussed in detail. But more importantly this book advises when to have hormone testing, what type of testing to have performed, and whether you are a candidate for bioidentical hormones and what all the information means to your optimal health. We even included prescriptions for bioidentical hormones in case your physician is not versed on the subject of natural hormone treatment. Our goal throughout *Sexy Hormones* is providing safe, effective treatments that get you feeling fabulous.

Sexual desire and satisfaction are affected by hormone havoc. Our feelings of being "sexy" are hormone driven. *Sexy Hormones* solves the mysteries of female sexual health. Sex is a central part of who we are. It is the basis for our relationships. Men are being prescribed the "little blue pill" in record numbers and you can't turn on your computer without being bombarded by spam to make "it" bigger, longer and stronger. Yet 43 percent of women have NO sex drive, many women are suffering with pain during intercourse and not much is being done in the research community to help these women. We have provided very frank information about female sexuality—everything from the anatomy of a woman's genitals to how to have an orgasm. We even include information on aphrodisiacs, tips and toys. Every woman should read this book and moms and grandmothers should pass this book on to their daughters. In essence we provide a complete guide to understanding *your* sexy hormones—enjoy!

Foreword

If you have read the book *The Secret* by Rhonda Byrne, you will know that the universe responds to the law of attraction. It is the very reason that you are reading this book right now. What we as humans put out into the universe will be what we will get back. Lorna Vanderhaeghe and I have been drawn together by a common factor—we are both trying to understand and learn how women can live healthy lives. In this book, we share our journey with you to help you understand the value and wisdom of preventive medicine.

You will learn about the proper use of vitamins, minerals, and herbs, as well as bioidentical hormones and their role in women's health. You will also come to understand how to balance the complicated lives and multiple roles that women have to play each and every day of their lives: be it as the inquisitive teenager, the young mother, the passionate wife, the caring sister, the loving daughter, the dependable co-worker, the respected boss, the constant housekeeper, the sexy girlfriend, and the wise grandmother.

Sexy Hormones outlines the investigation, diagnosis, and treatment of many of the women's conditions caused by estrogen dominance. Most important, we have included the proper tests to assess hormone status and the follow-up required when using bioidentical hormones. You will discover that conditions such as PMS, endometriosis, fibroids, ovarian cysts, and fibrocystic breast disease can all be prevented and treated. You will also discover the high rate of serious diseases, such as cancer of the breasts, ovaries, and uterus, can be significantly decreased with the knowledge of estrogen dominance and how to prevent it. Learn about the role of exercise and nutrition and how these two together can lead to good health. Did you know that if you exercise three hours a week, you will decrease your risk of breast cancer by 50 percent? Do you know the foods that cause cancer and the food that prevent cancer? Has your physician talked to you about the importance of supplements such as I3C and coenzyme Q_{10}?

Sexy Hormones gives you clear and thoughtful advice on how to prevent illness as well as how to enjoy your wellbeing. It includes tips on how you can enhance your life and make the time to come not just the next years of your life but also the best years of your life. You will find that you and only you are the master of your ship. You are the guiding light to your own health. Lorna and I are just here to remind you of your own intuitive wisdom.

The words in this book will echo true to you because they come from a place of truth. Lorna has dedicated her life to this quest. Her words ring true to me, and I have had the privilege of caring for women for 38 years as an obstetrician and gynecologist. During that time I was fortunate enough to have attended 10,000 deliveries and not once have I not marveled at the strengths and compassion that women have shown during pregnancy and labor. Helen Reddy was right when she sang, "I am invincible, I am Woman." Any man who has attended a woman in labor knows which is the stronger sex!

Lorna's message flows from her heart to the page. Her mind and her soul are within this book, and you can feel it. The words are the body of the book, but it is the soul of a woman that will know they are true. Although I am a man, my soul also understands my role in the message of this book, and I understand the responsibility I have in my life. I have been very fortunate for I have been allowed to do what I was truly meant to do. All that I have ever learned in the practice of medicine has come from women. I feel that Lorna and I are in harmony with each other. Sometimes when I read her notes, I would make comments beside the paragraph and laugh with approval as the next paragraph contained the very thought I had written. The reason our thoughts were synchronistic is because we both have heard the same words and felt the same things. Although we live on different sides of the continent, the message is universal and the solution is within us all. All each of us ever has to do is listen to our intuition and have an open mind to the concept of a healthy and balanced life.

With this book women can once again enjoy their sexuality and learn some new methods to keep this part of them alive and very well. *Sexy Hormones* outlines the use of bioidentical hormones such as progesterone, Bi-Est, estriol, and testosterone. Hormones should fit their receptors like a lock and key, and, if they fit properly, the body uses them and removes them within 12 hours. Synthetic hormones do not fit the lock, and the body has a hard time getting rid of them; the half-life of a synthetic hormone can be thirty-six hours. This means if you take synthetic hormones every day, you cannot get rid of them and they become toxic. Natural hormones are good for you, if used in the proper amounts and monitored with the proper tests. Although blood tests are very helpful, and I use them, the accurate testing is in the use of saliva testing, and the use of saliva testing is outlined for you here.

Sexy Hormones also details the basics of sexuality and orgasm, outlines the use of vaginal lubricants, and, of course, goes into detail about the use of vaginal estriol (the safe estrogen), as well as the use of clitoral creams that contain menthol and arginine, the amino acid needed for orgasm. You will also find out about the use of transdermal testosterone (the hormone of desire); this hormone can safely be applied to the lower half of the body and the doses can be increased while the blood levels are monitored. Natural testosterone not only increases sexuality, it also increases the sense of wellbeing, assertiveness, and muscle strength.

Sexy Hormones also passionately asks you to be good to yourself. Listen to the message. Be good to yourself, be very good to yourself. You deserve it! May all the days of your life be enhanced by the knowledge you receive from this book. This book is timely—"An army can be defeated, but not an idea whose time has come," and the message of preventive medicine's time has come. It is our fervent wish that with this knowledge we can save our children and their children's children from the estrogen dominance our generation has suffered. I lost my mother to breast cancer, and I live each day with the hope that I can prevent at least one woman from ever having breast cancer, believing that, "If you save one life, you save a whole civilization."

We hope the message in *Sexy Hormones* will be like a pebble tossed into a pond, and that it will ripple for all eternity. We hope that by picking up this book you will not only learn about the good health you have a right to have but that you will share this knowledge with someone you love as well. The universe wants you to be happy; it needs you to be healthy. You possess the ability to prevent illness; you possess the ability to live a happy, healthy, and sexy life. Enjoy each word we have written. It came from a place of love. May it find your heart—for truly what is written from the heart will go to the heart. It is women like Lorna Vanderhaeghe who continue to inspire me and make me want to be a better man. May this book also inspire you. Thank you for your gift, Lorna.

Dr. Alvin Pettle F.R.C.S, OBS and GYN

Introduction:
Hormone Havoc

What Dr. Pettle and I call "hormone havoc" results in some of the more common complaints of modern women—exhaustion, infertility, insomnia, fibroids, heavy menstrual bleeding, or drenching night sweats. This is just a partial list of what can happen when your hormones—in particular what we call your "sexy hormones"—are not performing as they should. You may have picked up this book because you are experiencing some of these problems.

What causes these symptoms? In a perfect world, all the interdependent parts and processes of your body are supporting each other for optimal function. Hormones regulate cell function and influence cellular activity, and they do this best when their levels are what we call "balanced"—the amounts of hormones in your system are not too low and not too high. They are "just right." This means that the level of each hormone is enough to do the job assigned without interfering with the work of any other hormone or body system.

When hormone levels are not "just right," body processes malfunction in grand or subtle ways, and the results wreak havoc on your sleep, your temper, your libido, and your life. This imbalance can happen at any time in a woman's life. Sometimes the imbalance is due to internal factors like too much estrogen being produced in relation to progesterone. Other times, estrogen from environmental sources may be creating hormone upheaval. Too much estrogen from either source creates a condition called estrogen dominance. In order to create hormone balance, hormones from the environment *and* hormones produced by the body have to be considered when making adjustments. It is startling for most people to learn that there is estrogen everywhere in the environment and that estrogen is affecting not only women, but men, our children, and babies too.

Environmental Hormones, Sexless Alligators, and YOU

In the early 1970s, biologists began counting alligators in Lake Apopka, Florida, an ideal place to hatch baby alligators. In the early 1980s, researchers would often see up to 2,000 alligators a night on the lake. But by the late 1980s, they were finding, at most, only 150 per night, and the alligators they found had some big (or small) worries. The males' penises were only one-quarter of the normal size, and their testosterone levels were so low the alligators were sterile and unable to do their part in making baby alligators. The researchers eventually discovered that some poisonous substances (for example, DDT breakdown products (metabolites)) had similar effects on mice, and it turned out that thousands of gallons of these same poisons (DDT-containing pesticides) had spilled into Lake Apopka in the 1980s. Lake Apopka's alligators were living in a sea of sex-hormone-destroying chemicals. What does this have to do with you? Well, we are all living in an estrogen stew.

Pesticides are estrogen-like in their chemical structure. The alligators had absorbed the pesticides from the water, and being estrogenic, the pesticide molecules were similar enough in structure to the alligators' own estrogen that the estrogen imposters were able to pose as natural estrogens. Substances that are man-made and similar in structure to the body's own estrogen are called "estrogen mimickers." Surrounded by estrogen-mimickers, the male alligators started to become more and more female-like; in fact they were becoming hermaphrodites—creatures that could not be classified as male or female because they had sex characteristics of both.

The estrogen mimickers not only created serious problems in the sexual development of the male alligators, they also interfered with the healthy development of the female alligators. As a result, there were no more baby alligators in Lake Apopka.

Estrogen mimickers do not restrict their impact to alligators. Florida panthers eat animals that have eaten other animals or fish that are contaminated with pesticides and other estrogenic compounds, and the panthers have their own reproductive problems: more infertile females and sterile males, lower sperm counts, and high levels of estrogens. In March 1994, toxicologist Dr. Charles F. Facemire of the United States Fish and Wildlife Service said that the male panthers had estrogen levels higher than those of most female panthers.

Canada and Russia's polar bears are also suffering the ill effects of estrogen mimickers. Polar bears eat a diet of fatty ringed seals almost exclusively. The seals provide energy, but they also pass along persistent organic pollutants, such as polychlorinated biphenyls (PCBs) and chlorinated pesticides, that have accumulated in their fatty tissue from eating contaminated fish and shellfish. According to scientists, these concentrations multiply five- to ten-fold with every step in the food chain, putting top feeders like polar bears, which eat the other animals, at the highest risk for health effects. High levels of the pesticide chlordane, PCBs, and other estrogenic compounds have been found in polar bears. Because these compounds are stored in fat reserves, female bears, fetuses, and cubs are at the highest risk from the toxic effects because the females fast for up to seven months of the year, using up fat stores loaded with toxins. During the first two years of the polar bear cubs' lives, they have PCB concentrations about twice that of their mothers, largely because these contaminants accumulate in the milk they feed on.

Environment Canada and researchers at the University of British Columbia have found these estrogenic compounds are interfering with testosterone metabolism in male polar bears as well. And Carleton University researchers announced that estrogen mimickers found in polar bear blood interfere with the transport of vitamin A and one of the thyroid hormones.

What does this mean for humans? Literally hundreds of chemicals found in the environment—PCBs, pesticides, polycarbons used in many plastics, chlorine-containing compounds, fire retardants, and synthetic estrogens and estrogen metabolites that enter the water supply courtesy of the urine of women taking oral synthetic estrogens—resemble human estrogens. They affect humans the same way they affect alligators, panthers, and polar bears. The Inuit women in northern Quebec, Canada eat marine mammals, and their breast milk has been found to contain PCB concentrations two to ten times higher than that of women in the southern part of the province.

The molecules of estrogen mimickers are identical enough to human estrogens to fit into the same cell receptor sites—the estrogen parking spots—that the body's naturally produced hormones would use. There is plenty of evidence that these environmental estrogens affect the human hormone system.

- In 1994, the research of Danish endocrinologist Dr. N. Skakkebaek indicated that since 1938, sperm counts in men in the United States and 20 other countries have decreased by an average of 50 percent, and testicular cancer rates have tripled.

- Women who eat meat high in estrogen mimickers are at higher risk of having sons with smaller testicles and penises and/or testicular and penis malformations.

- A German study published in 1994 reported that women with endometriosis were more likely to have high levels of PCBs in their blood.

- A study published in 1993 by New York's Mount Sinai School of Medicine found that women with the greatest number of DDE markers (a DDT metabolite) are four times more likely to get breast cancer.

- Girls as young as eight years old are now having periods (this is called precocious puberty), possibly due to high levels of estrogens in the environment.

Ana Soto, associate professor of Anatomy and Cellular Biology at Tufts University, points out that the body eliminates natural estrogen cyclically. Many estrogen mimickers, on the other hand, are not eliminated. Instead, they accumulate in fatty tissues such as those in the breast, where they remain even after menopause, when natural estrogen levels drop. In Israel between 1976 and 1986, breast cancer deaths (which had been continually rising for 25 years) dropped eight percent. In 1978, Israel had banned three organochlorine pesticides: DDT, alpha-benzene hexachloride (BHC), and gamma-benzene hexachloride (lindane). Before the ban these pesticides had been used in cowsheds. As a result, pesticide levels in Israeli milk soared up to 100 times. Within two years of the ban, DDT, BHC, and lindane levels in milk had dropped dramatically.

"Xenoestrogens" (pronounced *zeno-estrogens*) is the technical name for this class of man-made chemicals that mimic the effect of estrogens. When xenoestrogens (also called environmental estrogens) are absorbed by the human body, they are highly cancer-causing and hormone-disruptive. Xenoestrogens contribute to estrogen-dominant conditions, breast cancer, uterine cancer, fibrocystic breast disease, ovarian cysts, endometriosis, premature sexual development, uterine fibroids, heavy periods, and infertility.

Sources of Xenoestrogens

Everyone in North America is exposed to estrogen mimickers every day; check the following list of sources.

- **Pesticides**: Pesticides are used on animals, farms, lawns, and golf courses. (Golf courses use seven times the amount of pesticides that farmers use.) The term "pesticide" includes herbicides and fungicides, and all of these easily enter the body through the skin and lungs. And an enhancing effect is known to occur when using more than one pesticide in a single application, promoting greater toxicity and estrogen effect. Pesticides include: Methoxychlor (used on fruits and vegetables and, sprayed on beef and cows to kill insects), Kelthane (used on cucumbers, tomatoes, lettuce, strawberries, and apples), Kepone (used on bananas, tobacco, ants and roaches), Lindane (used on crops and in head lice treatments), Chlordane (used to kill termites, and on home lawns and gardens), and Atrazine (weed control).

- **Beef**: Cattle for beef production in both Canada and the U.S. are given zeranol or estradiol, as well as testosterone or trenbolone acetate. (It likely never occurred to you that beef cattle need hormone replacement therapy.) All of these hormones are estrogenic or, in the case of testosterone, convert into estrogens. Cows are big animals, and high levels of estrogens have been found in North American beef products.

- **Dairy Products**: *The International Journal of Cancer* published a joint study as part of the National Enhanced Cancer Surveillance System, and it reported a strong association between the consumption of cheese and the risk of getting testicular cancer. They found the increase stemmed from the high amounts of the hormones estrogen and progesterone in Canadian dairy products. Testicular cancer has been growing more prevalent over the last few decades, becoming the leading cancer among young men at a time when more people are ingesting dairy products. Researchers stated that dairy foods contain high levels of female sex hormones. Cows in the U.S. are also given bovine growth hormone (BGH) so they can produce more milk. BGH is banned for use in Canada.

- **Cosmetics**: Make-up, shampoos, conditioners, shaving creams, and deodorants using phthalates or parabens are another source of xenoestrogens. Preservatives used in skin lotions, suntan lotions, and body lotions, including parabens such as methyl paraben, ethyl paraben, proply paraben, and butyl paraben, are estrogenic. These preservatives are found in the vast majority of skin and body lotions. When purchasing natural progesterone creams, make sure you ask for a clean base that is free of parabens and phthalates. See www.ewg.org to find out if your cosmetics contain toxic estrogenic compounds.

- **Plastics**: Bisphenol-A and phthalates are used to make plastics. The bisphenol-A prevents plastic from breaking down in sunlight. Bisphenol-A is used to make drinking water bottles, plastic baby bottles, plastics used to pack food, and some dental composites. Bisphenol-A contamination has been found in the majority of canned foods because the tins are lined with it. Amounts as high as 27 times the minimum amount of estrogen used to stimulate breast cancer cell growth in test tubes were found in canned food. Be aware that heating plastics, for example, in your microwave or in the case of plastic bottles left out in the sunshine, releases these chemicals into the food or beverage that is stored in them. In one Dartmouth University study, the researchers found that microwaved plastic wrap that had olive oil on it produced a concentration of xenoestrogens 500,000 times the minimum amount of estrogen needed to produce breast cancer cell proliferation in a test tube. When you use plastic wrap on your food to stop splattering in the microwave, tiny droplets of these xenoestrogens are released onto your food. Never microwave anything in plastic or covered in plastic.

- **Cleaning Chemicals**: Ordinary household cleaners such as laundry and dish detergent break down into chemicals that include nonylphenol and octylphenol. Laundry detergent persists in clothes, even after the rinse cycle. As clothes are worn or sheets and towels are used, the skin is exposed to the estrogenic compounds. Bacteria naturally found on the skin break down the estrogenic compounds from the soap residues, and the estrogenic metabolites are then absorbed by the skin.

- **Dryer fabric softener sheets and fabric softeners** may contain one or several of the following chemicals: benzyl acetate, Benzyl alcohol, ethanol, A-terpineol, ethyl acetate, camphor, chloroform, linalool, or pentane. These are also broken down and absorbed by the skin.

- **Farmed fish**: Herbicides are used to keep sea lice under control in sea-based farms, and algaecides are used in above-ground fish farms. When choosing protein sources, opt for free-range poultry and eggs, and choose wild fish over farm-grown fish to avoid contamination from those chemicals.

- **Bleaching chemicals**: The chlorine-bleaching process used to whiten tampons, pads, and toilet paper produces the chemical dioxin as a by-product. Dioxins, fragrances and deodorants, and pesticides, which are all estrogenic, may be lurking in your tampons and pads. Tampons, unless stated to be cotton, are rayon, and rayon is a synthetic often made from wood pulp, which contains dioxin. You can purchase cotton pads and tampons that are 100 percent organic; if you do not, you may also be getting a dose of dioxin or pesticides.

- **Pharmaceuticals**: Synthetic estrogens (Prempro, DES, and Premarin), Cimetidine (Tagamet), and birth control pills are all toxic estrogens. The *Pharmaceutical Desk Reference* (PDR) lists gynecomastia (breast enlargement in men) as a side effect for Tagamet. Also, xenoestrogens have been found in spermicides. These estrogenic compounds are stored in fat cells. Furthermore, not only do these chemicals affect those who are prescribed them, but once the chemicals are flushed out of the body via the urine, they go into the general water system and affect us all as we eat the fish and shellfish or drink the contaminated water.

How Xenoestrogens Affect You

Chemicals enter your body when you eat, drink, or breathe and are distributed throughout your body via normal body processes. Chemicals that are not removed efficiently by your body's detoxification pathways (such as your liver) accumulate. Those that are fat-soluble, notably PCBs and pesticides, accumulate in your fat cells. Your fat stores are mobilized during times of stress, malnutrition, pregnancy, or even perspiration, and these chemicals are re-released into your blood circulation. The result can be one (or more) of a number of conditions you will see classed as "estrogen-dominant" conditions later in this book. They result when your body's level of estrogen is too high.

Hormones made by your body are neutralized by sex-hormone-binding substances that bind the majority of the hormones in your blood, thereby reducing their availability for initiating responses. It has been found, however, that numerous xenoestrogens, despite their chemical similarity, bind far less to the hormone-binding substances than do the hormones produced by your body, leaving more free xenoestrogens available to bind with estrogen receptor sites on the cells. Furthermore, it has been found that if several of these xenoestrogens are absorbed together, their effects are magnified, so exposure to even small quantities of a range of xenoestrogens can add up to a large impact. Many xenoestrogens, particularly fat-soluble ones, can also travel into the system of a fetus from the mother's blood.

Birth Control Pills are a Dangerous Xenoestrogen

The pill is prescribed for many "non-contraceptive" reasons (from acne to fibroids) with no consideration as to safety from breast cancer and blood clots. Women taking "low dose" birth control pill are getting more estrogen than what is recommended for menopausal women. "Low dose means lower than before," which is still a problem as the research shows.

Some of the common side effects associated with the birth control pill include spotting, nausea, headaches, decreased sexual desire, vomiting and other stomach complaints, weight gain, breast changes, water retention, vaginal or bladder infections, skin rashes, and changes in the eyes, causing some to become intolerant to contact lenses. The less common but more serious side-effects include: blood clots, heart attack, high blood pressure, high cholesterol, diabetes, elevation of cortisol (stress hormone) and prolactin levels, changes in thyroid hormones, and uterine and cervical cancer. Some researchers, including Dr. Louise Brinton, epidemiologist at the National Cancer Institute, say taking oral contraceptives for five years or more increases estrogen levels associated with breast cancer.

Taking a combined oral contraceptive increases the risk of developing a blood clot by three to four times if you are on a second generation pill, six to eight times if you are taking a third generation pill, and possibly over eight times for those on pills containing cyproterone (Diane 35). Women using progestin-only pills are at little or no increased risk of blood clots.

In addition to its birth control function, the Pill is prescribed for many peri-menopausal conditions, including endometriosis, acne, uterine fibroids, breast lumps, ovarian cysts, heavy periods, thickened uterine lining, and more. Estrogen replacement therapy (which includes the Pill) that is not monitored with appropriate testing is a significant cause of estrogen-dominant conditions.

The Pill, even the low-dose pill, contains seven times the estrogens often given to women to treat the symptoms of menopause. Women over age 35 cannot stay on the Pill long-term due to concerns about developing blood clots and cardiovascular problems, so what happens when women come off all this estrogen? The answer is more heavy periods, clotting, and enhanced fibroid growth, potentially ending in hysterectomy as the "treatment." (Just turning 40 and entering peri-menopause puts women at high risk for hysterectomy.)

Now research published in the *Journal of Sexual Medicine* shows the Pill has a very negative effect on testosterone levels that persists long after a woman has stopped taking it. Researchers measured levels of sex-hormone-binding globulin (SHBG) in women before and after they stopped taking the Pill. Sex-hormone-binding globulin is a protein that binds testosterone, making it unavailable to receptors, so women do not benefit from testosterone's effects. Testosterone's positive effects include maintaining a healthy sex drive, lubrication, the ability to achieve orgasm, increased endurance and muscle tone, and overall vitality. Researchers found that women who had taken the Pill had low unbound testosterone and more symptoms of low libido, vaginal dryness, and pain during intercourse than women who had never taken the Pill, and these levels remained low long after discontinuing the contraceptive.

The research involved 124 peri-menopausal women with sexual health complaints for more than six months. The three groups of women included 62 oral contraceptive continued-users, who had been on oral contraceptives for more than six months and continued taking them; another group of 39 women who had been on oral contraceptives for more than six months but who stopped taking them; and the last group of 23 women who had never used oral contraceptives. The researchers concluded that SHBG values in the oral contraceptive group who continued to use the Pill were four times higher than those in the group who had never used the Pill. Despite a decrease in SHBG values after discontinuation of oral contraceptive pill use, SHBG levels in those who discontinued the Pill remained elevated when compared to those who had never taken the Pill. The SHBG in those test subjects remained much higher even four months after discontinuing the pill.

With over 40 percent of North American women reporting no sex drive or sexual problems, this effect of the Pill should be discussed with every woman considering using it.

The researches also believe that it is possible that prolonged exposure to synthetic estrogens causes alterations in the way the gene for SHBG works in the liver in some women. In other words, long-term studies need to be performed to see if these increased SHBG levels due to using the Pill are permanent. As the authors of this book, we would go one step further and suggest that any woman who has used synthetic estrogens for longer than six months be tested to find out if she has elevated SHBG.

Doctor Recommends All Women Be Warned

Endocrinologist Dr. Claudia Panzer, lead author of this important study, also noted that "it is important for physicians prescribing oral contraceptives to point out to their patients potential sexual side effects, such as decreased desire, decreased arousal, decreased lubrication and increased sexual pain. Also, if women present with these complaints, it is crucial to recognize the link between sexual dysfunction and the oral contraceptive use."

Women Know the Pill Affects Sex Drive

For decades, women have reported a reduction in sex drive when taking the Pill. All too often those complaints were largely ignored. Researchers know that the birth control pill suppresses both ovulation and the male hormones produced by the ovaries in the middle of the menstrual cycle. Then SHBG binds the testosterone that is produced. Therefore, the Pill decreases testosterone's availability in two ways: one, by reducing overall testosterone production by the ovaries, and two, by increasing testosterone-binding SHBG.

More than a 100 million women worldwide use oral contraceptives. The Pill was introduced in the 1960s, but until recently, no one looked at the long-term health effects of elevated SHBG. Eighty percent of American women born since 1945 have used the Pill at some point. It is interesting how, even after 40 years of use, researchers are still uncovering potentially dangerous side effects of the Pill.

If you are taking the Pill for contraception, make sure you follow the recommendations on page 111 to protect yourself from the negative effects of the synthetic hormones and the metabolites produced by the Pill, which promote cervical cancer. Look at alternative types of contraception like the fertility monitors that are now available. The First Response Fertility Monitor can detect when you are ovulating, so you can use condoms or abstain from sex during that time frame.

Hormone havoc results when any one of the key sexy hormones—particularly estrogens—becomes either dominant or low. As you may suspect from reading this introduction, it is very easy to become estrogen-dominant.

Exposure to Xenoestrogens Self-Assessment

Place a tick mark beside every situation that applies to you, and then total the number of points indicated on the right.

❑	I am worried about paying my bills this month.	1
❑	I took birth control pills during my teens or early 20s. (A few months use may increase risk of breast cancer by 30 percent. Ten years use may double it.)	3
❑	I have taken or am taking synthetic HRT. (Premarin, Provera, Prempro).	3
❑	I do not exercise three times per week, which reduces fat stores of xenoestrogens.	2
❑	I have been diagnosed with depression, and tricyclic anti-depressants were prescribed. (Studies showed increase in mammary tumors in rats.)	2
❑	I dye my hair with dark-colored dyes (a source of xenoestrogens).	2
❑	I use commercial cosmetics containing parabens and other xenoestrogens.	3
❑	I wear dry-cleaned clothing (a source of xenoestrogens).	1
❑	I use bleached sanitary products (a source of xenoestrogens), e.g., tampons, pads.	2
❑	I eat pesticide- and herbicide-laden foods.	3
❑	I use nail polish that is not toluene or phthalate-free.	1
❑	My periods started before age 12.	2
❑	I had late onset menopause, starting after age 50.	2
❑	I eat a diet high in animal fat, dairy, and meat (sources of xenoestrogens).	3
❑	I smoke, with early or excessive use. (Cigarettes contain xenoestrogen chemicals.)	3
❑	I drink alcohol, with early or excessive use. (Alcohol raises estrogen; see page 176).	3
❑	I do not eat cruciferous vegetables. (These vegetables detoxify carcinogenic estrogens.)	3
❑	I am using tranquilizers. (Studies show an increase in breast tumors if tranquilizers are used regularly.)	2
❑	I am using ulcer medications. (Medication disrupts estrogen metabolism, which decreases good estrogen.)	2

❑   I am overweight or obese. (Fat stores estrogens.)   3
❑   I use or have used Flagyl for yeast infections.   2
        (Studies show an increase in mammary tumors in rats.)

Total Score Shows Increased Risk for Estrogen-dominant
Conditions due to Xenoestrogens: _____

0-18 lower risk
19-35 moderate to high risk
36-47 high risk

In the coming chapters, we are going to take you beyond your hormone-related symptoms to help you understand what some of the root causes might be and give you pointers on assessing your situation in order to find the culprit in your own case of hormone havoc. Then you can begin to work with your healthcare practitioners to fix the causes and put an end to the symptoms. Later chapters will tell you more about the care and feeding of your sexy hormones and how to program yourself for passion.

1

Hormone and Endocrine Basics

Hormones are complicated and discovering the root cause of a hormone-related problem can take some time. This is why many physicians will simply write a prescription for the birth control pill or Premarin as a temporary fix. Dr. Pettle and I are going to give you a simplified summary of the information you should know. The first thing you need to know is that because hormones are complicated, any "quick fix" you use to solve hormone-related trouble now is most likely going to cause more problems, either now and later.

Hormones are chemical messengers that tell other systems throughout your body what to do, how to do it, and when to do it. The messages they send could be to make you sleepy like melatonin does; or to rev up your energy supply to meet the next deadline, which is what occurs when cortisol is secreted; or raise your blood pressure, which aldosterone can do; or to release an egg, like luteinizing hormone signals, or get you in the mood for love (thanks to an increase in testosterone). Many hormones are secreted in the body—over 50 are known at the moment. There are thousands of body processes that occur because of your hormones. This "complicated" interaction means that if you tinker with one component of a hormone process, you may interfere with every process that is related to it. There can be a domino effect (or a "cascade effect") that can affect every hormone down the chain.

Remember this: hormones work together. When the correct amount of the right hormone is in the right place at the right time, you have beautiful, clear skin; strong bones; and a great sex drive. You have strength and stamina, are breast-cancer-free, and prior to menopause, you are fertile (as Nature intended you to be). You are reading this book because that may not be the case at this moment or you want to keep your hormones balanced and prevent hormone -related problems from occurring.

Hormone Messengers Control the Body

You were not born with a lifetime supply of hormones. Your body's organs, glands, and cells make these powerful messengers day in and day out from building blocks like cholesterol, amino acids found in protein, or components of fats in your diet. The three types of hormones are summarized in the table below.

Hormone Type	Source(s)	Selected Examples
steroid hormones	• cholesterol (lipids, mainly high density lipoproteins (HDL) and to a lesser extent low density lipoproteins (LDL)) • fatty acids (eicosanoids, e.g., linoleic acid, arachidonic acid, phospholipids)	progesterone, testosterone, estrogens (including estradiol, estrone, estrid), cortisol, prostaglandins, DHEA (dehydroepiandrosterone)
peptide (protein) hormones	• protein (amino acids)	insulin, luteinizing hormone, follicle-stimulating hormone, prolactin, growth hormone, dopamine, antidiuretic hormone
amine-derived hormones	• protein (amino acids tyrosine and tryptophan)	melatonin, serotonin, epinephrine, thyroxine

How do hormones do what they do?

Organs, glands, and cells in your body, mostly those in your endocrine system, secrete hormones into your bloodstream. Once it has traveled through the bloodstream, the hormone acts like a key that fits into a lock on specific target cell membranes. The lock is called the receptor. Sometimes the hormone (the key) fits the lock exactly, and other times it alters the action of the lock. Some of these "locks" can take more than one key (meaning several hormones can affect it).

The Hormonic Symphony

In women, the endocrine glands that most influence hormone balance are the adrenals, the pituitary, the hypothalamus, the thyroid, and the ovaries. And, although they are not part of the endocrine system, the liver and the large intestine also play major roles in hormone health. The liver is the key organ for clearing excess hormones. It also manufactures cholesterol, the starting material for all steroid hormones, and the liver decides if a hormone is going to convert to one hormone or another. A healthy liver is the key to hormone balance. The intestines are involved in hormone balance and detoxification. Together, these many glands and organs can be thought of as an orchestra playing a complex, beautiful, and ever-changing musical work, a "hormonic" symphony.

The pituitary regulates so many hormones that it can be considered the "concert master" of the hormone orchestra, taking its orders in the form of releasing hormones sent from the conductor, the hypothalamus. The pituitary sends out its instructions to the other endocrine glands and organs via various stimulating hormones. It is through the leadership of the hypothalamus and pituitary that the hormone symphony orchestra is able to continue playing beautiful music.

During times when hormone levels fluctuate dramatically, such as ovulation or through the transitional years from peri-menopause to post-menopause, the orchestra may go out of tune. Players such as the thyroid or adrenal glands may not be able to adjust to the new notes the body wants to play. The adrenals may be exhausted from prolonged stress before peri-menopause and be unable to meet the demand for more hormones when the ovaries shut down. Sometimes the concert master, the pituitary, cannot stimulate the glandular orchestra to play loud enough or in proper harmony. There is also an important interaction between the thyroid and the adrenals. When this partnership becomes stressed during the transitional years, pregnancy, or other physiological or emotionally stressful times, many women become symptomatic with hormone-related concerns.

Hormone Factories

As noted, hormones are mostly produced and secreted by the endocrine system. The main hormone producers in the body include the hypothalamus, pituitary, thyroid, parathyroid, adrenals, pancreas, ovaries, pineal, thymus, and the newly added fat cell. The key endocrine players are illustrated below. Some non-endocrine organs also produce and secrete hormones; these include the heart, lungs, brain, kidneys, liver, large intestine, skin, and placenta. All of these organs and glands, not just the ovaries, have a powerful influence over the health of hormones from birth to death.

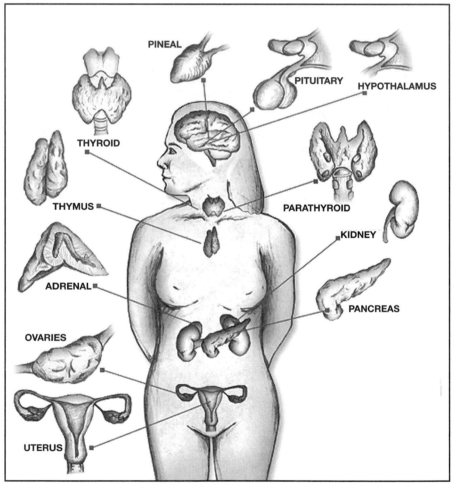

Permission granted by ZRT Laboratory http://www.zrtlab.com

Hypothalamus

The hypothalamus sits just below what is called the base of the forebrain, so it is in the lower part of the front of the brain. It manages the regulation of the body's internal environment by taking signals from the nervous system and sending out hormone messages to the pituitary gland, directing it to either start or stop a hormone process.

The Pituitary Gland

The pituitary gland is only about the size of a pea, but it has a front and a back —the anterior lobe and the posterior lobe—that each produce specific hormones in response to a signal from the hypothalamus. The instructions for action that go out to the kidneys, uterus, mammary glands, thyroid, adrenal cortex, ovaries, and bones and tissues come from the pituitary gland.

Adrenal Glands

The two adrenal glands are among the most important glands in the body. These small glands release the stress-response hormones that guide the body's reaction to a stressor, as well as small amounts of estrogen, testosterone, DHEA, cortisol, and progesterone. The accumulated effects of internal and external stressors have a profound impact on the adrenal glands, an impact that ripples out into the area of hormone health.

Each adrenal gland sits on top of one of the kidneys and contains two parts: the adrenal medulla and the adrenal cortex. In response to triggers from the hypothalamus, the adrenal medulla secretes hormones called epinephrine (aka adrenaline) and norepinephrine. These hormones are part of the "fight-or-flight" response that cause that fast, short-term increase in blood sugar levels; breathing rate; cardiac output; blood flow to the muscles, lungs, and brain; and cellular metabolism that can get you moving when you think you are in danger. The adrenal cortex is responsible for the production of a wide range of hormones called glucocorticoids, including cortisol, and the mineral corticoids aldosterone and testosterone. This release happens in response to a signal from the pituitary gland and results in a longer-term stress response that increases blood glucose as well as suppresses your immune response, in order to concentrate your energy on dealing with the stressor.

The secretion of hormones by the adrenal cortex in response to stress is one of the most important functions of the adrenals as these hormones help you adapt to the stresses of life over the longer term. Various adrenal hormones stimulate the conversion of protein to energy, so that energy levels remain high even after the glucose released for the fight-or-flight reaction has been used up. The adrenal hormones help maintain elevated blood pressure and create changes needed for dealing with such stressors as emotional shocks, infection, high workload, weather changes, environmental chemicals, or physical or emotional trauma.

Over time, particularly a period of continual exposure to stressors, it is possible for the adrenal glands to become exhausted and unable to secrete the necessary hormones. Adrenal exhaustion is a serious concern because the adrenal glands secrete both male and female sex hormones—the estrogens and androgens—and become the prime producers of estrogens and progesterone when the ovaries "retire." In today's world, most women (and people in general) have some degree of adrenal compromise. Women are generally working a full-time job, raising children, and juggling hundreds of other demands of daily life. Poor adrenal health undermines a woman's ability to make the transitions inherent in female life smoothly. In particular, it can compromise sleep quality, which in turn further compromises adrenal function.

Many medical doctors do not recognize adrenal exhaustion unless the glands become so compromised that disorders such as Addison's disease or Cushing's syndrome occur. Until adrenal exhaustion is recognized, the person will most likely have suffered for years from symptoms of under- or overactive adrenal function. Years of chronic stress eventually cause poor adrenal function, but prior to the organ becoming compromised, there are usually periods of over-activity that, if untreated, usually result in inadequate adrenal function.

Some people, however, stay in the overactive state for a prolonged period. Menopausal symptoms resemble those of Cushing's syndrome, a disease related to over-activity of the adrenal cortex. For example, hot flushes, night sweats, and insomnia, which are common menopausal symptoms, are also symptoms of Cushing's syndrome, which is caused by chronic exposure to excess levels of cortisol.

Thyroid Gland

The thyroid gland, located at the front of your throat, sets the rate of your body's metabolism, which means it regulates nearly every cell in your body. This butterfly-shaped gland receives messages from thyroid-stimulating hormone (TSH) from the pituitary and secretes thyroxine (T4) and triiodothyronine (T3), which travel through your bloodstream and affect the rate that your body metabolizes fats, proteins, and carbohydrates for energy at many sites. In other words, thyroid hormones set the rate for the way you use food as fuel, rev up your fat-burning furnace, and set your heart rate and temperature, among dozens of other important functions in the body.

Calcitonin, another hormone secreted by the thyroid, is involved in the balance of blood calcium levels. It lowers the amount of calcium and phosphate in the blood as necessary by inhibiting bone breakdown and accelerating the assimilation of calcium. Calcitonin stimulates movement of calcium into bone in opposition to the effects of parathyroid hormone (discussed below). Any change in thyroid function has far-reaching effects, including slowing down your fat-burning furnace, which causes you to gain weight; affecting your heart rate and your fertility; and promoting bone loss.

Because thyroid hormones regulate every cell—in every organ—keeping your thyroid healthy and your levels of thyroid hormones balanced is another key to vibrant health.

The Thyroid and Adrenal Connection

The thyroid—adrenal feedback interaction is orchestrated by the nervous system. Stressors on the body and the resulting chronic secretion of cortisol from the adrenal glands have a negative impact on the thyroid gland. When cortisol goes up, estrogens increase. Estrogens block the uptake of thyroid hormone. So stress on your adrenals has a negative effect on the thyroid, causing reduced uptake by thyroid hormone receptors and low thyroid hormone output. Adequate amounts of thyroid hormone are needed to make cortisol function properly and vice versa. So interdependent are these two hormones that they share many of the same deficiency or excess symptoms when they are not in balance. (See page 36 for symptoms of deficiency and excess of steroid hormones.)

When the adrenal glands are overworked due to stress, working too much, not enough sleep, or poor diet, the body converts progesterone into adrenal hormones, which depletes your body of progesterone. Thyroid hormones and progesterone feed information back to the pituitary, helping to balance other hormones and thereby help the adrenals—which, like the thyroid, are stimulated by the pituitary—with stress adaptation. When progesterone levels are low because of its conversion into stress-fighting hormones, the thyroid suddenly has to take on the task of sending hormones to the pituitary with little outside help.

As we noted, the thyroid determines your metabolic rate. If your adrenals are depleted, your thyroid will force them to maintain the proper rate. However, this type of pressure on your endocrine system over time leads your thyroid to decrease hormone production in order to conserve energy. When this first happens, symptoms of low levels of both adrenal and thyroid hormones occur. (See Chapter 4 for a complete list of symptoms.) If the symptoms are not addressed, over time they will come to be predominantly related to one gland or the other—usually your thyroid.

The Thyroid and Liver Connection

Some non-endocrine organs, such as the heart, lungs, liver, large intestine, and skin, also play a regular part in maintaining optimal levels of key hormones. A healthy liver is particularly important if you hope to avoid hormone havoc. Your liver can break down and eliminate excess hormones to help maintain the correct levels. It also manufactures the cholesterol that is used to make the key sexy hormones including testosterone, estrogen, progesterone, and DHEA.

The thyroid is influenced by the function of the liver. The liver governs the flow of fluids through the body. When the liver is congested or stagnant, swelling (edema) occurs. This congestion may occur in the thyroid area. When a noticeable enlargement of the thyroid occurs—called a goiter—this is also a sign of liver congestion.

Research indicates that thyroid problems are on the rise because of the widespread poor nutritional status of people today. Thyroid hormones are made from protein and minerals. Vitamin D made from sunshine on the skin is also a key nutrient for thyroid hormone manufacture. Vitamin D deficiency is common in the Northern Hemisphere. As well, the high levels of environmental toxins to which people are exposed affect liver function. The liver's ability to eliminate toxic compounds and so support good thyroid functioning depends on the strength of its detoxification systems, which, in turn, are directly influenced by diet and lifestyle.

The Parathyroid Gland

The parathyroid gland is made up of four small glands that are adjacent to your thyroid. It secretes parathyroid hormone (PTH), the hormone that stimulates bone cells to break down bone and release the stored calcium whenever your body detects a low concentration of calcium in your blood. PTH is thought to be more important than calcitonin for bone health as those who have had their thyroid removed but still have healthy levels of PTH maintain normal calcium metabolism. PTH is also involved in the absorption of food by the intestines and the conservation of calcium by the kidneys.

Pancreas

Your pancreas is a gland that is about six inches long; it sits behind your stomach and is connected to your small intestine. It assists in the work of digestion by secreting digestive enzymes, but it also takes on an endocrine function by secreting the hormones insulin and glucagon directly into your bloodstream. These two hormones are a tag team: insulin's job is to push glucose (sugar) into cells and decrease your blood level of glucose; glucagon increases the level of glucose in your blood when it gets too low. The pancreas monitors the levels of glucose in your bloodstream and secretes one of those two hormones to make the adjustments and keep your blood glucose levels where they should be. (When blood sugar levels are constantly too high, the pancreas can become exhausted from chronic insulin production, and this leads to the reliance on insulin drugs.)

Ovaries

When the pituitary gland sends out follicle-stimulating hormone and luteinizing hormone, the target organ is mainly the ovaries. The ovaries are the storage organ for the eggs, held inside the follicles. The average woman is born with over a million follicles, and each one contains an immature egg. By the time menstruation begins many, many of these follicles have degenerated and a woman may have half as many eggs as she had at birth. Every month up to 20 follicles begin maturing. An increase in follicle-stimulating hormone (courtesy of the pituitary gland) stimulates the full maturing of one egg (or, less often, multiple eggs).

Luteinizing hormone (LH) is the hormone that stimulates the release of the egg from the ovary. Fallopian tubes on either side of the uterus, not attached to the ovary, act as portals for the egg to the uterus, sweeping up the egg that has been released and ensuring its passage to the uterus. Meanwhile, the LH stimulates the spent follicle (now known as a corpus luteum) to release progesterone and some estrogen.

The Ovary and Thyroid Connection

There is a direct relationship between the ovaries and the thyroid gland. Next to the thyroid, the ovaries contain the greatest concentration of iodine in the female body, so when iodine is deficient you will feel the effects in both the ovaries and the thyroid. But most importantly, the ovary has hormone receptors for thyroid hormones. These receptors for thyroid hormones play a role in development of the egg and conception. Also, too much thyroid hormone activity may increase estrogen receptor function and too little thyroid hormone activity on the ovary can create menstrual problems and infertility.

Research published in the *Journal of Clinical Endocrinology and Metabolism* in 2007 evaluated the ovarian surface epithelial cells for hormone receptors, including those for thyroid hormone. The ovaries from women who had had a hysterectomy were used. Researchers found that the ovarian surface is a target for T3 thyroid hormone and that T3 hormone increased the action of estrogen receptors. They believed this discovery could help explain the link between hyperthyroidism (too much thyroid hormone) and ovarian cancer. But if your levels of thyroid hormone are low, this could have huge implications for the level of estrogens, as well as the functioning of your reproductive system and your sex drive.

In 2000, a group of Slovakian doctors found clear evidence of the ovary/thyroid connection when they used pure thyroid gland extracts to treat young, infertile women who had menstrual cycle dysfunction. By giving the infertile women pure thyroid hormones, doctors had improvement of the women's menstrual cycles, which ultimately led to conception. In previous studies, the doctors had discovered the presence of thyroid-stimulating hormone and T3 receptors in the ovary. They found that T3 had a direct effect on egg maturation. With up to 30 percent of North American women walking around with undiagnosed low thyroid, many women could be suffering with ovarian issues and infertility that could be cleared up with thyroid support.

There is also a clear connection between polycystic ovary syndrome (PCOS) and autoimmune thyroiditis. According to the March 2004 *European Journal of Endocrinology*, women with PCOS were almost seven times more likely to have autoimmune thyroid disease than women without PCOS. Women with PCOS rarely form a corpus luteum (which releases progesterone), and therefore these women do not manufacture appropriate levels of progesterone. Endocrine researchers have shown that low progesterone levels lead to an overstimulation of the immune system in women with PCOS, causing autoimmune thyroiditis and other immune abnormalities predominantly found in women, including MS and lupus.

The ovaries are the organs that get the "bad rap" during menopause and in other hormone-related disorders. They do play an important role, but, as we've noted, the ovaries are only one player in the large hormone orchestra.

Pineal Gland

The cone-shaped pineal gland is located deep in the brain. Its function is not well understood, however it is known to make melatonin and secrete it into the bloodstream. Melatonin is the hormone that regulates the sleeping and waking cycle.

Hormone Factory Summary

Endocrine Gland	Hormones Secreted	Key Functions/Effects
hypothalamus	stimulating and inhibiting hormones that turn processes on or off	• sends hormonal instructions to the pituitary gland
pituitary	human growth hormone (hGH) thyroid-stimulating hormone (TSH) follicle-stimulating hormone (FSH) luteinizing hormone (LH) prolactin (PRL) adrenocorticotropic hormone (ACTH) antidiuretic hormone (ADH) oxytocinoxtyocin (OCT)	• sends out hormones that stimulate activity in other endocrine organs such as the thyroid (TSH), the ovaries (FSH, LH), the mammary glands (PRL, OCT), the adrenals (ACTH), the kidneys (ADH), as well as stimulating bone and muscle growth and metabolism (hGH)
adrenal (cortex and medulla)	aldosterone cortisol, epinephrine (adrenaline), norepinephrine DHEA estrogen, DHEA, androgens	• regulates sodium and water • sustains the stress reaction by raising blood glucose levels and helping to break down protein • blood pressure and stress reaction
thyroid	thyroxine (T4) triiodothyronine (T3) calcitonin	• helps regulate the rate of metabolism
parathyroid	parathyroid hormone (PTH)	• helps regulate bone status and blood calcium
pancreas	insulin glucagon	• lowers blood glucose levels • raises blood glucose levels
ovaries	estrogens	• promotes formation of female secondary sex characteristics • stimulates endometrial growth • increases uterine growth • maintenance of vessel and skin • reduces bone resorption; increases bone formation • protein synthesis

ovaries	estrogens	• coagulation
		  – increases anti-thrombin and plasminogen
		  – increases platelet adhesiveness
		• lipid function
		  – increases HDL, triglyceride, fat deposition
		  – decreases LDL
		• balances salt and water retention
		• gastrointestinal tract function
		  – reduces bowel motility
		  – increases cholesterol elimination

ovaries	progesterone	• assists in thyroid function, in bone-building by osteoblasts, in bone, teeth, gums, joint, tendon, ligament and skin resilience, and in some cases healing by regulating various types of collagen, and in nerve function and healing • increases core temperature during ovulation • reduces spasm and relaxes smooth muscle • acts as an anti-inflammatory agent and regulates the immune response • reduces gall-bladder activity • normalizes blood clotting and vascular tone, zinc and copper levels, cell oxygen levels, and use of fat stores for energy • appears to prevent endometrial cancer (involving the uterine lining) by regulating the effects of estrogen
pineal (located in the brain)	melatonin	• helps control sleep/wake cycles, is an antioxidant, supports healthy immune function

The endocrine system does not act on its own when making hormones. It interacts with other systems in the body, maintaining communication while controlling and coordinating the body's work. For example, the nervous system routinely sends messages to the endocrine system to stimulate or inhibit the secretion of hormones, or the endocrine system sends messages to the nervous system to tell it to stop or start certain activities. With this in mind, it is clear that the nervous system, which includes the brain as well as thoughts and emotions, can have a powerful effect on hormones. And this effect, you will learn later, can play a role in reducing sex drive, or increasing stress hormones and much more.

The endocrine system can make hormones that are used both inside and outside the body. For example saliva is manufactured for use outside the body, as are vaginal secretions. You will learn later how important saliva is as a tool for measuring the action of certain hormones.

Your Fat Cells Are Also Hormone Factories

Fat cells (also called adipose tissue) are located in different places in men and women. Men tend to carry body fat in their chest and abdomen. Women carry it in their breasts, hips, buttocks, thighs, and waist. Estrogen and testosterone play a role in the deposit of fat on the body. And there are two types of fat: white fat and brown fat. White fat insulates you from the cold, cushions your structure, and is used as fuel for energy. Brown fat is very important for producing heat (thermogenesis). Brown fat cells contain mitochondria, the energy producers of the body, which is why they can generate heat.

There are also two types of obesity: one in which fat cells are too large (called hypertrophic obesity) and another in which the person has too many fat cells (called hyperplastic obesity). The size of fat cells can change throughout life, but the number of fat cells is determined by the late teens. Having too many fat cells is a product of the types of foods your mother consumed while she was pregnant and/or if she developed gestational diabetes, as well as the amount of food fed to you throughout your childhood. (Remember this if you are going to have children or have babies or toddlers.) During the third trimester of fetal development, and then later at the onset of puberty, fat cells are formed at increased rates. This is why healthy, appropriate prenatal and teen nutrition play a role in weight management as an adult.

From a hormone perspective, the size and number of fat cells also affect adult hormone balance. Scientists around the world have found that fat cells, swollen to capacity with stored fat, spew out vast amounts of hormones and chemical messengers that hasten death from heart disease, strokes, diabetes, and cancer. Fat cells are hormone factories, using androstenedione and the enzyme aromatase to make estrogens. These estrogens in the system are in addition to those produced elsewhere and can be a source of estrogen-dominant conditions.

Moderately obese people cut their lifespan by up to five years, and the severely obese see a reduction of at least ten years. Fat cells are now viewed as one of the most important endocrine cells in the body. Fat cells secrete approximately 25 signalling compounds—including estrogens, resistin, leptin, adiponectin, inflammatory proteins, tumor necrosis factor-alpha, interleukin-6, growth hormone, and more—that are sending out messages that can promote or weaken dozens of deadly health conditions and negatively affect your sexy hormones.

How else can fat cells harm your health?

- Doctors used to think that high blood pressure associated with weight gain simply occurred because the person had to push blood through more mass. Now, with the discovery that fat cells can manufacture a potent constrictor of blood vessels called angiotensinogen, researchers know that action of this chemical is a major contributor to high blood pressure in the overweight—and why the fat cells are killing them. Combine this blood-constricting hormone with the inflammatory factors produced by the fat cell, and artery walls develop a build-up of tissue that blocks blood flow, thus increasing the risk of stroke and heart attack.

- The growth hormone and estrogens produced by fat cells also fuel **cancer** cells. Obese women are at much higher risk of developing estrogen-dominant cancers, particularly breast cancer, and they are more likely to die from the disease because their fat cells pump out copious amounts of estrogens. Overweight women who have not gone through menopause have an increased risk of developing polycystic ovary syndrome, ovarian cysts, fibrocystic breasts, migraine headaches, uterine fibroids, endometriosis, and acne as a result of their bulging fat cells.

- Those xenoestrogens (estrogen mimickers absorbed from environmental plastics, cosmetics, hair dyes, pesticides, PCBs, parabens, glycols, and hundreds of other chemicals) discussed earlier are stored in fat cells. Even an extra 10 lbs. (4.5 kg) of fat increases these deadly estrogens that disrupt hormone balance in the body, congest the liver, and further increase rates of cancer.

The fat cell can be thought of as an active manufacturing facility of hormones with lots of fat-storage capacity that can maintain its size.

Fat Cells and the Liver

Any disruption of the liver detoxification pathway contributes to excesses or imbalances in hormones and toxins and fat gain. The liver is also responsible for conjugating (combining) estrogens and other steroid hormones, certain drugs, and chemical compounds. Too much estrogen is one reason why women have a difficult time losing fat around the abdominal area. A decreased rate of estrogen excretion because of poor liver detoxification contributes to what we commonly call "estrogen belly," which is simply too much fat around the middle, promoted by having too much estrogen due to faulty excretion of excess estrogens.

Too much fat on your body also increases your estrogen levels. This is because fat cells are not only involved in manufacturing estrogen via the enzyme aromatase but are also a storage site for estrogen. This sets up a vicious cycle of too many fat cells manufacturing and storing too much estrogen, which creates high levels of estrogen, which maintains increased fat and larger fat cells and causes hormone disruption.

Fat Cells and Insulin

Insulin, a hormone secreted by the pancreas, is another culprit contributing to "fatness." The standard, excessively high carbohydrate, low-protein diet disrupts the body's ability to regulate blood sugar adequately. When too much insulin is being pumped out to reduce abnormally high blood sugar (by storing it in fat cells), the body inevitably gains weight, becomes fat, and cells become very resistant to insulin (leaving glucose in the bloodstream) and fat loss. Everyone who is overweight has insulin resistance, and insulin resistance puts them at higher risk of heart disease, cancers, diabetes, polycystic ovary syndrome, facial hair growth, anxiety, and more.

Endocrine Summary

As you can see, the key organs of the endocrine system do not work alone. Just as hormones work together, so do the organs that produce them. The relationships among them, particularly related to the thyroid, ensure that you are feeling fabulous when a partnership is working and not well at all when a pair is out of tune.

The amount of hormone secreted by the glands and organs of the endocrine system is determined by the body's need for the hormone at any given time. It is important to understand, especially when we start discussing hormone therapies, that a single hormone can promote a cascade of events in the body. For example, one of the side effects of high-dose oral estrogen therapy or exposure to high levels of environmental estrogens is low thyroid function because estrogen blocks the uptake of thyroid hormone. Through complex feedback mechanisms, hormone production is regulated so that there is no over- or underproduction of particular hormones. When women start adding hormones, either from pills, creams, or patches, along with environmental hormones, they can create hormone imbalance if proper monitoring does not occur. Or conversely, when hormones are added in the correct dose and form, hormone harmony happens. Hormone balance can also be achieved with optimal nutrition and lifestyle changes.

There are times when the body's regulating mechanisms do not function properly, and hormone imbalances do occur. Stress factors, poor nutrition, weight gain, and transitional times such as puberty and menopause have a tremendous effect on the endocrine system's ability to maintain hormone balance. For example, a woman who has not taken care of herself during her 30s and 40s may find that her adrenal glands are so exhausted they cannot make her a good supply of estrogens when her ovaries retire at menopause. Or pregnancy may overwhelm the thyroid, and a woman may suffer post-partum depression or hair loss.

Each endocrine organ or gland secretes specific hormones that help maintain balance in the body by changing the activities of the cells of an organ or of cells in groups of organs; or the hormone may directly affect the activities of all the cells in the body. In the next chapter, we will outline what the steroid hormones—the sexy hormones—are and what they do.

2

The Hormones at the Heart of Hormone Havoc

Most women learned a little bit about hormones in sex education class, which was often delivered around grade five at school. Veiled in secrecy, the boys were sent to one room and the girls to another. During that one class you may have learned how babies were made and been told about monthly periods. If you were like most girls in the room, you walked away confused about what it all meant. The rest of your hormone lesson was learned from friends and less often parents—and most of what was learned was vague and often incorrect.

It is no wonder that most women suffer with unnecessary hormonal problems and may not even know it. Women suffering with terrible monthly periods think this is normal. Called "the curse," women are unaware that nasty periods are an early sign of hormone dysfunction, and that, if left alone, this dysfunction can lead to more serious hormonal conditions like uterine fibroids or breast cancer. This chapter will teach you everything you should have learned about your hormones at puberty but didn't.

The Making of Steroid Hormones

Steroid hormones—our "sexy hormones"—include estrogens, progesterone, testosterone, dehydroepiandrosterone (DHEA), and cortisol. As the graphic below indicates, all steroid hormones are made from cholesterol manufactured by the liver. In essence, cholesterol can be called the "mother" hormone. It provides the raw materials for three groups of steroid hormones including glucocorticoids (that regulate blood sugar), mineralcorticoids (that regulate blood pressure and water balance), and all the sex hormones.

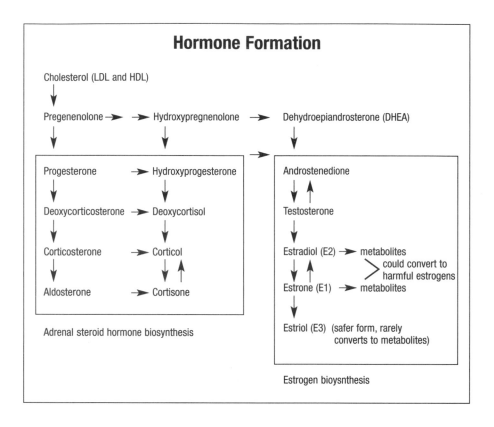

As the double arrows on the chart indicate, some steroid hormones can convert to another hormone and back again. Both high-density lipoprotein cholesterol (HDL or "good" cholesterol) and low-density lipoprotein cholesterol (LDL or so-called "bad" cholesterol) are raw material for these hormones. Low-density lipoprotein is used for hormone synthesis by steroid-hormone-producing cells in the ovaries, liver, fat cells, and brain; high-density lipoprotein is used for hormone synthesis in the adrenal glands.

Cholesterol-lowering Statins Affect Estrogen Levels

The number-one selling drug in North America is statin medication for lowering cholesterol, sold under the names Lipitor, Mevacor, and Zocor. There is little research involving statin medications and their effect on women's health. One study, published in the *Procedures of the American Society of Clinical Oncology*, found that the incidence of breast cancer goes up when women use statin medications. A total of 66,843 women over the age of 35 were included in this study. Statin use was identified from pharmacy data collected from 1997 until 2002. Statins were found to increase estrogen levels in women. The average age of women in the research group taking statins who developed breast cancer was 57.6 years. The researchers reported that women taking statin medications should be advised of the potential increased risk of breast cancer.

Statins also deplete the body of coenzyme Q_{10}, an important nutrient for the prevention and treatment of breast cancer. Anyone taking statin drugs should be supplementing with 200 mg of coenzyme Q_{10} for protection from the hormone-disrupting effects of the drug and the depletion of coenzyme Q_{10}. The reduction of cholesterol levels through aggressive diet and lifestyle changes makes more sense than taking a hormone-disrupting drug.

Women and men both produce estrogens and testosterone. The adrenal glands in men are their main source of estrogen. Women make and need testosterone too. Hormones in women are predominately produced in the adrenals and ovaries with the liver, fat cells, intestines, and the thyroid playing a role. A woman who has had a hysterectomy (removal of the uterus) with ovary removal, or a woman who has gone through menopause, relies on her adrenal glands for the majority of her hormone production.

Estrogens

There is no single hormone called "estrogen." Instead, estrogens are a group of hormones that play an important role in the normal sexual and reproductive development in women (and men). Estrogens are also called sex hormones. A woman's ovaries produce most estrogens, along with the adrenal glands, and to, a lesser extent, fat cells. The liver, intestines, and thyroid also play a role. (In men, the adrenal glands are their main source of estrogens.)

In addition to regulating the menstrual cycle, estrogens affect the reproductive tract, the urinary tract, the heart and blood vessels, bones, breasts, skin, hair, mucous membranes, pelvic muscles, and the brain. Secondary sexual characteristics, such as pubic and armpit hair, begin to develop when levels of estrogens rise.

The main estrogens and most widely recognized are estrone (E1), estradiol (E2), and estriol (E3). Each estrogen has different degrees of interaction with estrogen receptors, making them either strong or weak estrogens. You will hear estradiol being called a "strong estrogen" that has a greater estrogenic effect than estriol, which is classified as a weak estrogen. Estradiol is eight times more potent than estrone, and estriol has 1/80 the potency of estrone. The stronger the estrogen, the broader its effects on estrogen receptors. As you can see on the Hormone Formation graphic (page 18), estriol and estrone are made from estradiol.

Estrogen Metabolism

Estrogen metabolism is intricate. Estrogens can stay in their original form, convert to another estrogen, or convert to cancer-preventive or cancer-promoting estrogen metabolites (breakdown products). Some of the possibilities are shown on the Hormone Formation graphic (page 18) and described below. This is why estrogens—even your body's own estrogens—can either be a friend or an enemy. Before considering whether to use hormone therapy, even bioidentical hormones, read the following hormone facts to aid you in making good decisions about hormone therapies.

Estrone (E1) is converted from estradiol mainly in the liver, and from the precursor hormones androstenedione, progesterone, and dehydroepiandrosterone (DHEA) in fat cells and in some organs. Thus, women who have had their ovaries removed and those experiencing menopause are still able to secrete high levels of estrone. Estrone can also be turned into estrone sulfate, a stored form of estrogen. Breast cancer cells tend to have high amounts of estrone sulfate. Estrone sulfate can be turned back into estrone and then back to estradiol. Estrone can also convert to a dangerous metabolite called 4-hydroxyestrone, which is also thought to play a role in breast cancer initiation. Many researchers now believe that 4-hydroxyestrone is a dangerous metabolite of estrone and that estrone should not be given to women in the form of supplemental hormones.

Estradiol (E2) is produced directly by the ovary from cholesterol and is the principal estrogen secreted by the ovaries before menopause (when periods cease). Estradiol is also produced via androstenedione from the adrenal glands. Estradiol is converted to estrone in the small intestine, and this conversion is reversible, meaning it can be converted back to estradiol. Estradiol is involved in building up the lining of the uterus. It can be called a strong estrogen that has a powerful effect on estrogen receptors. Both estrone and estradiol can be converted to estriol.

Estriol (E3) is a weaker form of estrogen, meaning estriol affects only some estrogen receptors, and, of those it does affect, it has a weaker affinity. Although it has been commonly believed that most estriol results from the conversion of estradiol and estrone, primarily in the liver, researchers have concluded that there may also be direct secretion of estriol by the adrenals and ovaries or a direct conversion of androstenedione to estriol. Estriol is very high during pregnancy, which is thought to protect the fetus from estradiol.

2-Hydroxyestrone is a breakdown product (metabolite) of estrogens. It is thought to be a breast cancer-protective (good form of) estrogen. Estradiol and estrone can be metabolized into either 2-hydroxyestradiol or 2-hydroxyestrone. For example, estradiol may be metabolized to 2-hydroxyestradiol or back through estrone into 16 alpha-hydroxyestrone or to 2-hydroxyestrone.

New research has shown that estriol may be metabolized to **16 alpha-hydroxyestrone**. Estriol conversion takes place when liver health is compromised by drugs and toxins; when you are exposed to high amounts of xenoestrogens found in pesticides, cosmetics, plastics, milk, meat, and more; and when you are taking high doses of estrogens. Research has shown that having high levels of 2-hydroxyestrone is cancer-protective and having low levels of 2-hydroxyestrone and high levels of 4-hydroxyestrone or 16 alpha-hydroxyestrone is cancer-promoting.

16 alpha-hydroxyestrone and Breast Cancer

In one large study of over 10,000 peri-menopausal women at the State University of New York at Buffalo, researchers found that women who went on to develop breast cancer had significantly less 2-hydroxyestrone and more 16 alpha-hydroxyestrone metabolites than women who did not. They followed the women for 5.5 years and discovered that participants with higher levels of 2-hydroxyestrone were 40 percent less likely to develop breast cancer.

It is very important to know your ratio of 2-hydroxyestrone to 16 alpha-hydroxyestrone. You will learn about the 2-to-16 ratio urine test for breast cancer risk assessment on page 47. At publication we had not found a laboratory that tests for 4-hydroxyestrone. Certain foods and nutrients can inhibit this conversion to unhealthy estrogens, making your estrogens safer. See Chapter 7 for more information on foods that protect your hormones by keeping the conversion or breakdown of estrogens on the positive, healthy pathway in order to decrease or eliminate 4-hydroxyestrone and 16 alpha-hydroxyestrone. Indole-3-carbinol from cruciferous vegetables can help stop the breakdown of healthy estrogens to 16 alpha-hydroxyestrone and therefore help protect you from cancer.

16 alpha-hydroxyestrone and Cervical Cancer

Women with cervical dysplasia (noted by abnormal Pap tests) have higher levels of the estrogen metabolite 16 alpha-hydroxyestrone. A study in the *International Journal of Cancer* found a connection between the human papilloma virus (HPV) and high levels of 16 alpha-hydroxyestrone or a greater affinity for conversion of estrogens into this carcinogenic metabolite and the development of cervical cancer. Researchers suggested that the combined action of 16 alpha-hydroxyestrone and HPV promotes abnormal cell proliferation. HPV is the virus that causes genital warts, and it is associated with the development of cervical dysplasia and cervical cancer. Now scientists think the HPV virus actually uses 16 alpha-hydroxyestrone to promote cancer cell development.

The controversy over the health benefits and risks of estrogen therapy will continue because estrogens are broken down into these metabolites.

Is it safe to take any estrogens?

The answer is, "Absolutely, if you are on the correct dosage and the right type of estrogen." You should also be taking protective nutrients that stop 4- and 16 alpha-hydroxyestrone from forming, and your doctor should be monitoring you with symptom questionnaires and blood or saliva testing. You will read about the nutrients to make hormone therapy safer on page 83.

When looking at the safety of using estrogens, whether they are bioidentical estrogens or synthetic, it is the conversions of estrogens that are an important factor in either protecting you from or promoting breast cancer. This will determine what type of estrogens and the delivery system, i.e., creams or pills, that will be used in your treatment.

Estrogens and Other Hormones

The metabolism of estrogens is affected by other hormones. Estrogens are made from the male hormone testosterone, its precursor androstenedione, and an enzyme called aromatase. Fat cells are a source of aromatase (malignant (cancerous) breast tissue also produces aromatase). Fat cells are estrogen factories, but other hormones, particularly cortisol, can indirectly promote even more estrogen production in fat cells.

Cortisol causes fat cells to become larger and more resistant to fat loss.

Therefore, high levels of cortisol maintain fat cells, which are a cause of high levels of estrogen. Thus, women who are overweight tend to have more estrogen-dominant conditions (endometriosis, uterine fibroids, lumpy breasts, heavy periods, and more). And regardless of body weight, most women now live very stressful lives and this also increases cortisol, thereby increasing estrogens. The stress-estrogen-breast cancer connection is just now being understood.

Estrogens can also interfere with thyroid hormone production, which you will learn about later in this chapter. And too much estrogen, especially when taken orally, can increase a protein in the blood called sex-hormone-binding globulin (SHBG), leading to lower amounts of free testosterone, therefore reducing your sex drive. Many women who were prescribed high doses of estrogens for low libido actually had a further worsening of their desire for sex for this reason. Also, as we noted, women on the birth control pill, even the low-dose estrogen pill (which has seven times the amount of estrogen given to menopausal women), have lowered sex drives for the same reason.

How will you know if you have an excess or deficiency of estrogens in your system? Symptoms of excess estrogens range from anemia to weight gain; symptoms of a deficiency of estrogens include urinary incontinence and vaginal dryness. For a complete listing of symptoms of each and a chance to take stock of your estrogens status, turn to page 36.

Progesterone

Estrogens are end-point hormones and, other than the breakdown metabolites or changes to other estrogens, it does not form different hormones. Progesterone, as the Hormone Formation graphic shows, is a precursor hormone, meaning the body uses it to make other steroid hormones. Progesterone is produced in the corpus luteum of the ovaries. In the adrenal glands, progesterone is mainly used to make cortisol, but it can also form dehydroepiandrosterone (DHEA) and, subsequently, androstenedione, a precursor to testosterone (and estrogens). In the ovaries, a series of reactions leads from cholesterol to pregnenolone to progesterone to hydroxyprogesterone to androstenedione to testosterone, and finally to estrogens. (Yes, progesterone converts to estrogen.) No hormone is solely acting on its own. Remember: each hormone affects other hormones.

During pregnancy, progesterone produced by the placenta is essential to maintain a pregnancy to term; it keeps the uterus from contracting until labor begins. Progesterone levels during pregnancy increase 100-fold. Many women feel hormonally fabulous during pregnancy due to their high levels of progesterone.

There are progesterone receptors throughout the body, from the brain to the bladder. Doctors often tell women who have had the uterus removed that they do not need hormone replacement therapy for progesterone. They suggest these women need only estrogen because the doctors have been taught progesterone's only action is to prevent the build-up of the endometrium in the uterus. Doctors believe that since the uterus and its endometrium are gone, there is no reason to take progesterone. This is wrong because the doctor has forgotten that there are receptors in the brain, skin, thyroid, blood vessels, breast, bone, and more, that need and want progesterone.

Progesterone levels naturally decrease at menopause when the ovaries stop producing eggs, although the adrenals continue producing the hormone in lesser amounts.

Progesterone and Other Hormones

Cortisol and progesterone compete for the same receptor sites. When the body is under stress, cortisol levels go up, which can cause an overabundance of cortisol to monopolize the receptor sites that should be served by progesterone. Tests on a stressed woman may show normal levels of progesterone, but the hormone cannot do its job because cortisol is filling all the receptors.

Estrogen and progesterone act together to create harmony in the harmonic symphony. If estrogen levels get too low, then progesterone comes to the rescue by converting to estrogens. Too much estrogen, and you need more progesterone to keep these hormones in balance. With stress reducing progesterone's ability to connect with its receptors, and stress creating more estrogen, you see how all this stress is causing hormone havoc.

How will you know if you have an excess or deficiency of progesterone in your system? Symptoms of excess progesterone range from depression to oily skin; symptoms of a deficiency of progesterone include anxiety and a gain in abdominal fat. For a complete listing of symptoms of each and a chance to review your progesterone status, turn to page 36.

Testosterone

Testosterone is considered to be primarily a male hormone, but it also plays an important part in the overall hormone health of women. It is essential to a women's sex drive, maintains muscle, bone, skin, and the heart. The Hormone Formation graphic on page 18 shows that testosterone is one step on the way to estrogen. In women, testosterone is mainly produced in the ovaries; most is then converted to estradiol, but some remains as testosterone. Other male hormones include the precursor hormones androstenedione, DHEA, and dehydroepiandrosterone-sulfate (DHEAS). Testosterone can be made from these as well. As we noted, testosterone is converted to estradiol by aromatase in fat cells, and women tend to have a pronounced conversion because they have more fat cells, increasing estrogen and decreasing testosterone.

How will you know if you have an excess or deficiency of testosterone in your system? Symptoms of excess testosterone range from acne and oily skin to weight gain; symptoms of a deficiency of testosterone include no sex drive and vaginal dryness. For a complete listing of symptoms of each turn to page 36.

DHEA

DHEA is mainly produced in the adrenal glands and is found in the blood as the metabolite dehydroepiandrosterone-sulfate (DHEAS). DHEA and its metabolite DHEAS are used to make both testosterone and estrogens. When you are young, you have high levels of DHEA and DHEAS. These hormones reach their peak levels in your late twenties, and, from that point on, there is a steady decline. In Canada, DHEA as a supplement is not available over the counter in health food stores and pharmacies like it is in the U.S. It is a prescription drug in Canada and other countries around the world.

DHEA and cortisol are directly linked. High levels of cortisol cause a decline in DHEA. Increase DHEA, and cortisol levels normalize. Only if your saliva or blood tests come back indicating you are low in DHEA, do we recommend supplementing; DHEA is a very potent precursor hormone that is easily converted into testosterone and estrogens.

Symptoms of low DHEA or high DHEA are the same as for low or high testosterone For a complete listing of symptoms of each and a chance to take stock of your DHEA status, turn to page 36.

Cortisol

Cortisol is essential for regulating many metabolic and immune functions and will be mentioned throughout these early chapters because it affects many other hormones. Some of the important functions of cortisol include the regulation of glucose metabolism, immune system hormones, and cardiovascular functions, as well as regulating the body's use of proteins, carbohydrates, and fats.

Cortisol has a natural rhythm throughout your day. Your body should produce more cortisol in the morning than in the evening, giving you the energy you need to begin your day. Your cortisol levels should drop by 90 percent in the evening as you leave the stresses of the day behind. A recent study found that women who work outside the home and have family responsibilities tend to have elevated evening cortisol levels. Men, on the other hand, have lower cortisol levels in the evenings. The difference may reflect the additional responsibilities women have after they get home from their day jobs. It may also tell us why more women have difficulty sleeping, particularly during the peri-menopausal and menopausal years. Elevated cortisol levels at night will prevent sleep or cause very light sleep with frequent waking.

A study published in the *Journal of the American Medical Association* in August 2000 found that increasing age was also associated with an elevation of evening cortisol levels; it became significant only after age 50. Sleep became more fragmented, and REM sleep declined. Stress and aging both result in high cortisol levels, especially during the transitional years from peri-menopause onward that negatively affect sleep.

Changes in sleep quality are linked to specific changes in several other hormone levels as well. There is a vicious cycle of poor sleep and impaired adrenals. If the adrenals are weak, sleep will be poor; if sleep quality is poor, the adrenal glands become exhausted. Support your adrenal glands if you have sleep problems.

Cortisol is also known as your chronic stress hormone. Called a glucocorticoid, it is secreted from the adrenal glands in response to long-term stressors. In order to help you respond to long-term stressors, cortisol maintains increased blood sugar levels, breathing rate, cardiac output, and blood flow to muscles, lung, and brain.

Long-term stressors can be physical, psychological, chemical, or environmental, and cortisol is gaining attention as the hallmark of chronic elevated stress levels. Excess or deficiencies of this crucial hormone can cause a variety of physical symptoms, which, if not treated, will lead to more serious chronic disease states and even death. Your ability to adapt to long-term stressors depends upon optimal function of the adrenal glands and regulation of cortisol secretion.

If you are continually exposed to stressors, your cortisol levels will remain elevated. Research now correlates chronically elevated cortisol levels with blood sugar problems, fat accumulation, compromised immune function, infertility, exhaustion, chronic fatigue, bone loss, high triglycerides levels, and heart disease. Memory loss has also been associated with high cortisol levels. As you can see, continual exposure to stressors can have a negative impact on many areas of your health.

As noted, an additional problem of long-term elevations of cortisol levels is that the adrenal glands may wear out and no longer be able to produce even normal levels of cortisol. This leads to adrenal exhaustion. (See page 5 for more information about the adrenal glands.)

Other serious effects of chronic high levels of cortisol include the following:

- Recent research has found that approximately half of patients with **major depression** have high levels of cortisol and that high cortisol levels might be a cause rather than a symptom of depression as previously thought. Lowering cortisol is one solution to the terrible problem of depression. In the U.S. and Canada, a 353 percent increase in the number of prescriptions filled for anti-depressant medication has occurred in the last two years.
- A study published in the *Journal of the National Cancer Institute* found that women with advanced **breast cancer** who had abnormally high daytime levels of cortisol compared to women with advanced breast cancer who did not have high levels were significantly more likely to die sooner than patients with normal levels. The researchers also found that women with increased cortisol levels had fewer immune cells, known as natural killer cells, and this reduced immunity was associated with the higher mortality rate. The study also reported that women with abnormal cortisol patterns during the day were more likely to have sleep disruptions at night, which increases the risk of breast cancer. Research has shown that melatonin, produced during sleep at night, helps to reduce the risk of breast cancer.

Cortisol and Other Hormones

Continuous stress causes chronically high cortisol levels, which increase estrogens, as you learned earlier. And cortisol competes with progesterone for the same receptor sites, so high levels of cortisol can cause symptoms of low progesterone, even when the blood and saliva progesterone levels read normal. Cortisol reduction through stress management is imperative for hormone balancing. Just taking progesterone to correct an imbalance does not always work because cortisol is a powerful hormone that will muscle its way into the progesterone receptors.

Beyond interfering with progesterone, high cortisol (as a result of stressors or high insulin levels) causes a cascade effect, beginning with a corresponding drop in the hormone dehydroepiandrosterone (DHEA). DHEA helps to increase muscle mass, improve immune function, is a precursor to other hormones, and has been called the anti-aging hormone. Just follow the hormone disruption that occurs from too many stressors or high insulin: both cause increased cortisol, which interferes with progesterone receptors and decreases testosterone and DHEA. The reduced effect of progesterone increases estrogens. High estrogens promote low thyroid and weight gain, and the cycle starts all over again with too many fat cells getting too big, producing more estrogen and insulin, which increases the secretion of cortisol.

How will you know if you have an excess or deficiency of cortisol in your system? Symptoms of adrenal stress range from insomnia and salt cravings to blurred vision to ulcers. For a complete listing of symptoms of adrenal stress and a chance to take stock of your adrenal status, turn to page 36.

Thyroid Hormones: The Great Equalizers

The thyroid gland and the hormones it secretes should be called the great equalizers. Located at the front of the throat, the thyroid sets the rate of body metabolism, thereby regulating every one of your trillion cells. Any change in thyroid function has far-reaching effects on all of your hormones. The steroid hormone cortisol is essential to healthy thyroid function. This is why a lot of discussion in this book will be around the adrenal-thyroid connection. If the adrenals become exhausted, the thyroid function goes low (hypothyroid), and hormone havoc follows. Cortisol is necessary for thyroid hormone to work well, and thyroid hormones are needed for cortisol to do its job.

Thyroid stimulating hormone (TSH) is secreted by the pituitary. TSH stimulates the production of thyroid hormones and the growth of thyroid cells. (Excess TSH causes thyroid enlargement or goiter. If you notice when you swallow it feels like there is something in your throat or your neck seems to be getting wider or your throat looks like it is protruding, a TSH test is needed immediately.)

Calcitonin is a thyroid hormone involved in the balance of blood calcium levels. It lowers the amount of calcium and phosphate in the blood as needed, by inhibiting bone breakdown and accelerating the assimilation of calcium. Thus, the thyroid is involved in bone health and diseases such as osteoporosis.

Thyroxin (T4) is the most abundant thyroid hormone. It is made from tyrosine and iodine. Triiodothyronine (T3) is the most active thyroid hormone and has up to ten times the activity of T4 and binds to receptors with a stronger action. Up to 80 percent of T4 is converted to T3 by organs, including the liver, kidney, and spleen. T4 is a precursor hormone used to make T3.

At any given time, most T3 and T4 molecules in the body are bound tightly to blood proteins. Only a small amount of each circulates as "free" hormones that are physiologically active. Free T3 or T4 hormone levels are seldom measured by medical doctors, yet these levels are the most accurate for determining thyroid function. Ask for a Free T4 and Free T3 test when having a thyroid hormone test. Do not just settle for a TSH as this does not provide the full picture of thyroid health.

You learned earlier that too much estrogen inhibits thyroid hormone, and too much cortisol causes too much estrogen. All hormones interact, which is why we believe it is important that a healthcare practitioner work with you to ensure proper hormone levels if you are supplementing with hormones.

How will you know if your thyroid is over- or underactive? Symptoms of thyroid problems range from heart palpations to constipation. Turn to page 38 for a complete listing of symptoms related to thyroid problems plus common thyroid tests.

The next chapter outlines not only the smooth functioning of sexy hormones but also consolidates hormonal imbalance symptom charts. We have included many self-assessment questionnaires as well and explanations of the most common tests you should have performed to evaluate the status of your hormones.

3

The Ins and Outs
of Hormone-Testing

The first step in discovering if your health problem is hormone-related is to take the time to assess the state of your hormone levels. There is a variety of assessment tools available, and each one can supply valuable information. We suggest that you begin by taking a look at your menstrual history and cataloguing your symptoms using the charts in this chapter, and then consider getting data from saliva, urine, and blood tests to verify any conclusions before you start treatment.

Reviewing Your Menstrual History

Even if you have stopped menstruating, it is important to know what a "normal" menstrual cycle is because your symptoms or lack of them are a very good barometer of your hormonal health. When you are completing the hormone questionnaires below, you will be asked about your past periods. Periods can provide valuable evidence about your past, present, and future hormonal health. Plus, one day you might have to explain periods to an important woman in your life—like your daughter—and you will want her to have the correct information so she does not have to suffer like many others have. Periods also give you clues to help you decide what type of treatment you need, be it bioidentical hormones or nutritional and lifestyle support.

The Normal Menstrual Cycle

At puberty, the hypothalamus increases production of a hormone called gonadotropin-releasing hormone (GnRH). As with all other hormone processes, GnRH carries its instructions to the pituitary gland in order to get the processes of maturation and reproduction in motion. In this case, the pituitary triggers the release of follicle-stimulating hormone (FSH) and luteinizing hormone (LH). These hormones stimulate the development of secondary sexual characteristics and then the monthly female reproductive cycle begins.

The menstrual cycle is divided into the follicular phase and the luteal phase, and it is regulated by complex interactions among the hormones secreted by the hypothalamus, the pituitary, and the ovaries. A cycle normally lasts 28 days, as shown in the graphic below, but some women have shorter and others have longer cycles. If you have a 25-day cycle and it is regular, meaning it comes every 25 days, then that is normal for you.

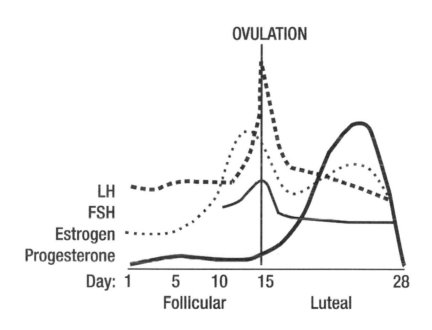

Days 1 to 14: Follicular Stage

Day 1 of your cycle is the first day of your period, and it is also the first day of the follicular phase of your cycle, which lasts until ovulation. Follicle-stimulating hormone (FSH) is secreted from the pituitary gland, which in turn stimulates a rise in estradiol and estrone (both of which are estrogens). Once the follicle develops, estradiol levels rise to a peak around day 13.

Menstruation usually occurs during the first five days of the follicular phase of your cycle. This monthly bleeding takes place because fertilization of an egg did not occur, thereby triggering a corresponding decline in estradiol, estrone, and progesterone levels. These hormones maintain the endometrial lining, the capillary-rich tissue that lines the wall of the uterus in which a fertilized embryo implants itself. If no embryo implants, estrogen and progesterone levels fall, and the endometrium sloughs off, tearing capillaries and causing bleeding. Low estrogen levels promote FSH secretion, stimulating ovarian structures called follicles to begin secreting more estrogen.

Eggs (ova) continue to mature during the follicular stage. After the menstrual period and until another egg (ovum) is released, FSH stimulates the ovarian follicles to produce estrogen to support the growth of the endometrium once again. The rising estrogen levels trigger a mid-cycle luteinizing hormone (LH) surge, which causes ovulation (release of an egg) sometime between days 12 and 15 of the cycle. The ovulatory phase, when the egg can be fertilized by the sperm, usually lasts 48 hours. At ovulation, the follicle that has been nurturing the growing egg ruptures, and the egg is released, to be swept up by special structures at the ends of the fallopian tubes that lead to the uterus.

Days 14 to 28: Luteal Phase

The luteal stage occurs after the egg is released. Once the egg is released, the ruptured follicle turns into a corpus luteum. Progesterone levels are higher relative to levels of estradiol and estrone in this phase, as the corpus luteum secretes large amounts of progesterone until day 21. Progesterone is needed to prepare the endometrial lining for implantation of a fertilized egg. If fertilization does not occur, as you can see on the graph, all hormone levels drop around day 25, and the uterus gets ready to shed the endometrial lining, beginning menstruation about 28 days after the beginning of the last bleed. The luteal phase is important because this is where large amounts of progesterone are manufactured. If you do not ovulate, your progesterone levels could be low.

Pregnancy

If the egg is fertilized, it will implant in the uterus (in the endometrium), and levels of progesterone and estrogens will stay high in order to maintain the pregnancy. Estriol, the safer form of estrogen, is very high during pregnancy. It is believed that the high levels of estriol are there to protect the fetus from the mother's high circulating estradiol, estrone, and estrogen metabolites. High levels of progesterone and estrogens also inhibit the release of FSH for the duration of the pregnancy.

The menstrual cycle continues for roughly 30-35 years, from puberty to menopause, unless pregnancy, breast feeding, or hormonal problems interrupt it. (Menopause means one year with no menstrual cycle.) Any extreme ups and downs in the estrogen/progesterone ratio, when either hormone is excessive or deficient, results in unwelcome symptoms. So many suffer with debilitating symptoms that a lot of women think it is normal to have painful, long, heavy, clotting periods; PMS; weight gain; and swollen, sore breasts. It is common but not normal, and bad periods are an early warning sign that hormones are out of balance.

The Liver, the Large Intestine, the Thyroid, and the Menstrual Cycle

The menstrual cycle is affected by more than the pituitary gland. Other organs that affect the menstrual cycle via their effects on levels of female hormones such as estrogen are the liver, the large intestine, and the thyroid. The liver's main function is to detoxify the body, and the more toxic the large intestine and other organs, the larger the burden on the liver. An overburdened liver has a decreased ability to break down excess sex hormones, especially estrogen. This can cause excess levels of estrogen in your system, leading to estrogen-dominant conditions like endometriosis, uterine fibroids, ovarian cysts, fibrocystic breasts, acne, heavy periods, and more. (See Chapter 5 for a closer look at estrogen-dominant conditions.)

In addition, adequate thyroid gland function is necessary for the production of progesterone. Both progesterone and thyroid hormone can be considered primary regulatory hormones. Both of these hormones regulate metabolism, have a normalizing, anti-stress action on the pituitary gland, and are consumed or affected by stress. Each has a supportive action on the other.

Menstruation Symptom Chart

Record the symptoms of your next monthly cycle in the chart below, using the following key: 0 = none, 1 = minimal, 2 = moderate, 3 = intense, 4 = severe; in the first row, simply records the supplies used. You can photocopy the chart and record on it monthly to see how your treatment is progressing also. Recording this information will allow you to see which days are the worst days and when symptoms start to abate.

MONTH	1	2	3	4	5	6	7	8	9	10	11	12	13	14	15	16	17	18	19	20	21	22	23	24	25	26	27	28
Tampons or pads / day																												
Flow																												
Cramps																												
Breats Sore																												
Fluid Retention																												
Muscus Secretion																												
Constipation																												
Headace																												
Sleep Problems																												
Anger																												
Anxiety																												
Depression																												
Sex Drive																												
Energy																												
Stresses																												

Comments

_____

_____

_____

_____

_____

_____

_____

_____

_____

_____

_____

_____

_____

_____

_____

_____

_____

_____

_____

Reviewing Your Symptoms

In addition to using the menstrual chart to gauge whether your hormones are in balance, you will also want to consider the following symptoms, which could indicate an imbalance in levels of estrogens, progesterone, testosterone or DHEA, cortisol, or thyroid hormones; adrenal exhaustion; or to see if you are experiencing peri-menopause or menopause symptoms. As you read in Chapter 2, hormones affect one another and an excess or low level of one hormone, for example testosterone or cortisol, can affect the level of another hormone, such as DHEA.

Symptoms can often tell you most of what you need to know about your hormones. In the days before sophisticated diagnostic tests, your doctor had to be very good at listening to descriptions of your symptoms in order to form an opinion of what might be causing your health problems. If you have more than three of the symptoms in a section, hormone imbalance may be present, and laboratory tests, such as saliva hormone, and/or urine and/or blood tests, can help provide a clearer picture of your hormone issues.

Excess progesterone

(for treatment options see Chapter 5)

- ❑ breast swelling and pain
- ❑ depression or low mood
- ❑ excess facial hair
- ❑ feeling tired, drowsiness
- ❑ hyper insulinemia (overproduction of insulin by the pancreas)
- ❑ low libido
- ❑ oily skin

Low progesterone

(for treatment options see Chapter 5)

- ❑ anxiety
- ❑ difficulty handling stress
- ❑ elevated cortisol levels
- ❑ estrogen dominant conditions (uterine fibroids, fibrocystic breasts, ovarian cysts, PCOS, breast cancer, thickening of the uterine lining, endometriosis)
- ❑ headaches
- ❑ heavy periods
- ❑ low bone density
- ❑ recurring miscarriage
- ❑ water retention
- ❑ weight gain on abdomen

Excess estrogen

(for treatment options see Chapter 5)

- [ ] acne
- [ ] anemia
- [ ] asthma intensifies
- [ ] depression
- [ ] estrogen-dominant conditions (uterine fibroids, fibrocystic breasts, ovarian cysts, PCOS, breast cancer, thickening of the uterine lining, endometriosis)
- [ ] fatigue
- [ ] fluid retention
- [ ] gallstones
- [ ] irritability
- [ ] loss of sex drive
- [ ] memory loss
- [ ] period problems (irregular, long or short, or heavy periods)
- [ ] PMS
- [ ] raging hot flashes and night sweats that do not abate with treatment
- [ ] weight gain

Low estrogen

(for treatment options see Chapter 5)

- [ ] brain fog
- [ ] painful intercourse
- [ ] recurring urinary tract infections
- [ ] urinary incontinence
- [ ] vaginal dryness
- [ ] thinning of the vaginal wall (vaginal atrophy)

Excess testosterone/DHEA

(for treatment options see Chapter 5)

- [ ] acne, oily skin
- [ ] facial hair growth
- [ ] hair loss
- [ ] high DHEA
- [ ] ovarian cysts and/or polycystic ovary syndrome (PCOS)
- [ ] resistance to insulin (diabetes)
- [ ] weight gain

Low testosterone/DHEA

(for treatment options see Chapter 5)

- [ ] fatigue
- [ ] high cortisol
- [ ] loss of strength and stamina
- [ ] low DHEA can be a result of low testosterone
- [ ] low or no sex drive
- [ ] memory decline
- [ ] muscle wasting and weakness (chin muscles start sagging)
- [ ] osteopenia
- [ ] osteoporosis
- [ ] sleep problems
- [ ] vaginal dryness

Overactive thyroid function

(for treatment options see Chapter 5)

- ❑ breathlessness
- ❑ fatigue
- ❑ hair loss
- ❑ heart palpitations
- ❑ heat intolerance
- ❑ increased bowel movements
- ❑ insomnia
- ❑ light or absent menstrual periods
- ❑ muscle weakness
- ❑ nervousness
- ❑ staring gaze (bulging eyes)
- ❑ trembling hands
- ❑ warm, moist skin
- ❑ weight loss
- ❑ goiter (enlarged thyroid)

Low thyroid function

(for treatment options see Chapter 5)

- ❑ a metallic taste in the mouth
- ❑ anemia
- ❑ anxiety/nervousness
- ❑ chronic fatigue, weakness, lethargy
- ❑ cold hands and feet, cold intolerance, low body temperature
- ❑ constipation
- ❑ cracking in the heels and skin
- ❑ depression and irritability
- ❑ doughy abdomen
- ❑ dry, coarse skin, hair, or both
- ❑ edema (swelling of eyelids or face)
- ❑ elevated cholesterol levels
- ❑ feeling unable to breathe deeply
- ❑ goiter (enlarged thyroid)
- ❑ hair loss
- ❑ headaches and dizziness
- ❑ heart palpitations
- ❑ high TSH, over 2.0
- ❑ hormonal imbalances (fibroids, ovarian or breast cysts, painful and/or heavy periods, endometriosis, PMS, frequent menstrual cycles)
- ❑ impaired memory
- ❑ infertility and/or recurring miscarriage
- ❑ insomnia
- ❑ low basal temperature (see Home Thyroid tests, page 51)
- ❑ low progesterone-to-estrogen ratio
- ❑ low T3, T4, or T7
- ❑ night sweats
- ❑ poor concentration
- ❑ poor vision
- ❑ presence of thyroid antibodies
- ❑ racing thoughts
- ❑ severe menopause symptoms that last for years without relief
- ❑ shortness of breath
- ❑ slow pulse
- ❑ slower metabolism (may show up as weight gain, either general or on the hips)
- ❑ sudden change in personality

Adrenal stress (for treatment options see Chapter 5)

- ❏ alcohol intolerance
- ❏ asthma/bronchitis
- ❏ blurred vision
- ❏ cold extremities
- ❏ cravings for stimulants, including salt, sugar, junk food, coffee or other caffeinated beverages
- ❏ depression
- ❏ digestive problems
- ❏ dizziness upon rising
- ❏ edema of extremities
- ❏ environmental sensitivities
- ❏ excessive perspiration
- ❏ excessive urination
- ❏ eyes light-sensitive
- ❏ food allergies
- ❏ headaches
- ❏ heart palpitations
- ❏ high cortisol
- ❏ hypoglycemia
- ❏ increase/loss of skin pigment (in the most advanced cases of adrenal exhaustion you will look like you have a suntan)
- ❏ inflammation and joint or muscle pain including arthritis, bursitis
- ❏ insomnia (where you fall asleep but it is disrupted after a few hours and it's difficult to fall back to sleep)
- ❏ irritability
- ❏ knee problems
- ❏ low back pain
- ❏ low energy, excessive fatigue
- ❏ low thyroid
- ❏ muscle twitches
- ❏ nervousness/anxiety
- ❏ poor concentration
- ❏ post-exertional fatigue
- ❏ recurring infections
- ❏ shortness of breath
- ❏ tired feet
- ❏ ulcers

Excess cortisol

(for treatment options see Chapter 5)

- ❑ hair loss
- ❑ high blood pressure
- ❑ high insulin
- ❑ insulin resistance (diabetes)
- ❑ irritable, anxiety
- ❑ low DHEA
- ❑ low progesterone levels
- ❑ low sex drive
- ❑ low thyroid
- ❑ mood swings and depression
- ❑ osteoporosis
- ❑ poor immune function
- ❑ weight gain
- ❑ "wired but tired" feeling

Low cortisol

(for treatment options see Chapter 5)

- ❑ allergies
- ❑ burned out feeling
- ❑ difficulty handling stress
- ❑ feel like you are pushing yourself through the day
- ❑ increased infections
- ❑ low blood pressure
- ❑ morning tiredness
- ❑ muscle stiffness
- ❑ no sex drive
- ❑ sensitivity to cold

Symptoms of peri-menopause

(for treatment options see Chapter 5)

- ❑ 35 or older
- ❑ a reduced libido
- ❑ endometriosis
- ❑ fibroid breast cysts
- ❑ gained ten pounds and abdomen is bloated
- ❑ headaches
- ❑ heavy periods, clotting or longer periods
- ❑ hot flashes and/or night sweats
- ❑ insomnia (early sleep is disrupted after a few hours, and it's difficult to fall back to sleep)
- ❑ keep forgetting things
- ❑ PMS symptoms
- ❑ skin outbreaks/acne
- ❑ thinning hair
- ❑ uterine fibroids

Symptoms of menopause

(for treatment options see Chapter 5)

- ❑ 45 or older
- ❑ have not had a period for 12 months or longer
- ❑ do not have a desire for sex
- ❑ feeling anxious, irritable, and tire easily
- ❑ gained weight
- ❑ hot flashes and/or night sweats
- ❑ intercourse is painful
- ❑ leaking urine
- ❑ memory problems and brain fog occurs
- ❑ insomnia (either can't fall asleep or wake up throughout the night)
- ❑ skin is excessively dry and wrinkled
- ❑ vaginal dryness or vaginal infections

Lab Test Help for the Hormone Puzzle

To determine a baseline for your hormones and for information when monitoring hormone replacement therapy, it makes sense to assess your hormone levels. Dr. Pettle and I do this with menstrual history, symptom questionnaires, and blood and/or saliva hormone testing. We receive thousands of emails, phone calls, and letters every month from women who have never had any basic diagnostic tests or hormone testing performed before being prescribed synthetic hormones. Nor have these women had any follow-up testing to ensure that the prescribed synthetic hormones were not creating an imbalance. If you are one of those women who took Premarin for decades without monitoring, you know what we mean.

Tests Recommended for Women Prescribed Synthetic HRT

The *Canadian Compendium of Pharmaceuticals and Specialties* (CPS) states that before using any synthetic estrogen alone or in combination with synthetic progesterone, all patients should undergo the following medical tests:
- thyroid tests (TSH, Free T3, Free T4, and thyroid antibodies)
- blood calcium levels
- blood glucose levels
- endometrial biopsy or pelvic ultrasound to measure endometrial lining thickness
- Papanicolaou smear (Pap test)
- lipid panel test (triglycerides, total cholesterol, HDL, LDL)
- liver function tests
- serum levels of 25-hydroxy vitamin D (see page 114 on vitamin D for thyroid health and cancer prevention)
- complete physical examination, including blood pressure evaluation and examinations of the breasts and pelvic organs

After the baseline examination is done, the first follow-up examination should be done within six months of the beginning of treatment, to assess the response to synthetic hormone use. Thereafter, says CPS, examinations should be done once a year and should include at least those procedures listed above. It is also important, emphasizes CPS, that patients be encouraged to examine their breasts frequently. How many women were given these tests before HRT was prescribed? In reality, not very many!

These basic tests should be performed for all women taking hormones, even those women prescribed bioidentical hormones, because hormones work differently in a healthy individual than they do in someone with poor liver function, a low thyroid function, or cardiovascular disease. These tests just make sense. Add the results to the appropriate saliva, blood, or urine hormone tests, and your physician will be able to help you make the best treatment choice.

Blood Hormone Tests

The standard blood test for determining menopause is the FSH test. FSH levels go up at menopause (menopause means one year with no periods). However, FSH levels may also be elevated in peri-menopausal women who are still menstruating regularly. The confusion of this traditional lab test means that even though these women are still having regular periods, they are told they are in menopause—when they are not. A woman in her late forties or older who has not menstruated for one year does not need an FSH test to tell her she is in menopause; it is not that difficult to figure out because the definition of menopause is one year with no periods. What is difficult, however, is determining what hormonal changes are related to the symptoms of peri-menopause versus menopause.

Blood levels of estradiol, FSH, LH, progesterone, progesterone 17OH, testosterone, and DHEAS can give an overall indication of hormonal imbalances, but they have their limitations because they measure hormones bound to blood proteins, which are the inactive hormones. Also, blood tests do not measure estriol levels. Estriol can be measured by a 24-hour urine test or by a saliva test. Blood hormone test results should be used *along with* an evaluation of symptoms and saliva hormone testing for a more accurate picture of hormone health. Menstruating women should note the day in the cycle when blood is drawn, or the information will not be useful. Some of the most common blood hormone tests performed by your medical doctor are listed below.

Estradiol Blood Test

17b-Estradiol is the dominant form of estrogen in a woman's body. It is normally produced by the ovary, the adrenal gland (limited amount), and by peripheral conversion of adrenal androgens. This blood test is a poor indicator of low levels of estradiol in women, mainly because the female reference range used when evaluating the test is too broad. Those with low levels fall in the "normal" range, and elevated estrogen values in female adults are also difficult to distinguish from normal. Medications containing estradiol also confound the results. When low levels are detected in women, this can be indicative of ovarian failure, menopause, pituitary failure, or Turner's syndrome. All in all, blood levels of estradiol alone do not give an accurate picture.

FSH Blood Test

Follicle-stimulating hormone (FSH) is the pituitary hormone that controls the maturation of eggs in the ovary. Levels go up during ovulation, ovarian failure (the inability of the ovary to respond to gonadotropic hormone), and the transitional years around menopause and in post-menopause. FSH is low in cases of infertility and pituitary insufficiency (low levels of pituitary hormones). FSH levels vary throughout a normal menstrual cycle, so taking the test on days 10 to 15, during ovulation, will provide the most accurate results. Infertility clinics use day 3 to measure FSH, and if it is above 10, this is a sign of poor fertility.

LH Blood Test

Luteinizing hormone (LH) is made by the pituitary gland. It controls the production of estrogen in the ovary and the formation of the corpus luteum. LH is elevated in ovarian failure and in the transitional years around menopause and post-menopause. If LH is low, this can be due to pituitary insufficiency, especially in peri-menopausal women.

Progesterone Blood Test

Progesterone is normally low in the first half of the menstrual cycle, rising during the latter third of the menstrual cycle (days 15 to 25) if ovulation has occurred and a corpus luteum developed. A progesterone test is most often used to determine if ovulation has occurred. The best days to test are days 20 to 22.

Progesterone 17OH Blood Test

17OH progesterone is made by the adrenal gland. High blood levels of progesterone 17OH are associated with problems of adrenal metabolism whereby excess male hormones (androgens) are produced. This blood test is used to evaluate possible causes of excessive body hair (hirsutism), weight gain around the hips, and acne in women.

Testosterone Blood Test

Elevated levels of testosterone in women are associated with hirsutism. Low levels of testosterone in women are a possible cause of low libido. As you read in the Prologue, elevated SHBG can be caused by the birth control pill and have negative effects. A basic blood testosterone test looks at bound testosterone— that is testosterone bound by sex-hormone-binding-globulin protein (SHBG).

Tests of free (bioavailable) testosterone measure the blood testosterone concentration without being influenced by sex-hormone-binding-globulin.

Dihydrotestosterone Blood Test

Dihydrotestosterone (DHT) is primarily made in the hair follicles, adrenal glands, and, in men, in the prostate and testes. Testosterone is converted into DHT using the enzyme 5-alpha reductase. DHT has a much stronger action on testosterone receptors than testosterone does.

A blood test for levels of DHT is used to diagnose the causes of head hair loss (Androgenetic Alopecia or "Male Pattern Baldness"), upper lip hair growth in women, and suspected polycystic ovary syndrome. DHT is elevated in women with these conditions. In some cases, DHT is also involved in stimulating the growth of excessive body hair in women.

DHEAS Blood Test

Dehydroepiandrosterone (DHEA) is a precursor hormone made from cholesterol by the adrenal glands, adipose tissue (fat cells), the brain, and in the skin. DHEA is used to make androstenedione, testosterone, and estrogen. Dehydro-epiandrosterone sulfate (DHEAS) is the sulfated version of DHEA. This conversion, which is reversible (meaning it can go back and forth between DHEA and DHEAS), takes place primarily in the adrenals, liver, and small intestine. In blood, most DHEA is found as DHEAS, with levels that are about 300 times higher than free DHEA. When DHEA is taken orally, it is converted to DHEA sulfate when passing through intestines and liver. Testing DHEAS provides information on how much DHEA is stored, and it is more stable than DHEA. Blood tests for DHEAS can detect excess adrenal activity or adrenal cancer. Women with polycystic ovary syndrome can have elevated levels of DHEAS.

Cortisol Blood Test

Many doctors do not include cortisol in their hormone test panel unless the person has obvious adrenal disease, such as Addison's (cortisol deficiency) or Cushing's Syndrome (excess cortisol), yet cortisol is an important indicator for many conditions. Cortisol is secreted from the adrenals, and healthy adrenals are essential for hormone balance. Any disturbance in cortisol can lead to hormone-related problems.

Elevated cortisol in the evening or afternoon can disrupt your sleep. Low morning cortisol makes you feel like you are pushing yourself through the day. High cortisol can cause hair loss and/or bone loss and is associated with high blood pressure, diabetes, low sex drive, weight gain around the middle, and increased risk of breast cancer. Cortisol blood tests can be either done as an AM/PM cortisol test or they can be done several times per day. Many doctors will ask for an AM cortisol blood test as this is easier for the person to do, rather than having to return to the laboratory several times in a day. (Cortisol is also measured in the saliva and urine. Testing is covered by many health plans.)

Saliva Hormone Tests

Over two decades of published clinical data has proven that saliva hormone tests are very sensitive. In fact, they are much more accurate at predicting if hormones are moving out of the blood to receptor sites on tissues than blood hormone tests are. Like blood tests, saliva hormone tests for women can also measure estrogens (saliva measures estriol and estrone levels accurately), progesterone, testosterone, cortisol, and DHEAS. The one exception is free testosterone, which can only be measured in blood tests. Unlike blood tests, saliva hormone tests measure the amount of steroid hormone not bound to carrier proteins in the blood. Saliva hormone testing is also convenient and non-invasive compared to blood draws done in labs, especially when hormones have to be tested at different times throughout the day.

Each woman is unique, and we prefer saliva hormone testing labs that provide a detailed interpretation with results that not only look at hormone levels in saliva but cross-reference the data with the symptoms provided on the symptom questionnaire. These questionnaires are included in the saliva hormone test kit and must be filled out. We recommend continued close monitoring of hormone levels when supplementary hormones are first prescribed and then every six months to one year thereafter. Saliva hormone testing is accurate when monitoring bioidentical hormone therapies.

Blood versus Saliva Hormone Testing

Several dozen well-designed, published studies have shown a correlation between saliva hormone levels and hormones produced by the body. When looking at hormones produced by the body, blood and saliva levels are similar. It is when hormones are provided in a supplement form that the blood and saliva do not show the same results, and those results are also affected by whether the hormone was delivered by mouth or skin.

Research published in the *Journal of the North American Menopause Society* showed that when hormones are supplemented via the skin, blood levels do not match saliva levels, but it is the blood levels that do not give a true indicator of how much hormone has actually made its way to the tissues.

Several other studies show that when supplementing hormones, blood hormone levels fail to show the hormones' ability to change symptoms. In fact, many Premarin studies showed that even though blood tests showed estrogen levels went up, there was little improvement in hot flashes. What a woman wants to know is this: "Are the hormones safe?" and "Does the hormone actually make a difference to my symptoms?" In 2005, a major review article on routes of administration of estrogens found that although blood testing showed an increase in blood levels when women were supplemented with estradiol, the patients did not experience any effect on the symptoms of menopause.

When it comes to predicting how blood levels of testosterone correlate to improvement in sexual function, again the level in the blood tells little of how supplementing the hormone will affect symptoms. Saliva hormone testing, on the other hand, gives a better picture of how much hormone is actually moving through the body to the receptors where it can have its effects. That said, how hormone levels in body fluids, whether it be blood, urine, or saliva, relate to the actions of the hormones at the receptor level is still far from being understood.

Rocky Mountain Analytical Labs in Canada and ZRT in the United States are excellent laboratories that we have used for hormone testing. We prefer these labs because they provide a written interpretation of the test results for you and your doctor. As well, there are other outstanding saliva hormone testing labs that your doctor may already be using. Saliva hormone testing orders in Canada must be signed by a regulated health professional. This includes, but is not limited to: medical doctors, naturopaths, pharmacists, and chiropractors. All test requisitions must be signed by one of the health professionals listed above before testing will proceed.

In Canada, you can contact Rocky Mountain Analytical labs at www.rmalab.com and in the U.S., contact ZRT Laboratory at www.zrtlab.com to learn about their specific tests and procedures. Meridian Valley Labs also provides high-quality tests. They can be reached at www.meridianvalleylab.com.

Urine Hormone Tests

Urine testing is another method of evaluating hormone status, but it has its limitations. Standard tests require a 24-hour urine collection, which can be challenging for people who are busy and rarely at home for 24 hours. Hormones that are in the urine have already been processed by the liver, and these are the hormones the body is excreting. Urinary hormone testing can survey a wide range of hormones and metabolites.

Urine Breast Cancer Risk Test

Several salivary hormone laboratories offer urinary hormone tests for breast-cancer risk assessment. These tests look at the levels and ratio of the estrogen metabolites 2-hydroxyestrone and 16 alpha-hydroxyestrone (see page 46 for more information). These metabolites are directly related—if more 2-hydroxy-estrone is made, less 16 alpha-hydroxyestrone is usually made, and vice-versa. 2-hydroxyestrone is to be deemed the good estrogen metabolite, whereas evidence suggests that 16 alpha-hydroxyestrone is the bad estrogen metabolite. 16 alpha-hydroxyestrone increases cellular growth and proliferation and cancerous transformation in estrogen-responsive tissues. Other researchers believe that cancer in the uterus, cervix, prostate, liver, and kidney may be affected by the 2-to-16 alpha-hydroxyestrone ratio, as well as by other estrogen metabolites. A higher 2-to-16 ratio is better than a lower one. This is one test we believe every woman should have performed annually, with no exceptions. We believe this test to be as important as other breast cancer diagnostics. You only have to provide a single sample of urine (not 24-hours' worth). On page 172 we discuss which nutrients keep this ratio in the breast-cancer protective zone.

Do You Need Hormone Lab Tests?

As we said earlier, if you have more than three of the symptoms in any of the sections on pages 36-40, you may have a hormone imbalance, and a saliva hormone test and/or blood and/or urine tests may help provide a clearer picture of your hormone issues.

Case Study: Lorna V

While writing this book, I had my hormones tested at dozens of saliva hormone testing laboratories, along with blood and urine testing, to get an idea of the types of testing being done all over North America and the results provided. Some saliva hormone testing laboratories provide detailed hormone evaluations along with the test results. This is helpful when determining treatments. Rocky Mountain Analytical laboratories provided excellent, detailed reports based on the symptom questionnaire I filled out and returned with the saliva kit. Below is my saliva hormone evaluation.

I am peri-menopausal, and the test was within one hour of waking in the morning on day 20 of my cycle. The following chart with my results will give you an idea of what "almost-normal" saliva test results reveal.

Hormone Tested	Actual Result	Normal Reference Range
estradiol pg/ml	high end of normal 8.5	1.0–9.0 mid luteal
estrone* pg/ml	within range 6.3	2.0–10 female endogenous range
estriol* pg/ml	below range 2.7	5.0–20 female endogenous range
progesterone pg/ml	within range 98	25–250 mid luteal
testosterone pg/ml	within range 26	15–45 female testosterone endogenous
DHEAS ng/ml	within range 6.4	2.0–11 female DHEAS endogenous
cortisol AM ng/ml	within range 4.9	2.0–11 sampled within 1 hour of waking

The following written report was included for both me and my physician.

Progesterone to Estradiol

Lorna's ratio of progesterone to estradiol is 11.5.

On average, the most commonly observed ratio in regularly cycling women in the luteal phase is in the range 8–30, with 15 being the middle value. Symptoms indicate minimal or moderate estrogen-progesterone imbalance at this time. If symptoms of estrogen dominance, such as water retention, weight gain at the hips, migraines, irritability, and breast tenderness develop or worsen, the situation should be reassessed.

What I learned from the tests that were performed is that I have to work on improving my estradiol-to-estriol ratio or my total estrogen-to-progesterone ratio. I will increase my dose of EstroSense (see page 83 for information on EstroSense) from two capsules per day to four per day and retest.

Cortisol to DHEAS

Lorna's ratio of A.M. cortisol to DHEAS is 0.8.

This ratio normally increases with age. Based on a large in-house analysis of more than 15,000 samples at ZRT Laboratory in Portland, Oregon, the ratio at age 20 is approximately 0.6; at age 45, it is 1.0; at age 60, it is 1.5; and at age 75, it is 2.3. This is because levels of DHEAS decline with age, whereas morning cortisol stays the same or increases slightly. If the ratio is higher than expected, based on the patient's age, this may be indicative of unbalanced adrenal function (cortisol too high or DHEAS too low). Factors that can contribute to imbalance include acute or chronic stress, obesity, metabolic syndrome/diabetes, and hypothyroidism. If the ratio is lower than expected for age, and DHEAS is within normal limits, this may simply be an indicator of healthy aging (i.e., preservation of DHEAS output with age); however, a lower-than-expected ratio for age may also be due to low cortisol, high DHEAS, or both.

My cortisol to DHEA ratio was surprisingly excellent or, as the report says, a sign of healthy aging. Considering I did these tests while writing this book and traveling, I was pleased that the diet and nutrient program I am doing is working.

Estriol

Lorna's estriol is low or low-normal.

Low estriol symptoms would be vaginal dryness and urinary incontinence, although these symptoms are not present currently. If low estriol symptoms develop, the situation should be reassessed.

Estriol to other Estrogens

Lorna's estriol quotient (EQ) Estriol (E3) to Estrone (E1) + Estradiol (E2) is 0.2.
In-house data indicate that the average estriol quotient in peri-menopausal women sampled days 19–21 is 0.4.

The estriol quotient in post-menopausal women who are not using supplemental estrogen is 1.4. A May 2006 survey of women supplementing with BiEst or TriEst creams indicates that 60 percent of them had an EQ of less than 1. Twenty percent had an EQ between 1 and 2, and 20 percent of the EQs were greater than 2. Note that no studies pertaining to the risk of breast cancer and the salivary estriol quotient have been published; therefore it is up to the practitioner to draw his or her own conclusions regarding the meaning of this EQ result.

I will also be having regular urine breast-cancer risk assessments performed by Rocky Mountain to keep an eye on my breast cancer risk as I age.

Tests for Adrenal Function

A test of postural (orthostatic) blood pressure is an easy, in-clinic assessment of adrenal function. A blood pressure reading is taken once while the patient is in the reclining position and twice when the patient is brought to a standing position. In a normal response, the blood pressure will be approximately 10 mg/hg higher in the standing position than in the lying position. With adrenal insufficiency, the blood pressure will drop 5 mg/hg or more when the patient moves from the lying to standing position. Generally, the orthostatic blood pressure is a reliable indication of the adrenal state, with a few exceptions: athletes and people taking cortisone. Competitive athletes are constantly pushing their adrenal glands to the point that the adrenals are constantly in overdrive, making it difficult to assess adrenal function based on this measurement only. Those taking prednisone or other forms of cortisone will not be able to use this simple test as the drugs mask normal adrenal function.

Blood Sugar Imbalance and Adrenal Function

One of the most common conditions that we see in people of all ages is functional dysglycemia (blood sugar dysregulation). Glucose (blood sugar) is the main fuel for the brain and is required by all the cells of the body. Thus, it is important to maintain balanced blood glucose levels, adequate for meeting demand. Women in particular have difficulty with the metabolism of carbohydrates. The result is dysglycemia.

Blood sugar illnesses such as diabetes and hypoglycemia are well-recognized and easily diagnosed by looking at fluctuations in blood glucose levels and the associated symptoms. Sub-clinical blood sugar dysregulation, called dsyglycemia, however, often cannot be confirmed by fasting blood glucose tests. Symptoms are very similar to those produced by the more serious blood sugar imbalances, though not as dramatic. The main symptoms include, but are not limited to, anxiety, fatigue, irritability, and poor concentration. Symptoms generally occur two to three hours after carbohydrate ingestion.

There are laboratory blood tests that may be helpful in assessing dysglycemia: the two-hour postprandial (post-meal) blood glucose test, the four- or six-hour glucose tolerance test, or the more sensitive four- or six-hour glucose and insulin tolerance test. The fasting blood glucose test (the most routinely done) is a single, isolated measurement and cannot provide information on overall blood glucose regulation.

Testing Thyroid Function

It is common for the thyroid to be functionally, or even clinically, low in women who experience hormone-related problems such as premenstrual syndrome (PMS), infertility, ovarian cysts, fibroids, endometriosis, fibrocystic breasts, menstrual pain, heavy bleeding, or menopausal symptoms.

Home Thyroid Test

Monitoring your basal temperature is a simple, inexpensive method to evaluate thyroid function. Your thyroid sets the thermostat for your body and regulates the rate of metabolism in nearly all of your cells. Therefore, a reliable window on thyroid function is the basic body temperature.

- Plan to measure your temperature as soon as you wake up in the morning, before rising.
- Shake down the basal thermometer the night before, and leave it at your bedside.
- Immediately on waking, put it under your arm and leave it in your armpit for 10 minutes.
- Women who are menstruating should take the test on the second, third, or fourth day of their period.
- The temperature should be recorded every morning for at least one week.

Normal basal temperature averages between 36.5 and 36.7° C (97.7 and 98.6° F). Having an average temperature below the normal range could indicate a hypothyroid state; a temperature above this range could indicate a hyperthyroid state.

If a blood test indicates your thyroid-stimulating hormone (TSH) level is above 2.0, your basal temperatures are low, and you experience some or many of the symptoms indicated for the condition (see page 38), you most likely are suffering from functional low thyroid.

If a blood test indicates your TSH is under .05 and you have taken your basal temperature and it is higher than normal, this indicates your thyroid is working too hard and is overactive (hyperthyroid). This condition usually precedes hypothyroidism because when the thyroid has worked too hard for too long, it becomes tired and has to slow down.

Clinical Low Thyroid

A diagnosis of clinical hypothyroidism (low thyroid) is made when a TSH blood test indicates TSH levels are higher than 5.5 to 6.0. The range of normal for most TSH tests, depending on which state or province you live in, is 0.5 to 5.5 or 6.0. This allows for a very broad definition of what is normal. High TSH levels indicate hypothyroidism because the pituitary is pumping out TSH in an effort to stimulate the thyroid into action. The range of normal for TSH is too broad and many labs are adjusting their reference ranges to show that a TSH above 2.0 is indicative of low thyroid function.

Functional or Suboptimal Low Thyroid

When laboratory tests show results that fall in the normal range, yet the patient has the classic symptoms of low thyroid, we consider this to be suboptimal function of the thyroid.

Suboptimal thyroid function can be diagnosed when the TSH is above 2.0, and the person has the classic symptoms of hypothyroidism (for the self-test for low thyroid see page 51). Many women deal with symptoms for a decade before the TSH test gives them a reading of 5.5 or higher, indicative of clinical low thyroid. Physicians have to stop relying solely on test results and start looking at the symptoms the patient is presenting. Estrogen, cortisol, and progesterone also have to be evaluated when looking for a low thyroid diagnosis. *Therefore, if your Thyroid Stimulating Hormone test result is 2.0 or higher, this suggests low thyroid.*

This problem with ranges holds true in any health situation and is particularly the case when it comes to diagnosing thyroid imbalances. The "normal" levels for thyroid tests are so broad that most patients with suboptimal thyroid function are not diagnosed. It is a mystery to us why the normal range for TSH is so wide, given the extreme sensitivity of the thyroid to even minute variations in TSH levels.

Two Non-Hormone Tests that Can
Save Your Life

In addition to testing for hormone imbalances, there are two other key tests that you should have regularly throughout your life—not just your reproductive life—your whole life after puberty.

Ovarian Cancer Test Life Saver

Ovarian cancer, the fifth most diagnosed cancer, accounts for almost five percent of all cancer deaths and is called "the silent killer." Vague symptoms make this cancer difficult to detect, allowing the cancer to invade other tissues. With an almost 60 percent death rate, women need to understand the symptoms so they can seek treatment early. Lorna lost an ovary and fallopian tube to a huge tumor nine years ago. She had symptoms for months, but nothing really "worth visiting the doctor" about—until one afternoon she developed severe pain and ended up in the operating room of the local hospital.

Symptoms of ovarian cancer can mimic common illnesses and are often vague. According to the Canadian Cancer Society, the symptoms of the early stages of ovarian cancer include a mild discomfort in the lower part of the abdomen, a sense of incomplete evacuation of stool, gas, a frequent urge to urinate, indigestion, feeling full after a light meal, low back pain, and vaginal discharge. More advanced ovarian cancer symptoms may cause build-up of fluid in the abdomen, making clothes fit tightly even though no weight has been gained, pain during intercourse, abnormal bleeding, diarrhea or constipation, abdominal pain, nausea and vomiting, and fatigue. These symptoms can also be caused by many other conditions, but if you have a combination of them for more than three weeks, you should have your doctor do some tests to rule out ovarian cancer.

The diagnostic tests are simple: a transvaginal ultrasound, a CA-125 blood test, and a pelvic exam. Most general practitioners will send you to a gynecologist.

Many doctors are not doing a CA-125 blood test for ovarian cancer because they believe it is not a reliable test. This is incorrect, and the U.S. National Ovarian Cancer Association recommends the test be done on women with the above symptoms and annually in women who are post-menopausal. In 1983, Harvard University found elevated levels in 80 percent of women with Stage 3 and Stage 4 ovarian cancer. In women with Stage 1 cancer, it is not as reliable, with only 40-50 percent having elevated levels. Test results can also be elevated in women with endometriosis and uterine fibroids. A normal level is less than 35u/ml, and a normal test has also been found in a small number of women with Stage 1 and Stage 2 ovarian cancer. However, the CA-125 is the best test we have when combined with a transvaginal ultrasound. Surgery, a laproscopy, is the only definitive method to detect ovarian cancer. The CA-125 blood test is covered under provincial medical plans in Canada and by most HMOs in the U.S.

Some doctors recommend birth control pills to stop ovulation as a form of ovarian cancer prevention. We feel this is a poor option due to the elevated breast cancer risks. A vegetarian diet with good protein sources, along with vitamins A, C, E, and selenium and zinc, combined with the plant nutrients indole-3-carbinol and d-glucarate, have been shown to lower the risk of developing ovarian cancer. Prevention is the key, but diagnostics for early detection need to improve so that the death rates start to decline. According to the latest statistics, one-third of North American women have not had a pelvic exam and Pap test in the last three years. If ovarian cancer is to be diagnosed in the early stages, you need to do your part and have proper gynecological exams every year. If you have one elevated CA-125 blood test, you should have this test annually as well.

Cervical Dysplasia and Cervical Cancer

The American College of Pathology states that four out of five women who died of cervical cancer had not had a Pap smear in the previous five years. According to Health Canada, the highest incidence of cervical cancer and the highest death rates occur in women over the age of 55, a group that often stops having annual Pap tests. Pap smears save lives by discovering abnormal cells called cervical dysplasia early enough to prevent loss of life from cervical cancer. All adult women from the age of 18 should have an annual Pap test to ensure their cervixes are healthy—but what can be done when the test comes back abnormal?

The main risk factors that promote abnormal cervical cells include using the birth control pill; increasing age; infection with the Human Papilloma Virus (HPV), the virus that also causes warts; smoking; and nutritional deficiencies of folic acid, vitamin A, and vitamin C.

We definitely do not want to ignore abnormal Pap tests. In North America, Pap results are graded as CINI, CINII, CINIII, or CINIV or CIS. A CINIV or CIS is cancer. Most women are not treated until they have an invasive CINII or CINIII. The Bethesda system of grading Paps is also used and tests are graded as Low Grade SIL (equivalent to a CINI) and High Grade SIL (includes CINII, CINIII and Cancer). Always ask what grade your Pap test is. Too many women are advised they have an abnormal test result, told to come back in six months for another test and not given any suggestions for how to get their cervical cells to return to normal. Yes, some abnormal cells return to normal with no treatment, but what if simply taking a nutritional supplement could ensure a normal Pap?

We know that HPV is implicated in the majority of cervical dysplasia and cervical cancer cases. New research has shown that indole-3-carbinol (I3C) can reverse abnormal cervical lesions before they have a chance to develop into cancer. In one of many studies, 30 women with CINII and CINIII cervical lesions took 200 mg of I3C daily for six months. 50 percent in the treatment group had complete regression of their lesions. None of the placebo group (those getting fake pills) had any change in their lesions.

Cervical dysplasia and cervical cancer can be prevented. Have your annual Pap smear, and make sure your mom has hers as well—too many women after menopause are not having annual tests. Pap tests save lives! Smart women take their multivitamin with minerals every day and include indole-3-carbinol. These simple steps can help ensure all women have normal Pap smears.

Beyond Hormone Testing

There is no hormone test on the market, whether it be blood, urine, or saliva, that can tell your doctor a hormone dosage. Hormone therapy should always be guided by a combination of diagnostic techniques—first and foremost for consideration is your symptoms. Hormone testing is only an aid to the diagnostic process.

If you come to the conclusion, through observation and testing, that you have less than optimal hormone levels, a variety of treatment options are available, including nutritional and lifestyle changes, with or without additional treatment with bioidentical hormones. We will look at these options in the following chapters.

4

The Truth About
Hormone Therapies

Hormone therapies have been promoted with great fanfare and promise of low-risk solutions. Here are the facts behind those promises.

The Story of Synthetic Hormones

Premarin, the miracle synthetic estrogen for the treatment of menopause symptoms, hit the marketplace in 1942 and went on to become one of the top-ten selling drugs in North America by the 1960s. In 1966, with financial backing from Wyeth-Ayerst, (manufacturers of Premarin), Robert A. Wilson, an M.D. and gynecologist, wrote the book *Feminine Forever*. The basic attitude underpinning the promotion of synthetic estrogen is summed up in the following words from *Feminine Forever*, "The unpalatable truth must be faced that all post-menopausal women are castrates…. From a practical point of view, a man remains a man until the very end." A multibillion dollar business was built on the premise that menopause made women less feminine. The brainwashing of doctors and women was so effective that even today women who have been taking synthetic estrogens will tell us that they do not want to go off them because they do not want to age faster, wrinkle, and generally become less feminine.

Wilson's book and its effect on the sales of Premarin was the beginning of a lucrative, dangerous love affair between synthetic estrogen and women in menopause. By the 1980s, women taking synthetic estrogen were found to have a fourteen-fold increase in endometrial cancer (cancer in the endometrial lining of the uterus) and a 30 percent increase in breast cancer. Once this information was released, synthetic estrogens lost their appeal—albeit only for a short time.

Then the dilemma of cancer problems was purported to have been "solved" by introducing synthetic progestin, also known as medroxyprogesterone acetate, into the mix. Then a woman who still had her uterus would be "safe" from endometrial cancer, and a woman who had had her uterus and ovaries removed during a hysterectomy could keep taking unopposed estrogens. No one discussed the breast cancer or heart health risks in those women taking estrogens alone, and it is still largely ignored today.

Women were told they could safely take synthetic estrogens with synthetic progestin (commonly called hormone replacement therapy or HRT) because progestin stopped the over-stimulation of the uterine lining caused by estrogens. Despite the use of synthetic progestin, the looming risk of cancer continued to haunt HRT.

Pre-mar-in: Pregnant Mare's Urine

Many physicians consider Premarin to be a natural hormone because it is derived from horse urine and is not synthesized in a laboratory. But Premarin is made up of horse estrogens, not human estrogens. It would be like using Ford parts for your BMW. They might just fit your vehicle, but it won't run well.

HRT was about to hit its demographic sweet spot as baby boomers entered menopause. Future sales were projected to be in the multi-billions. Although HRT was originally developed for estrogen deficiency during menopause, doctors also prescribed HRT to prevent cardiovascular disease and bone loss, relieve depression, reduce urinary incontinence, stop colon cancer and Alzheimer's, and keep women young forever. HRT became the panacea drug for all sorts of women's conditions and was touted as the "fountain of youth" even though the safety of HRT was still being debated and no randomized, controlled clinical trials were ever conducted to verify that HRT could be used for all those conditions. Furthermore, its safety in healthy women had never been proven. That is, until the findings of the Women's Health Initiative (WHI) estrogen-and-progestin and estrogen-alone studies were released.

The HRT Bomb Dropped

The WHI studies were supposed to put to rest all the debate about the safety of synthetic HRT for healthy women. Then one sunny day in July 2002 front-page headlines in every major newspaper across North America dropped the bomb—HRT was potentially deadly for some women. The WHI estrogen-and-progestin trial was halted five years and two months into the study due to serious safety concerns. This study, which was supposed to last eight years, involved 16,608 healthy, post-menopausal women aged 50–79 years, who were at low risk for heart disease. The women received 0.625 mg of synthetic estrogens (Premarin) along with 2.5 mg of synthetic progestins (Provera) or a placebo for 5.2 years. Premarin contains synthetic estradiol plus several horse estrogens, such as equilin and equilenin. The trial used synthetic medroxyprogesterone, which does not act the same way as the body's own progesterone.

Researchers conducting the study concluded that the combination of synthetic estrogens and progestins posed a significant health risk to women and that the benefits, such as the reduction of hot flashes and night sweats and improved bone or colon health, did not outweigh the risk of heart attack, stroke, and/or breast cancer. The study found the combination of synthetic estrogens and progestins was linked to:

- a 26 percent increase in the incidence of invasive breast cancer
- a 41 percent increase in the incidence of stroke
- 29 percent increase in heart attacks
- doubled rates of blood clots in legs and lungs
- a 76 percent increase in Alzheimer's dementia, according to further evaluation of the WHI study in 2003
- breast tissue so dense it was challenging to detect breast cancer on a mammogram
- increased hearing loss, according to a 2004 analysis of the data
- 37 percent reduction in the incidence of colorectal cancer, and 33 percent fewer hip fractures, which were the only positive notes

Then in March 2004, an extension of the WHI Premarin-only arm of the study was halted due to an increased risk of developing blood clots, stroke, and dementia.

Many have suggested that the number of women affected was quite small, yet George Gillson, M.D. Ph.D, coauthor of *You've Hit Menopause, Now What?*, states,

The HRT-attributable risk of invasive breast cancer (the "extra" risk over and above the natural incidence) was 8 per 10,000 persons per years of use, in the combined HRT arm. Extrapolating to a hypothetical, but reasonable, assumption that two million Canadian women use this form of drug therapy for five years, we can easily calculate that the number of excess cases of invasive breast cancer will be 16,000 under these circumstances. This is not a small number by any stretch. In actuality, large numbers of women have probably been harmed by what has passed for hormone replacement therapy over the past 30 or so years, due to apparently "small" risk increases.

In April 2007, a study published in *The Lancet* found that women who take synthetic HRT (estrogen and progestin) are 20 percent more likely to develop (and die from) ovarian cancer than women who have never taken HRT. The results are from the Million Women Study, covering 1.3 million British women from 1996 to 2001. Data from 948,000 post-menopausal women were evaluated; 30 percent of those in the study were current HRT users, 20 percent had used it previously, and 50 percent had never used HRT. The 20 percent increased risk was found more predominantly in those who were current users and who had used HRT for up to five years. Smoking and oral contraceptive use was equal among all groups. Ovarian cancer is a silent killer. The researchers recommended that if women decide to use synthetic HRT for menopausal symptoms, they should do so for the shortest period of time and use the lowest dose possible.

What Was a Woman to Do?

Almost immediately after the early end of the WHI estrogen-and-progestin study there was a huge drop in the number of prescriptions written for synthetic hormones. The backlash was fast—many women threw their hormones in the garbage, and doctors recommended their patients stop taking them. According to IMS Health Canada, the leading provider of market intelligence on the pharmaceutical and healthcare industry, prescriptions for HRT, which in their data included estrogens, progestins, the combination of both, and the birth control pill, dropped by double-digits during 2003. There was a decrease of 26.8 percent in the number of prescriptions, but, because IMS included the Pill in its data, the drop for estrogens/progestins and/or both for HRT was much larger.

In the U.S., an even higher percentage of women stopped taking HRT. In 2004, a study published in the *Journal of the American Medical Association* revealed that HRT prescriptions decreased by over 37 percent, from 91 million prescriptions in 2002 to 57 million in 2003.

Data for U.S. HRT prescriptions from January 1995 through July 2003 found that between:

- 1995 to 1999: A 57 percent increase in HRT prescriptions occurred when combination HRT was introduced, with up to 90 million prescriptions filled by 1999.
- 1999 to June 2002: HRT prescription rates flat-lined as new evidence surfaced about the dangerous effects associated with combination HRT.
- July 2002 to July 2003: After the cancellation of the WHI estrogen-and-progestin study, the rate of HRT prescriptions declined by 38 percent, dropping to approximately 58 million.

These declines were for oral HRT prescriptions; vaginal HRT formulations did not decline, and lower-dose estrogens prescriptions increased by 6 percent in the second half of 2002.

No one should have been surprised by the results of WHI study. Negative reports about blood clots, breast cancer, heart attacks, and more had appeared in dozens of studies prior to July 2002, but the cancellation of the estrogen-and-progestin and estrogen-alone WHI studies got the media's attention.

Many women stopped HRT cold-turkey and suffered; others reduced their dosage of HRT. Some women were cutting sections out of their HRT patches to reduce the dosage, and many sought to replace their HRT with herbal remedies with limited success. A body that has been used to a steady supply of hormones for years or decades will experience severe withdrawal and menopausal symptoms as a result of an abrupt halt in hormones—even in women who are 75 years of age and long past menopause. The lack of information to help women get off their synthetic hormones or switch to natural remedies or bioidentical hormones was and still is appalling. (See page 144 for some possible scenarios for doing just that.)

Since the end of the WHI estrogen-and-progestin and estrogen-only studies, there has been total confusion over what women should do. Suzanne Somers's 2006 book *Ageless: The Naked Truth About Bioidentical Hormones* sought to provide solutions but, unfortunately, has compounded the questions as healthcare professionals and journalists now have heated debates in the media on the subject of bioidentical hormones and the validity of saliva hormone testing.

In the previous chapter, we gave you our recommendations on saliva hormone testing (see page 45). In this chapter, we will navigate the ins and outs of alternatives to synthetic hormone therapies to help you assess the option of bioidentical hormones and understand how to use them safely and effectively. In the remaining chapters, we will talk about nutritional and supplement support for a variety of hormone-related health problems and then give you some tips on how to harness all your recovered energy and passion.

Commonly Prescribed Synthetic Hormones

Brand name	Delivery method	Ingredients
Celestin	oral	conjugated estrogens
Depo Estradiol	injection	estradiol
Depo Provera	injection	progestin
Estratab	oral	estrogen along with horse estrone and equilin
FemPatch	patch	estradiol
Megace	oral	megestrol acetate
Methyltestosterone	oral	synthetic testosterone
Premarin	oral, vaginal cream	estrogen along with horse estrone and equilin
Provera	oral	progestin

What are Bioidentical Hormones?

The term "bioidentical hormones" (or natural hormones) refers to hormones that are compounded by a pharmacy and are identical in chemical structure to the hormones produced by the body. They fit hormone receptors perfectly, and, unlike estrogen mimickers, they do the job Nature intended sex hormones to do.

You may think that bioidentical hormones are new to the marketplace, but they have been produced commercially on a large scale for decades. Several prescription drugs, including Estrace tablets; Estrace vaginal cream; all the estrogen skin patches, including Estraderm; topical gels; and Estring, a vaginal ring, would fit this category. Prometrium is an oral form of bioidentical, micronized (crushed into micron-sized particles) progesterone. Bioidentical, micronized progesterone is also available in cream form.

All bioidentical hormones originate from either soy or diosgenin (wild yam) plant sterols that are then put through several chemical steps in a lab and altered to become a hormone that is identical to the hormones manufactured by the body. While some are available by prescription in predetermined dosages in the form of tablets or topical creams or gels, most bioidentical hormones are purchased as pharmaceutical grade ingredients to be mixed by a pharmacist, based on a dosage specific to the patient's needs as determined by a healthcare practitioner.

In the U.S., many Internet companies are selling non-prescription, bio-identical hormones. For the purposes of this book, we will focus on prescription-dispensed, bioidentical hormones, either sold through regular pharmacies or compounding pharmacies. And we will sometimes recommend DHEA, which is sold freely in the U.S. over the counter or by prescription in Canada.

How Hormones are Delivered

Before we discuss individual hormones and the research behind them, we will take a moment to explain how the way a hormone is taken affects its performance. The way hormones are supplied to your body is called the delivery system. Bioidentical hormones can be delivered in an oral form, or as creams, patches, gels, or rings. Depending on your hormone problem, your doctor will recommend the correct delivery system for your symptoms and health status. The delivery system will affect how the hormone works and any potential side effects. Below are the pros and cons of some delivery systems. After reading this section, you will understand why custom-compounded, bioidentical hormones offer you a unique way of getting what you need.

Oral Delivery

Oral delivery of hormones was originally thought to be the best way to take them, but subsequent research has revealed that all orally delivered hormones—synthetic or bioidentical—are altered by the gut and sent to the liver, where they are further altered. Conversion of hormones to other metabolites occurs in the liver and digestive system.

You read earlier that the conversion of estrogens can be a positive or a negative event, especially when treating a woman with estrogen replacement therapy. Remember that the liver can convert estradiol, estrone or, to a lesser extent, estriol into 16 alpha-hydroxyestrone, a potentially cancer-causing estrogen metabolite. When a dose of estrogen is given orally, 10 percent stays as estradiol; the other 90 percent becomes estrogen metabolites, with over 50 percent stored as estrone sulfate. Estrone sulfate has the potential to feed estrogen-receptor-positive breast cancer cells. Therefore, swallowing either prescribed bioidentical or synthetic estrogens may not be the solution to your hormonal problems because the liver does not break down oral estrogens the same way it breaks down ovarian- or adrenal-produced estrogens. In addition, physicians often prescribe dosages of oral hormones that are too high, giving the liver even more raw materials to convert to more toxic estrogens.

When it comes to oral progesterone, we know that 80 percent of it is converted to pregnanolone and hydroxypregnanolone or one of several other metabolites. One reason why some women get drowsy after taking oral progesterone is because of these metabolites. This could be viewed as a positive if the woman has insomnia, but not so if she is already feeling lethargic.

Not only does oral delivery have an effect on the conversion of progesterone, but, more importantly, bioidentical progesterone and synthetic progestins are each treated very differently by the liver. The synthetic progestins delivered in the Pill and HRT do *not* behave like progesterone produced by the body and can have negative effects on breast tissue and other organ systems. A new study showing that synthetic progestin metabolites do have the potential to be problematic supports our recommendations that only bioidentical hormones should be used, and transdermal delivery is generally thought to be the safest, most effective route. Remember: research is always evolving so sometimes what is considered to be correct will need to be updated as new science is published.

HRT and Other Hormones

In addition to working to detoxify the body, the liver is involved in cholesterol synthesis, insulin regulation, thyroid hormone conversion, blood clotting, and more. Women taking Premarin (estradiol and horse estrogens) often develop low thyroid function because estrogens block the uptake of thyroid hormone via the liver.

Estradiol taken orally does help elevate good cholesterol (HDL). Some women and their doctors prefer oral delivery because it seems to be more convenient than transdermal delivery, but most often doctors who have extensive experience with bioidentical hormones prefer skin delivery systems because they bypass the liver and gut.

Creams, Gels, and Patches

It is easy to bypass the actions of the liver. The skin is the largest detoxification organ of the body. It is also the biggest component of the immune system. Skin membranes are fat-loving and hormones are fat-soluble, making them an excellent pairing when delivering hormones. Like hormones produced in the ovaries or adrenal glands, when hormones are applied to the skin, they travel via the blood to the heart and on to the necessary receptors throughout the body, bypassing the liver. The exception is hormones applied to the abdomen, which have been found in concentrations in the liver. Do not apply hormones to the abdomen or breasts.

Not only do transdermal hormones bypass the liver, but lower doses of hormones can be used to achieve the same effect as higher doses delivered orally. You may be told by your medical doctor there is no science to back up our recommendations, but there is clear, published scientific evidence showing the effectiveness of transdermal-delivered hormones.

Most compounded hormones for skin delivery have penetration enhancers called liposomes, esters, or fatty acids added to the base of the **cream** or **gel** to ensure hormones enter the capillaries (tiny blood vessels) in the dermis of the skin. Make sure your hormone base does not contain parabens or glycols, which are known to be xenoestrogens. Hypoallergenic bases are also available for those with topical allergies.

Transdermal patches provide a controlled release of the hormone over many days. This consistent delivery over time makes for a more convenient way to use hormones, which many women appreciate. We would not recommend transdermal patches for hormones that require a break in application, for example, progesterone that requires a five-day halt in application to let hormone receptors rest. At the time of publication, not all hormones are available as transdermal patches.

Vaginal delivery of hormones is most often reserved for those women with urinary incontinence, urinary problems related to low levels of estrogens, vaginal dryness, and thinning of the vaginal wall because the effect of the estrogens will be more localized. Progesterone is used vaginally to help maintain a pregnancy and to thin an overly thick uterine lining. The mucous membrane of the vagina is very permeable and absorbs hormones readily.

There are other delivery methods, such as sublingual drops, rectal suppositories, injections, rings, and implants, but we have focused on the most common ones that we will recommend for treatment of hormonal problems in the next chapter.

Research on Bioidentical Hormones

We constantly hear claims that there is no research on bioidentical hormones. Granted we would always like to see more research, especially larger and longer-term studies. But to say there is no research is incorrect.

Research is an expensive business. It currently costs up to US$20 million to get a new drug approved for use—money that is spent mainly on researching the compound's validity, toxicity, safety, and effectiveness. Thus, a company must be able to make substantial sales from the drug in order to justify its investment. If a company cannot expect to make a high profit on a drug because it cannot be patented—that is, the company cannot claim the drug as its property alone and shield itself from competition—then it makes little economic sense to do the necessary studies. Bioidentical hormones—hormones that have the same molecular shape as hormones produced by the human body—cannot be patented. Hormones whose molecular shape has been altered from the human pattern by the pharmaceutical firm can be patented. As a result, any company that produces bioidentical hormones would be in for stiff competition from other companies. This is why there are few investments and even fewer studies on the effects of bioidentical hormones compared to studies on patentable hormones. What little we do know about bioidentical hormones indicates that, when used appropriately, they are much safer than synthetic hormones. But because bioidentical hormones do not have the potential for proprietary protection, they are not manufactured or promoted en masse the way synthetic hormones are. It is simply a matter of economics.

Most physicians have little time to search medical journals for new double-blind, placebo controlled trials. Also, bioidentical hormone therapy is not taught in most medical schools, nor is it promoted by any large pharmaceutical companies. Doctors are heavily marketed to by major drug companies through salespeople, advertising, medical conferences, free samples, and other common marketing techniques that have created an atmosphere in which physicians virtually equate estrogen replacement with synthetic hormones, primarily Premarin.

Studies on Bioidentical Estriol

Bioidentical oral estrogen supplements typically consist of estriol alone or estriol in combination with smaller percentages of the stronger estrogens. Examples include Tri-Est, which is most often prescribed as 80 percent estriol, 10 percent estradiol, and 10 percent estrone, or Bi-Est, which is 80 percent estriol, with 20 percent estradiol. Bi-Est and Tri-Est are also available in transdermal form, which is the delivery system that we prefer in most cases.

In *Clinical Obstetrics and Gynecology* in 2001, Dr. Maida Taylor published a review article, called *Unconventional Estrogens, Estriol, Bi-Est and Tri-Est*, in which she evaluated all the research at that time on bioidentical hormones. Her conclusions were that they appeared safer but should be monitored by a physician and given in appropriate dosages. No controlled trials of Bi-Est and Tri-Est had been performed at the time of publication. On the other hand, estriol, the major component of Bi-Est and Tri-Est, has many good studies showing its positive effects, especially for mitigating urinary incontinence and vaginal dryness and thinning. Estriol's unique and perhaps most important role, one that is still being explored, is to oppose the growth of cancer cells, including cancer promoted by its more potent sisters estrone and estradiol.

We know estriol plays far more than just a defensive role. In Europe, estriol has been used for over four decades to successfully treat hot flashes, night sweats, thinning of the vaginal wall, and urinary problems. Estriol only remains "safe" when given in appropriate doses. It is all about balance, as research has shown that high doses of oral estriol can negate the positive effects. Vaginal estriol, on the other hand, is without these risks.

- **Bioidentical Estriol for Hot Flashes**: In one major trial, 22 practicing gynecologists from 11 large hospitals in Germany treated 911 peri-menopausal women with bioidentical estriol and evaluated them regularly for five years. They found this form of estriol to be extremely effective for common peri-menopausal symptoms. No significant side effects were reported, and no thickening of the endometrial lining of the uterus was noted upon annual biopsy.

- **Bioidentical Estriol for Urinary Incontinence**: Another Swedish study of 40 post-menopausal women with urinary incontinence for up to a decade showed a 75 percent improvement with vaginal bioidentical estriol treatment. Eight of the participants who had lost the ability to regulate their urination returned to normal. Think of the number of women suffering with urinary incontinence who could be helped with vaginal bioidentical estriol.

- **Bioidentical Estriol for Bone Density**: Japanese studies using bioidentical estriol to improve bone density have shown a positive effect, which may be due to diet and/or genetics because studies with conflicting results have been published in the U.S. The more potent bioidentical estradiol reduces post-menopausal bone loss. Because Bi-Est and Tri-Est each contain a combination of estriol with estradiol, it is possible that these formulations will have positive effects on bone, but it has not been researched yet.

• **Bioidentical Estriol Counters Strong Estrogens**: Bioidentical estriol, in normal, low doses does not cause proliferation of the endometrial lining and does not cause proliferation of breast tissue. It also blocks and counters the action of the stronger estradiol and estrone. Estriol in oral form would have to be taken in double the dose of bioidentical estradiol or synthetic estrogens to cause proliferation of the lining of the uterus.

Further research shows that the best use of bioidentical estriol is in combination with natural progesterone.

Studies on Bioidentical Progesterone

Remember this: progesterone is natural, and progestin is synthetic. We never recommend progestin. Even doctors may be confused on this point because while writing this book we were shocked at the number of studies that mistakenly called synthetic progestins "progesterone," even in the titles of the research papers. In order to be called progesterone, the hormone has to be either made by the body or be bioidentical.

Initially, progesterone therapy was only used to counteract the negative effect estrogens have on the endometrial lining, but you know from earlier chapters that progesterone is needed for far more than protecting the uterine lining.

According to a Canadian study published in *Clinical Therapy*, oral bioidentical progesterone, called Prometrium, is better tolerated than the synthetic progestin medroxyprogesterone acetate, also known as Provera. In this study, patients taking estrogens and Prometrium reported improvements in menstrual problems (such as vaginal bleeding, breast tenderness, abdominal cramps, and bloating) and cognitive problems (such as clumsiness, poor concentration, and poor memory) compared to those in the group using synthetic estrogens and progestins. Provera caused a long list of unpleasant side effects, including breast tenderness, weight gain, depression, and break-through bleeding (abnormal bleeding that occurs throughout the cycle).

Soy Interferes with Progesterone

Helene Leonetti, M.D., in a study published in *Obstetrics and Gynaecology*, reported that women using bioidentical transdermal progesterone had an 83 percent reduction in hot flashes. This study also looked at bone density and, disappointingly, found no change in bone density after one year of treatment. Since the publication of her study, newer research published in 2004 in the *European Journal of Nutrition* may have revealed a possible reason for progesterone's lack of effect on bone. The European study was divided into four groups: one group received soy milk containing isoflavones, which have extremely high estrogenic activity; another group received transdermal progesterone; another received the combination of soy and transdermal progesterone; and another group was given a placebo. The results were eye-opening.

All participants had a DEXA scan, the gold standard to determine bone density, at the beginning of the study, and all took comparable calcium, minerals, and vitamins. The study lasted two years, and another DEXA was performed at the end of the trial. No change was found in the bone of those taking soy with isoflavones alone or progesterone alone, but the group receiving transdermal progesterone and soy isoflavones together experienced a significant *loss* of bone. Think about the amount of soy North American women eat. Soy is added to most packaged foods today. You have to make a concerted effort to avoid soy in light of this study showing bone loss in women who combined progesterone with soy.

Helene Leonetti's study did not ask patients to eliminate soy from their diet. Now that we know that soy and progesterone together cause bone loss, Dr. Leonetti's study should be redone with the exclusion of all soy in the group of women who are using natural progesterone for bone health. You will learn in Chapter 6 which types of soy are a problem not only for bone health, as we have seen in this study, but also for breast health. Regular, genetically modified soy available in North America is not the same as the soy Asian women consume in their diet. Hence the reason why studies on bone health in Asian countries have shown positive results, whereas in North America they have shown conflicting evidence.

Good Cholesterol and Bioidentical Progesterone

Bioidentical progesterone does not negate the benefits that estrogens have on our good cholesterol the way synthetic medroxyprogesterone does. Synthetic progestin interferes with estrogen's positive effect on good cholesterol.

The Post-menopausal Estrogen/Progestin Interventions (PEPI) trial involved 875 post-menopausal women who were randomly placed in one of four treatment groups: placebo; estrogen (Premarin) only; Premarin and Provera; or Premarin and natural progesterone (oral Prometrium). This study looked at the level of "good" HDL cholesterol, systolic blood pressure, fibrinogen (a blood component related to clotting), and insulin. Estrogen studies have shown that when women take estrogens, their good cholesterol levels rise, which is viewed as a protective effect against coronary artery disease. The results in the PEPI trial clearly showed that when synthetic Provera was added to Premarin, good cholesterol levels dropped back to almost baseline. By contrast, when natural progesterone was added to Premarin, there was no loss of good cholesterol.

Evidence also suggests that there is an increased risk of breast cancer when synthetic progestins are added to estrogen therapy. This is reflected in the WHI estrogen-and-progestin trial, but also in the women enrolled in the PEPI trial. In the PEPI trial, women taking synthetic progestin/estrogens had higher breast density than women taking progesterone and Premarin.

No More Waiting for Research

Some doctors will continue to wait for more research before prescribing bioidentical hormones, but the research already shows that bioidentical progesterone is better than synthetic progestin for keeping good cholesterol healthy. Dr. Pettle and I are satisfied that bioidentical progesterone also works to protect against endometrial lining thickening, and we know that it reduces menopausal symptoms. There is nothing to be gained by waiting when it comes to prescribing bioidentical progesterone.

When it comes to estrogen therapy, we also know estriol, used appropriately, is best, and transdermal delivery is often a better choice than oral therapy. Bi-Est or Tri-Est are more similar to a woman's own estrogens. Estrogen therapy requires monitoring and should always be given with progesterone, even in women who do not have a uterus because there are progesterone receptors throughout the body.

Bioidentical Hormones to Restore Balance

For up to 80 percent of women the recommendations for herbal remedies and other nutrients in the next chapter will provide relief from peri-menopausal and menopausal symptoms, but for the other 20 percent of women, supplemental hormones will be required. This section will outline the types of bioidentical hormones. In the next chapter, the most common hormone-related conditions will be presented with treatment protocols. You filled out the questionnaires in the previous chapter, so you know what your symptoms are pointing to. You may have had a saliva hormone evaluation and blood or urine tests performed as well. Now you are wondering what to do with all this information, especially if your doctor is not an expert in hormone balancing.

Bioidentical Hormone Profiles

We recommend that all the women using bioidentical hormones be tested on a regular basis with the tests recommended on page 41. In addition, every woman should be taking nutrients like EstroSense (see page 83), when using the recommended bioidentical hormones. This is to ensure that hormones are processed through detoxification and elimination as necessary to protect women's breasts, cervix, and ovaries. EstroSense is essential when women are taking any form of estrogens because the ingredients in EstroSense halt the conversion of good estrogens into harmful estrogen metabolites.

Bioidentical Estrogens

As we mentioned at the beginning of this chapter, compounded bioidentical estrogens are originally derived from soy or diosgenin plant sterols; then, through several chemical steps in a laboratory, these plant sterols are formed into bioidentical hormones. Many women well into post-menopause exhibit ample levels of estrogen—sometimes higher levels than younger, peri-menopausal women. Progesterone is recommended more often than estrogens, but there are times, especially with vaginal dryness or urinary symptoms, that estrogens are required. There are several types of bioidentical estrogens that we recommend.

Bi-Est
Bi-Est is a combination of two estrogens: estriol (E3) and estradiol (E2). These two estrogens are two of the three naturally occurring estrogens found in the female body. Bi-Est is compounded as 80 percent estriol and 20 percent estradiol. Prescriptions may look like this:

Bi-Est: 1.25 mg = 1.0 mg estriol + 0.25 mg estradiol

or

Bi-Est: 2.5 mg = 2.0 mg estriol + 0.5 mg estradiol

The success of any hormone therapy is to restore the body's natural hormone levels, thus restoring balance. When a woman enters menopause, estrone (E1) becomes dominant because her ovaries have stopped producing estradiol. Estrone is produced by the adrenals and in the fat cells of the body. Because estrone can be produced in fat, depending on the individual's number of fat cells and diet, estrone levels can remain high. Estrone can also be made from estradiol. Because women have an abundance of estrone at menopause, most often only estriol and estradiol in combination will be prescribed.

Tri-Est

Tri-Est is a triple estrogen combination containing either: 80 percent estriol, 10 percent estrone, and 10 percent estradiol or 90 percent estriol, 5 percent estrone, and 5 percent estradiol. Doctor Jonathan Wright, M.D of Tahoma, Washington, an avid promoter of bioidentical hormones, was the first doctor to recommend combining estriol and estradiol. There are many possible combinations. Like Bi-Est, it is compounded into either capsules for oral use or transdermal cream. Many doctors today prefer Bi-Est because it does not contain estrone. Common prescriptions for Tri-Est are:

1.25 mg = 1.0 mg estriol + 0.125 mg estrone + 0.125 mg estradiol

or

2.5 mg = 2.0 mg estriol + 0.250 mg estrone + 0.250 mg of estradiol

If you are currently using Premarin, your physician could write you a prescription for Tri-Est as 2.5 mg of oral Tri-Est, taken twice a day, which is approximately equal to 0.625 mg of conjugated equine estrogen (Premarin).

Estriol

Estriol is the estrogen that is most beneficial to the vagina, cervix, and vulva. In cases of vaginal dryness and atrophy, which predispose a woman to vaginitis and cystitis, topical estriol is the most effective and safest estrogen to use. As mentioned earlier, estriol is recommended for the treatment of urinary tract infections and urinary incontinence and leakage (see page 66 for this information).

In an open, multi-center, controlled study, 629 women suffering from stress and urgency urinary incontinence were treated with vaginally administered estriol at a dose of 1.0 mg daily for three weeks, and 1.0 mg bi-weekly for a further three weeks. All data for 552 of the patients were available at follow-up after six weeks of treatment. Up to an 82 percent improvement in symptoms of stress urinary incontinence was noted. Voluntary urinary control and symptoms of urgency were improved in more than 80 percent of patients. Frequency was reduced in almost 50 percent. Vaginal lubrication was improved in 77 percent of patients, and painful intercourse was no longer present in 88 percent. Vaginal atrophy improved in approximately 40 percent of cases. A quality of life score revealed an overall improvement in 72 percent of women.

The recommended dosage for intra-vaginal estriol is 0.5 mg to 1 mg once daily for three weeks, with 0.5 mg to 1 mg once weekly for six months. If you use this treatment, you should be examined to determine if vaginal atrophy is improving. If it has improved, you can discontinue use of estriol or use it 0.5 mg to 1 mg once every other week for another six months.

Bioidentical Progesterone

Bioidentical progesterone is available in cream and capsules. Until a process of micronization of progesterone was developed, progesterone was not easily absorbed by mouth. Micronized progesterone is available at a compounding pharmacy, and it does not have the side effects found with synthetic progestins. Micronized progesterone does not inhibit estrogen's positive effect of improving good cholesterol, so it is the best progesterone to take with estrogens. Approximately 90 percent of oral progesterone is converted into progesterone metabolites. So if you are taking a typical oral dose of 100 mg of oral progesterone, approximately 10 mg will enter your bloodstream as unchanged progesterone. The metabolites of progesterone do not have the kind of negative effects that the metabolites of estrogen have.

Progesterone is used when a woman is taking estrogen, to protect her uterine lining from thickening and developing endometrial cancer. It is also recommended when estrogen levels are elevated or a woman has estrogen-dominant conditions. For peri-menopausal women who used to have regular menstrual periods, but who now have amenorrhea (an absence of menstrual periods), progesterone is also used to restore menstruation.

Wild Yam is NOT Progesterone

Over the last decade, wild yam creams have been mistakenly promoted as a natural source of progesterone. Wild yam, in its natural state, is actually phytoestrogenic. Through several chemical processes, the saponins in wild yam, primarily diosgenin, can be converted into steroid hormones such as corticosteroids, estrogens, androgens, and progesterone. But it must be emphasized that natural diosgenin found in wild yam is not equivalent to progesterone (or other hormones) made by the body until it has gone through the chemical process mentioned above. Natural wild yam's effects occur not because it contains steroid hormones but rather because the natural phytohormones have similar effects to the steroid hormones. The body does not mistake the precursors for its own hormones but instead uses them in a similar manner, if needed.

Several brands of wild yam creams are available. All vary in strength and quality, and most are advertised as either "wild yam extract" or "derived from" wild yams. In the U.S., the wild yam creams that contain natural progesterone are labelled USP progesterone, meaning that USP progesterone is added to the wild yam cream. The wild yam cream then is a pharmaceutical product containing added progesterone. USP micronized progesterone is bioidentical to natural human progesterone. In Canada, it is illegal for a wild yam cream to contain USP progesterone, which is classed as a drug. In truth, wild yam creams that do not contain any added USP progesterone do not have a progesterone effect.

USP Progesterone Cream

USP stands for United States Pharmacopeia, which is the international standard of purity for substances used in the manufacture of drugs and cosmetics. In the case of progesterone, USP simply confirms that the progesterone is identical to the molecule produced by the human body. Progesterone is the most fat-soluble hormone, and as such, it lends itself to delivery through the skin very well.

When you go to get a prescription for compounded progesterone you may find that some physicians still believe that progesterone cream will not protect the endometrial lining when taken with estrogens—but we know it does and the research also shows progesterone is protective. One study performed by gynecologist Dr. Helene Leonetti, comparing progesterone cream to Provera (a synthetic progestin in tablet form) taken along with Premarin (synthetic mare's estrogens), found that after six months there was no difference in the uterine lining biopsies taken in both groups. This means that natural progesterone had the same effect as Provera. We know that progesterone cream is well-absorbed, based on dozens of clinical studies so we will not debate this here. Progesterone can also be delivered via the vagina and as a nasal spray.

The average menstruating woman produces between 25 and 40 mg of progesterone per day. Most doctors prescribe progesterone cream in dosages ranging from 20 to 40 mg per day. Formulations can be made in a variety of strengths, from one percent (10 mg per 100 ml) up to 30 percent or more. A 4 percent progesterone cream will deliver 40 mg of progesterone per ml. The most commonly prescribed progesterone cream is 2 percent, delivering 20 mg progesterone per ml. As with estrogens, topical progesterone is not broken down by the liver the way oral progesterone is, so dosages are much less.

The cream can be applied at a variety of sites, rotating among neck, inner arms, inside of thighs, and the palms of the hands. It is important to take a break for five days from the progesterone treatment each month. Progesterone receptors can become overloaded, and although you may test normal for progesterone, symptoms may suggest that you are progesterone deficient because your receptors have been over-sensitized and are non-responsive. The exceptions are in women with fibroids, when the doctor is focusing on reducing blood flow, and in cases of anemia. In these cases, the doctor may have you use progesterone cream every day without a break.

Menstruating women use about 20 mg per day for 14 days before the expected day of the period, stopping the day or so before the period arrives. So if you have a 28-day cycle, you will start the progesterone cream on day 14. If you have a 21-day cycle, you would start the cream on day 11. The cream is applied morning and night in a divided dose (i.e., 10 mg in the morning and 10 mg at night).

Women with premenstrual syndrome use 20 mg per day from day 10, stopping the day or so before the period arrives. The cream is applied morning and night in a divided dose (i.e., 10 mg in the morning and 10 mg at night).

Women with breast cysts use 40 mg per day; 20 mg in the morning and 20 mg at night, from 14 days before the expected day of the period. Again, take a break when the period arrives.

Post-menopausal women use 20 mg per day for 25 days of the calendar month with a five- to six-day break. The cream is applied morning and night in a divided dose (i.e., 10 mg in the morning and 10 mg at night).

Prometrium
Prometrium, put on the market in 1998, is a micronized oral progesterone. The standard dose of Prometrium when used continuously is 100 to 200 mg per day. For those on a cyclical therapy with estrogens, the dose is 200 mg per day, taken at bedtime for 12 days before menstruation begins. For women who have amenorrhea (loss of menstrual periods), a dosage of 400 mg at bedtime for 10 days often works to restore menstruation. We recommend you take Prometrium at night because it can cause drowsiness in some women.

Because Prometrium contains peanut oil, those with peanut allergies should not use it. In this case, your doctor should prescribe oral micronized progesterone that does not contain peanut oil. Prometrium should not be taken by women who have or have had blood clots, liver disease, or have cancer of the breast, vagina, or ovaries, or if they are nursing, without the guidance of their doctors.

Too much progesterone will cause breast swelling and pain, low libido, depression or low mood, fatigue, headaches, a tired or groggy feeling, water retention, and overproduction of insulin by the pancreas. As with anything, too much of a good thing can be bad. If symptoms of excess progesterone appear, advise your doctor, cut your dose, and take a break, allowing receptors to recover from being over-sensitized.

Bioidentical Testosterone

Testosterone, called the hormone of desire because of its powerful effect on libido, is also important in building strong muscles, bones, and ligaments, as well as increasing energy and easing depression. Low levels of testosterone have been known to cause fatigue, irritability, depression, aches and pain in the joints, thin and dry skin, osteoporosis, weight loss, and the loss of muscle tone. Low levels of testosterone in women are seen in those with high levels of cortisol. Often stress reduction and an increase in weight-bearing exercise will bring testosterone levels back to normal. Later chapters will discuss all the lifestyle and nutritional recommendations that will enhance sexy hormones and bring that vitality back into your life. If these lifestyle changes do not achieve the desired result, low-dose bioidentical testosterone could be the answer. Dosages for women are generally one-tenth of those used in men.

Testosterone is not effective when taken orally; it is best in a topical gel or cream. As you read in the Prologue, the birth control pill is known to have a negative effect on testosterone's action, both reducing overall production of testosterone and binding it so that it is not useful to receptors.

The recommended dosage for testosterone gel or cream is 0.5 to 1.0 mg of testosterone, applied daily in the morning for two weeks, then reduced to one application per week. This often works to return desire in a healthy relationship. (Dr. Pettle has had to use dosages of up to 10 mg per day, but these should be used only under the careful monitoring of your physician.) Testosterone should be applied just above the clitoris. Testosterone taken in high doses for long periods of time can result in hair growth in the area of application. Thankfully testosterone works quickly, and there is usually no need for high-dose, long-term use.

Bioidentical DHEA

Dehydroepiandrosterone (DHEA) and its breakdown product dehydroepiandrosterone sulfate (DHEAS) are precursors of both male hormones (androgens) and
estrogens. When you were younger, you had high levels of DHEA and DHEAS.
These substances reached their peak levels in your late twenties, and, from that
point on, there has been a steady decline.

Given that DHEA is a precursor hormone to both testosterone and estrogens, it is essential to establish a baseline level for all the major hormones
before taking DHEA, and then monitor the levels while using it. Hormone supplementation will affect every person differently and will affect the same person
differently at different stages of life. Back in the late eighties and early nineties,
DHEA was popular as an anti-aging hormone. High doses of DHEA were
being used without proper testing to see if the person was deficient in the first
place and what their levels were after supplementation. This is another hormone where more is not better. Low doses of DHEA, even 5 mg, can have a
dramatic effect on all other hormones in the body.

Along with its ability to control age-related disorders, DHEA helps repair
and maintain tissues, control allergic reactions, and balance the activity of the
immune system. It controls the inflammatory immune factors IL-1 and IL-6
and cortisol, while enhancing gamma-interferon and interleukin-2, our cancer-
and virus-fighting cytokines. DHEA acts as an anti-inflammatory and stimulates natural killer cell activity. As you know, when you are experiencing stress,
your adrenal glands secrete cortisol, the stress hormone, causing a drop in
DHEA. Conversely, when DHEA is increased, cortisol and inflammatory
immune factors are controlled.

Those with diabetes or atherosclerosis are often low in DHEA. Research
has demonstrated that the number of antibodies attacking the "self" cells is
reduced with DHEA, thereby controlling autoimmune disorders such as
rheumatoid arthritis and lupus. A report published in *Science News* stated that
DHEA was added to prasterone (a drug for lupus) after it was found to elicit
fewer symptom flare-ups in women with lupus. If you live in Canada, DHEA is
not available for sale over the counter; it has to be prescribed through the drug
release program. Have your DHEAS level checked through standard blood
testing to see if it is in the normal range.

A word of caution: if you have fibroids, do not take DHEA. It is likely that
the DHEA will choose the estrogen pathway and increase the size of the
fibroids already growing due to excess estrogen. We have seen women take
DHEA and have their fibroids grow to the size of grapefruits in months.

Commonly Available Bioidentical Hormones

Brand name	Delivery Method	Ingredients
Androderm	patch	testosterone
Androgel	gel	testosterone
Bi-Est	oral, cream	estradiol and estriol
Climara	patch	estradiol
Estrace	vaginal cream or oral	estradiol
Estraderm	patch	estradiol
Estradot	patch	estradiol
Estring	vaginal ring	estradiol
Estriol	vaginal	estriol
Estrogel	gel	estradiol
Ogen	vaginal cream	estrone sulfate
Prometrium	tablets or cream	progesterone
Testoderm	patch	testosterone
Tri-Est	oral, cream	estriol, estradiol, and estrone

Some of these bioidentical hormones are available by prescription in predetermined dosages in the form of tablets, topical creams, or gels. Bioidentical hormones can also be custom-compounded in a pharmacy, based on a dosage specific to the patient's needs as determined by a healthcare practitioner. In the U.S., natural progesterone cream is also available over the counter in health food stores and pharmacies, whereas in Canada, this cream is strictly a prescription drug. (Canadian consumers may find wild yam creams on the shelves of health food stores, but these are NOT progesterone creams. See page 72 for more information.)

Canada has stringent regulations regarding the prescribing and dispensing of all hormones. Bioidentical hormones are drugs, and compounding pharmacies are highly regulated. Custom-compounded hormones provide certain benefits, such as individualized doses and mixtures of products and dosage forms that are not available commercially by prescription.

Finding a Bioidentical-Friendly Doctor

If your doctor declines to help you in your quest for bioidentical hormone therapy or saliva hormone testing, contact the organizations below. Canadian doctors also belong to these organizations.

- **ACAM**
  1-888-439-6891
  http://www.acam.org

- **American Holistic Medical Association**
  http://www.holisticmedicine.org

Compounding Pharmacies

Compounding pharmacies specialize in custom-compounded medicines, not just hormones. This is one of the oldest professions. Long before medical doctors and drug stores, the town's local chemist would mix up tonics and herbal and plant remedies for folk. These "chemists" have come a long way since then and are now highly regulated professional pharmacists.

In the U.S., there has been plenty of negative press about compounding pharmacies providing substandard preparations. In October of 2005, Wyeth-Ayerst, the maker of Premarin and Prempro (the hormones used in the WHI estrogen-and-progestin and estrogen-alone studies), filed a citizens' complaint with the U.S. Food and Drug Administration (FDA), requesting that the FDA prohibit compounding pharmacists from providing bioidentical hormones to patients. Thankfully Wyeth's attempt to shut down the making of hormone supplements for women by compounding pharmacists has failed. Wyeth-Ayerst was hit hard by the results of the WHI estrogen-and-progestin and estrogen-alone studies in 2002. They made over US $2 billion from their Premarin family of drugs, but by 2004 sales had dropped to US $880 million, almost a 56 percent decline.

Let us be clear: compounding pharmacists are professionals. Like any profession, there are people who are excellent at their job, and there are those who are not. If your physician has worked with the compounding pharmacy, he/she will have knowledge of the competency of the pharmacist.

To find a compounding pharmacist near you in Canada, call the Professional Compounding Centers of America at 1-800-331-2498. In the U.S., contact the

International Academy of Compounding Pharmacists at www.iacprx.org. You can search by zip code.

Where to Buy Bioidentical Hormone Creams

- Wiler / PCCA Canada
  744 3rd Street
  London, ON N5V 5J2

- **York Downs Pharmacy in Canada**
  3910 Bathurst Street
  Toronto, Ontario M3H 5Z3
  York Downs Pharmacy ships all over Canada
  North American Toll Free 1-800-564-5020;
  Toronto area 416-633-2244
  www.yorkdownsrx.com

- **College Pharmacy Compounding Specialists**
  North American Toll free: 1-800-888-9358 or
  Colorado Springs: 1-719-262-0022
  3505 Austin Bluffs Parkway, Suite 101
  Colorado Springs, CO 80918
  www.collegepharmacy.com

5

Treatments to Tame
Hormone Havoc

There are several strategies for treating hormone imbalance that is related to disorders such as difficult periods, problems related to peri- and post-menopause, estrogen-dominant conditions (such as fibroids and endometriosis), exhausted adrenal glands, low thyroid, or urinary tract infections (UTIs). All treatment recommendations must be combined with excellent nutrition, as outlined in Chapters 6 and 7. It is also essential to take a well-formulated multinutrient combination, essential fatty acids, and bone nutrients.

We will suggest a combination of plant or herbal extracts with or without bioidentical hormones. Some women will want to use only herbal or plant-based therapies to deal with their hormone problems, so these options will be presented first in the treatment recommendations. Not all women need bioidentical hormone therapy, while others suffer terribly without adequate supplemental hormones. Therefore, many conditions presented will conclude with a discussion of how to use bioidentical hormones as part of the treatment plan. Suggestions for treatment will be the safest, least toxic, and least invasive available. You should work with your healthcare provider to establish the lowest possible dose of bioidentical hormones and the most appropriate method of delivery based on your overall health.

Hormone Havoc During Peri-menopause

For many women, peri-menopause is a more challenging time than the menopausal years. In some women, hormones can start to shift as early as age 35; other women do not experience hormone fluctuations until five years before menopause. (The average onset of menopause is around 52 years of age.) Prior to that, the relatively consistent up-and-down rhythm of hormones during the perimenopausual years can start shifting as wildly as it did during puberty—estrogen becomes high, progesterone low, and, at other times, as you can see on the graph below, there are steep increases and drops in estrogen.

FEMALE ESTROGEN CYCLE

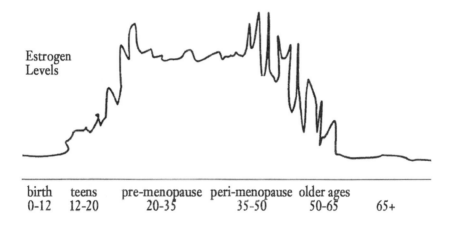

Adapted from *Estrogen's Storm Season* by Jerilynn Prior to order CeMCOR, 2775 Laurel St., Vancouver, BC, Canada V5Z 1M9

During the peri-menopausal years, some women notice symptoms of hormone changes such as breast tenderness or lumps (cysts), heavy or long periods, mood changes (including PMS, which may not have been a problem in younger days), fatigue, uterine fibroids, endometriosis, problems staying asleep, thinning hair, occasional sweats at night, weight gain around the middle, skin outbreaks, low libido, or they may be diagnosed with chronic fatigue, fibromyalgia, or joint pain.

Periods are a barometer of hormone health, and although period problems can plague any age, period changes are the most common symptom of peri-menopause. Women who experienced period problems when they were younger often have more difficulty during the transitional years. (See page 31 for details of a normal menstrual cycle.) Other women experience nearly the same complaints they had when their periods were just starting up during the teen years—light, heavy, long, clotting, missed, later, earlier—but most often, the problem is heavy periods that become debilitating due to the subsequent development of anemia. Anemia causes heavier bleeding, and it also promotes hair loss. Anemia often runs hand-in-hand with low thyroid, so it is important that thyroid function is checked with a hemoglobin and ferritin blood test (See page 42 for relevant tests). If confirmed, the anemia must be treated immediately with double the dose of non-constipating Floradix (by Flora Distributors). It can take up to a year to rebuild iron stores, so make sure you have ferritin tested, not just hemo-globin, in order to monitor your iron stores.

A thickened uterine lining caused by exposure to too much estrogen and not enough progesterone is often at the root of heavy periods. The next most common cause of heavy periods is uterine fibroids (see page 96 for treatment suggestions). Remember: estrogen makes cells grow and thicken the uterine lining; estrogen also makes fibroids grow. Progesterone shuts off or inhibits excess estrogen. High levels of estrogen from both environmental estrogens and surges of estrogen from ovaries, adrenals, and fat cells, which in turn suppress progesterone, are now known to be at the root of peri-menopausal symptoms.

Estrogen Storm

Jerilynn Prior, M.D., professor at the University of British Columbia, wrote a 32-page peri-menopausal review back in 1998 and an excellent book called *Estrogen's Storm Season: Stories of Perimenopause*, published in 2005, about the fact that estrogen dominance or surges of estrogens, causing a corresponding drop in progesterone, are the predominant hormone imbalances seen in peri-menopausal women. In her book she states that women can be estrogen-dominant well into their 60s.

She states, "Symptoms of vaginal dryness or atrophy and urinary problems are the only true symptoms of estrogen deficiency." Even though Dr. Prior's very thorough work and other published studies point to estrogen dominance, medical doctors are still prescribing the Pill and estrogen replacement for women with symptoms of estrogen overload. If a classic peri-menopausal prob-lem like heavy periods caused by uterine fibroids is treated with added estrogen alone, most women will have a worsening of heavy bleeding. When this "extra estrogen" therapy does not work (which most often it does not), the women will be recommended for microwave uterine ablation or hysterectomy (see page 104 for more information about unnecessary hysterectomy).

Other Symptoms of Peri-menopause

Some women experience night sweats, mood swings, heart palpitations, sleep disturbances, and hot flashes during peri-menopause. Night sweats are a sign of low thyroid. Insomnia, where you fall asleep easily but wake up later and can't return to sleep, is a symptom of exhausted adrenals. Mood swings, hot flashes, and heart palpitations go along with the estrogen surges women develop during peri-menopause (due to too much estrogen and corresponding low proges-terone). EstroSense (see page 84 for more information), Vitex, and a good mul-tivitamin, along with the diet recommendations in Chapters 6 and 7 can ease these peri-menopausal symptoms.

If you are having symptoms like night sweats that are associated with low thyroid, follow the recommendations on page 118. If you have insomnia, sup-porting and nourishing the adrenals will be the first line of treatment. See page 107 for adrenal support recommendations or later on page 118 for sound sleep recommendations.

Protect the Reproductive System and Make Periods Effortless

Medical professionals have to start looking at conditions of younger and/or peri-menopausal women differently. Cysts, fibroids, endometriosis, thickened uterine lining, and more are all caused by abnormal cell growth. The woman may or may not develop cancer as a result of this abnormal cell growth, but the conditions are still about cells growing when and where they should not. There are outstanding nutrients, herbs, and plant extracts that stop abnormal cell growth while protecting women from breast cancer and other estrogen-dominant con-ditions and balancing the estrogen-to-progesterone ratio. These are described below. Every woman from the age of menstruation until death should be taking the following nutrients every day to protect her cervix, breasts, ovaries, and uterus, and for menstruating women, to make periods effortless. These nutrients are sold separately or are found together in EstroSense, which is described below.

The key nutrients for safe hormone balancing that do not contain any estrogenic compounds include Indole-3-carbinol, d-glucarate, green tea extract, curcumin, milk thistle, sulforaphane, Vitex (chaste tree berry), and evening primrose or borage oil.

INDOLE-3-CARBINOL

Indole-3-carbinol (I3C) is a plant nutrient found in cruciferous vegetables like broccoli, Brussels sprouts, cauliflower, kale, and cabbage. Research has shown that I3C helps to break cancer-causing estrogens down into non-toxic forms, and it eliminates harmful estrogen mimickers. I3C does this by improving detoxification of the cytochrome P450 enzyme system, thereby removing excess estrogens and/or xenoestrogens.

In the stomach, I3C is converted into many active compounds, one of which is diindolylmethane (DIM). Although DIM appears to be an important metabolite of I3C, most of the past and ongoing studies are performed on I3C itself, which is why we prefer I3C. I3C breaks down into a number of beneficial indole products, aside from DIM, which may also have protective effects on estrogen metabolism. If you are taking DIM only, you will not benefit from all the protective effects of I3C and its full complement of metabolites.

Indole-3-carbinol:
- makes periods effortless, with normal flow, no pain, and shorter duration
- improves the ratio of good estrogens (2-hydroxyestrone) to toxic, cancer-causing forms of estrogens (4-hydroxyestrone and 16 alpha-hydroxyestrone)
- protects women on the Pill from the toxic estrogens (16 alpha-hydroxyestrone) produced in the liver. Every woman on the Pill should be taking I3C.
- protects against estrogen-dominant cancers (breast and ovarian)
- reduces tumor development in the endometrium and cervix
- reduces the thick uterine lining that causes heavy periods
- works with tamoxifen (a drug used to block estrogens) to inhibit the growth of estrogen-dominant cancers more effectively than tamoxifen alone
- improves abnormal Pap tests. HPV (human papilloma virus), which can lead to cervical cancer, uses the toxic form of estrogen (16 alpha-hydroxyestrone) to develop into cancer. In one research study, 30 women with CINII and CINIII cervical lesions took 200 mg of I3C daily. These women were followed

for six months. There was also a control group getting fake pills (placebos). Fifty percent of those women in the treatment group had complete regression of their lesions, and their Pap smears returned to normal. Many women taking I3C had a CINIII improve to a CINII. None of the placebo group had any improvement, and some in the placebo group had a worsening of their lesions (for example, a CINII progressed to a CINIII).

Indole-3-carbinol is effective at keeping the balance of healthy estrogens in the body while supporting liver hormone function. Remember that fat cells manufacture estrogen, and excess estrogen contributes to weight gain. By using I3C, you can help support proper estrogen function in your fat cells. I3C should also be taken if you have cellulite.

Several studies have recently evaluated I3C dosages. The Strang Cancer Prevention Center in New York looked at different dosages of I3C in women and compared the results to those taking a placebo. The urinary estrogen metabolite ratio of 2-hydroxyestrone to 16 alpha-hydroxyestrone was used. Remember, this is a test also used to determine breast cancer risk (see page 47). Researchers looked at 50, 100, 200, 300, and 400 mg doses. They determined that 300 mg per day of I3C was protective against cancer. Other studies have looked at dosages as high as 800 mg and found no difference in effectiveness once a level of 300 mg was reached.

Recommended dosage: 150–300 mg per day. Or keep it simple, and use EstroSense, 2 to 4 capsules per day with food.

> EstroSense contains I3C, D-glucarate, decaffeinated green tea extract, curcumin, milk thistle, sulforaphane, rosemary, and lycopene in the appropriate dosages recommended here. EstroSense is readily available at all North American health food stores.

D-GLUCARATE

D-glucarate is found in all fruits and vegetables, with the highest concentrations found in apples, grapefruit, and broccoli. It is a very important nutrient that helps detoxify excess estrogens and protects from the toxic estrogens made by the liver. D-glucarate helps rid the body of toxic substances by way of conjugation (combining toxic substances with carriers in order to be safely removed from the body) in the liver (Phase II detoxification) so that dangerous substances are combined and safely excreted from the body. D-glucarate is a powerful, fat-flushing nutrient as well.

D-glucarate:
- reduces total triglyceride levels by an average of 12 percent, thus reducing the risk of cardiovascular disease and helping the body to metabolize fats
- removes excess estrogens and xenoestrogens
- supports the liver
- inhibits tumor formation caused by chemical cancer-causing agents
- resulted in a 50 to 70 percent reduction of breast tumor formation in animal studies

D-glucarate is a powerful detoxifier of excess estrogens. Every woman using hormones of any type should include D-glucarate in her nutrient program.

Recommended dosage: 150–300 mg per day. Or keep it simple, and use EstroSense, 2 to 4 capsules per day with food.

GREEN TEA EXTRACT

Green tea extract is a powerful antioxidant containing polyphenols, catechins, and flavonoids, which have been shown to be protective against estrogen-dominant conditions and related cancers, especially breast and ovarian. Green tea extract has been extensively studied for its weight-loss benefits, but it also keeps estrogens in check.

Green tea extract:
- increases the activity of other antioxidants
- inhibits cancer by blocking the formation of cancer-causing compounds
- increases detoxification of cancer-causing agents
- prevents breast cancer
- eliminates xenoestrogens
- supports the liver in metabolizing fats and hormones
- aids weight loss and cellulite reduction

Thousands of research studies have confirmed the beneficial effects of green tea and green tea extract. According to Michael Murray, N.D., in his book *How to Prevent and Treat Cancer with Natural Medicine*, "Both green and black teas are derived from the same plant, *Camellia sinensis*. Of the nearly 2.5 million tons of dried tea produced each year, only 20 percent is green tea." Green tea, as science has confirmed, is the healthier choice because it contains compounds called polyphenols, known for their powerful healing effects.

The manufacturing process is what makes the difference between green and black tea. Green tea is produced by lightly steaming the fresh-cut leaf, stopping fermentation. Oolong tea is partially fermented, and black tea is fully fermented. During the fermentation process, enzymes convert the polyphenols that provide fabulous healing actions to compounds with much less activity. Green tea is not fermented, therefore it provides higher levels of healing polyphenols.

Green tea extract is an extract of the active ingredients in green tea, including epigallocatechingallate (EGCG) and epigallocatechin (EGC). These are powerful polyphenols that are close cousins to the flavonoids found in broccoli, cabbage, grapes, and red wine. The extract in capsule form is a highly concentrated way of consuming green tea.

Green Tea for Peri-menopausal Arthritis

Several studies have been published in Sweden, Taiwan, and the United States describing green tea's efficacy in inhibiting the COX-2 enzymes that cause inflammation in those with arthritis. Not only was green tea found to be as good as COX-2 anti-inflammatory medications like Celebrex and Vioxx (without the side effects), but green tea also contains 51 other anti-inflammatory compounds. The USDA Phytochemical Database also identified 15 anti-ulcer compounds in green tea, supporting evidence that long-term use can also inhibit ulcers caused by prolonged use of non-steroidal, anti-inflammatory medications, including ibuprofen. Women often complain of joint pain around the time of peri-menopause and menopause, and this is a time when many women are diagnosed with fibromyalgia and/or arthritis due to hormone fluctuations. Green tea can help calm inflammation at this time of transition, while also balancing hormones.

Recommended dosage: 100–200 mg per day; ensure the green tea extract has at least 60 percent polyphenols (an important active ingredient). Or keep it simple, and use EstroSense, 2 to 4 capsules per day with food. Drink green tea throughout the day instead of coffee, as coffee elevates estrogen levels and wreaks havoc with cortisol.

Kick Caffeine with Green Tea

Worried about getting too much caffeine from green tea? Three cups provides about the same amount of caffeine as one cup of drip coffee. Three cups of green tea also provides approximately 240 to 320 mg of polyphenols. Green tea contains L-theanine, which counteracts the

negative side effects of the caffeine found in green tea, including hypertension and sleep disturbances. L-theanine is very well researched and has been shown to promote relaxation without drowsiness, improve learning and concentration, support immune function, lower cholesterol, and reduce stress and anxiety. Now you know why you can drink several cups of green tea and not develop the caffeine jitters.

CURCUMIN (Turmeric)

Curcumin is the yellow pigment of turmeric, one of the chief ingredients in curry. It is a powerful anti-inflammatory agent, and it works to inhibit all steps of cancer formation— from initiation to promotion and progression. Curcumin also helps to eliminate cancer-causing estrogens and environmental estrogens via the liver. Curcumin increases detoxification.

Curcumin:
- halts initiation, promotion, and progression of cancer
- enhances progesterone action and decreases excess prolactin.
  In rat studies, rats fed a diet of curcumin had a reduced incidence of both estrogen- and progesterone-positive mammary tumors, a reduction in prolactin, and they also had reduced weight in their ovaries and uterus (a positive protective effect)
- is a potent antioxidant; it blocks free-radical production
- enhances glutathione, the most powerful detoxifier of the liver
- promotes detoxification of the liver, cleansing it of cancer-causing substances, including xenoestrogens
- inhibits tumor growth directly—stops abnormal cell growth
- halts the destruction of neurons associated with the development of Alzheimer's. (Alzheimer's is not found in India, where curcumin is eaten daily.) Many women took estrogen replacement therapy because they were told it would help keep their memory intact.

The WHI estrogen-and-progestin hormone study revealed the exact opposite for women who were taking synthetic estrogen and progestin. Curcumin is a better solution.

Recommended dosage: 50 100 mg per day; ensure the curcumin supplement contains 95 percent curcuminoids. Use the spice turmeric in cooking too. Or keep it simple, and use EstroSense, 2 to 4 capsules per day with food.

MILK THISTLE

Milk thistle, called the protector of the liver, is extremely important for proper estrogen balance in the cells of the body. Its active ingredients include silybin, silydianin, and silychristin, collectively known as silymarin.

Milk thistle:
- enhances detoxification of toxic estrogens from the liver
- detoxifies a wide range of hormones, drugs, and toxins
- improves estrogen balance by metabolizing estrogen into the good estrogens
- stimulates growth of new liver cells
- acts as a powerful antioxidant and free-radical scavenger, several times more potent than vitamin E and vitamin C
- promotes bile flow for healthy digestion and gut health
- increases intracellular glutathione (necessary for detoxification) by 35 percent in healthy persons
- is effective in treatment for psoriasis, suppressed immune function, gallbladder disease, hepatitis, atherosclerosis, and liver disease
- reduces cellulite
- reduces the toxic effects of chemotherapy
- inhibits breast cancer cell growth

Recommended dosage: 50–100 mg per day; ensure your milk thistle contains at least 80 percent silymarin. Or keep it simple, and use EstroSense, 2 to 4 capsules per day with food.

SULFORAPHANE

Sulforaphane from broccoli sprout extract has been shown to stimulate the body's production of detoxification enzymes that eliminate toxic estrogens and balance estrogens in the body. It is also a powerful antioxidant and cancer-fighting nutrient. In its precursor form, sulforaphane glucosinolate (SGS), it functions as an indirect antioxidant. Indirect antioxidants induce the activity of the Phase 2 detoxification enzymes. The highest level of SGS is found in broccoli sprouts. One ounce of broccoli sprouts provides as much SGS as 1.25 lbs (560 g) of mature, cooked broccoli. That is 20 times the concentration.

Sulforaphane:
- helps liver detoxification in a similar manner to calcium D-glucarate, which is important for detoxifying excess estrogens and environmental estrogens
- neutralizes dangerous carcinogens before they can damage DNA and promote cancer
- blocks the formation of mammary tumors in rats treated with a potent carcinogen, according to research performed by Dr. Paul Talalay, who founded the Brassica Chemoprotection Laboratory at John Hopkins University. The number of rats that developed tumors was reduced by as much as 60 percent, the number of tumors in each animal was reduced by 80 percent, and the size of the tumors that did develop was reduced by 75 percent. Furthermore, the tumors emerged later, and they grew more slowly.
- inhibits the formation of pre-malignant lesions in the colons of rats according to scientists at the American Health Foundation
- induces cell death in test tube studies of human colon-carcinoma cells according to researchers in Toulouse, France. These results have not yet been validated in humans.

Recommended dosage: 200–400 mcg per day. Or keep it simple, and use EstroSense, 2 to 4 capsules per day with food.

VITEX (Chaste Tree Berry)

Vitex, also called the progesterone-enhancing herb, contains no hormones, has no direct hormonal activity, and is not phytoestrogenic. It contains flavonoids, iridoid, glycosides, and terpenoids. Its main active ingredients, aucubine and agnusides, work on the pituitary gland to stimulate the production of luteinizing hormone (LH), which in turn increases progesterone and helps regulate the menstrual cycle. The LH increases the level of progesterone in the luteal phase of the menstrual cycle, thereby shifting the ratio of estrogen-to-progesterone in favor of progesterone. The increase in progesterone created by Vitex is thus achieved indirectly; the plant does not have direct hormonal action.

Vitex also inhibits excessive production of prolactin, which is found in women with polycystic ovary syndrome, women with male facial hair growth, and in women who are infertile. Prolactin levels have also been found to be elevated in women with low thyroid.

Vitex is a very well-researched herb. It has a strong reputation in the traditional treatment of menstrual abnormalities, PMS, menopausal complaints, and infertility. In 1997, a team of German researchers conducting a double-blind, placebo-controlled study found that Vitex was more effective in the treatment of PMS complaints (breast tenderness, edema, tension headaches, constipation, depression, skin problems) than vitamin B6, which is commonly used for PMS. Another study found that 90 percent of its 1,542 female participants had relief from the symptoms of premenstrual syndrome (PMS). Further double-blind research performed in Germany confirmed that Vitex can lower prolactin levels in women. Another study showed that hormonal acne was reduced using Vitex.

Vitex's full effects develop over time. Those with PMS notice symptom relief within one to two menstrual cycles. Normalizing prolactin levels can take many months using Vitex. Use of Vitex should be discontinued during pregnancy or breast feeding.

Vitex is recommended for:
- irregular or heavy periods
- cramps
- polycystic ovary syndrome
- reduction of ovarian cysts
- PMS
- breast tenderness
- bloating
- depression and mood swings

- regulation of ovulation
- infertility
- endometriosis
- uterine fibroid growths
- menopausal symptoms such as hot flashes and night sweats
- acne related to hormonal imbalance
- normalizing prolactin levels

Recommended dosage: 2 to 4 capsules per day with food.

Oils Containing GLA

Evening primrose, borage, and black current seed oil are omega-6 oils. Omega-6 oils should be considered as two types: omega-6 oils that contain gamma linoleic acid (GLA) and those that do not. Those oils that have GLA, including black current seed, evening primrose, and borage, are classified as "good" omega-6 oils and have been shown in clinical studies to be breast-cancer protective. Those that do not contain GLA, including corn, safflower, canola, and soy, have been found to be disease-promoting and are called "bad" omega-6 oils.

Borage oil naturally contains more GLA than evening primrose oil, so you will note the difference in recommended dosages. Echium oil, from the plant *Echium plantagineum*, is both an omega-3 and omega-6 oil that is rich in GLA and stearidonic acid. For more information on echium oil, see page 155.

GLA Eases Cramps and Breast Pain
A deficiency in gamma linoleic acid (GLA) is a major cause of PMS. A healthy body creates GLA by converting dietary linoleic acid found in many oils, such as organic hemp oil, sunflower oil, or safflower oil. Borage, evening primrose, black current seed, and echium oils naturally contain GLA and are therefore the preferred sources to supplement your diet. The body then takes GLA and through several steps makes prostaglandins, which are hormone-like compounds made in every cell of the body. Prostaglandins function as regulators, either enhancing or inhibiting a variety of responses, including inflammation, muscle contraction, blood vessel dilation, and blood clotting.

Enzymes can also take GLA and produce arachidonic acid. The hormone-like prostaglandins produced from arachidonic acid have a pro-inflammatory action (causing blood vessels to constrict) and encourage blood clotting. These properties are important when the body suffers from a wound or an injury because without them you would bleed to death from a cut. However, an excess of the hormone-like prostaglandins from arachidonic acid can be harmful and contribute to disease. Arachidonic acid is found predominantly in organ meats, dairy products, eggs, and chicken, to name a few sources.

Before monthly menstruation, arachidonic acid is released and a cascade of prostaglandins is initiated in the uterus. The inflammatory response initiated by these prostaglandins results in vasoconstriction and contractions, causing the pain, cramps, nausea, vomiting, bloating, and headaches that may be found in those with PMS.

Painful menstruation and breast pain are worse in women who have low levels of the anti-inflammatory prostaglandins. Symptoms of PMS have been specifically attributed to these deficiencies and by simply adding "good" GLA-containing oils like black currant, evening primrose, echium and/or borage oil, pain and PMS symptoms are reduced. The prostaglandins that worsen the pain in the breasts and other tissues are found in excess in women suffering from PMS, in whom the conversion of GLA to good prostaglandins is often impaired.

Both the deficiency of anti-inflammatory prostaglandins and an imbalance of healthy fats (too many bad fats and not enough good ones) may result in increased sensitivity to pro-inflammatory hormones. Some symptoms of PMS, especially breast pain, are due to high consumption of saturated fatty acids found in red meat, milk, and processed foods, resulting in not enough GLA. Women with breast cysts and pain have abnormal fatty-acid profiles, with increased proportions of saturated fatty acids and reduced proportions of essential fatty acids. (For more information on fatty acids, see Chapter 6.)

A trial done at the breast clinic at the University of Hong Kong evaluated evening primrose oil for the treatment of cyclical breast pain. Among the 66 women who were referred to the clinic for disturbing breast pain, 97 percent responded to treatment with GLA after six months. The authors recommended that evening primrose oil be a first-line treatment for women experiencing cyclical mastalgia (breast pain).

Research has shown that GLA can help stimulate serotonin, the "happy" hormone so GLA deficiency may also be responsible for menstrual depression.

GLA Relief from Bloating, Depression, Flushing, and Pain

The enzyme that converts fats into GLA is impaired in many people, but it appears to be particularly low in women and the elderly. Supplementation with GLA has been found to relieve symptoms during the transitional years from peri-menopause through to post-menopause, including night-time flushes, breast pain, inflammation, fluid retention, depression and irritability, and skin wrinkling.

GLA is not Estrogenic

There has been total confusion in doctors' offices about evening primrose and borage oil. Some doctors and pharmacists are misleading women, advising them that these oils are estrogenic, i.e., breast cancer-promoting, and should be avoided. The reports that originally started this misinformation linked omega-6 oils to breast cancer. The misleading studies did not consider the *type* of omega-6 oils that the participants were using. Nor did they reveal whether the oils consumed were refined, genetically modified, or organic. Studies that *did* consider the type of omega-6 oil found that evening primrose oil and borage oil reduce the risk of breast cancer, eliminate breast pain (a risk factor for breast cancer), and improve fibrocystic breast disease. For example, a British study published in 2000 found women with breast cancer who received GLA along with tamoxifen demonstrated faster clinical response than those on tamoxifen alone.

Evening primrose oil and borage oil contain GLA and are safe, non-estrogenic "good" fatty acids that every woman should consume. Lorna has been taking 4,000 mg of borage oil a day for two decades to reduce skin wrinkling and promote hormone health.

Recommended dosage: Dosage varies for each woman, but the general recommendation for breast or period pain is 4,000 mg of borage oil or 8,000 mg of evening primrose oil, every day with food.

Estrogen-dominant Conditions

Who needs nutrients that balance hormones and detoxify environmental estrogens? All women need these nutrients, but especially women with estrogen-dominant conditions. These conditions include uterine fibroids, endometriosis, hormonal acne, breast and ovarian cancer, ovarian cysts, period problems, polycystic ovary syndrome, fibrocystic breast disease, or premenstrual syndrome. It also includes those women whose peri-menopause is characterized by flooding periods; women who are overweight who carry more harmful environmental estrogens and estrogens in their fat cells; and women who have cellulite or high cholesterol. (Any abnormal bleeding should be evaluated with an ultrasound and/or uterine biopsy before embarking on any treatment.)

By this point in the book, you understand that there is much, much more to hormone health than just deciding for or against hormone replacement therapy (HRT). Nevertheless, this decision is an important one. Every woman has a different hormone history, different genetic strengths and weaknesses, a unique personal situation, and is at a unique place on the journey to optimal health. No one can make the decision for you whether to use HRT. The treatments below aim to give you the information and resources you need to make an informed decision for yourself.

Uterine Fibroids and Heavy Bleeding

Uterine fibroids (myomas) are non-cancerous growths that occur on the walls of the uterus. Composed of connective tissue and muscle, these round, firm growths can be microscopic or grow to the size of a large grapefruit. They can appear in groups and typically grow slowly. Fast-growing fibroids may be malignant and should be checked with a uterine biopsy. At least 40 percent of women over age 35 will experience fibroids at some time. Because fibroids are affected by high estrogen levels, some growths tend to shrink at menopause; others increase in size at menopause and become malignant.

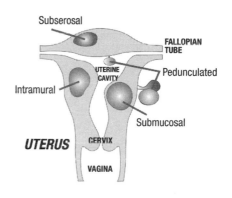

If fibroids cause heavy bleeding or pain or put pressure on other organs, they can be removed surgically in a procedure called a myomectomy, which removes only the fibroid. Fibroids can return after this surgery if lifestyle changes are not made, and there is no reduction in excess estrogens. The number-one reason for a hysterectomy in North America is uterine fibroids.

Fibroids can cause menstrual problems, including heavy, irregular, or painful periods and mid-cycle bleeding. Vaginal discharge, pain, or bleeding with intercourse, frequent urination, problems with bowel movements, and compromised digestion can also occur. Heavy bleeding as a result of fibroids can cause anemia and fatigue.

Suggested Non-drug Treatments for Fibroids and/or Heavy Periods

All recommendations in the book should be combined with excellent nutrition and a good multivitamin with minerals.

Recommended daily treatment:
- EstroSense: 2 capsules at breakfast and 2 capsules at dinner. See page 83 for EstroSense information.
- Vitex (Chaste Tree Berry): 2 capsules with food
- Borage, echium, or evening primrose oil: 4,000 mg per day of borage oil or echium oil or 8,000 mg of evening primrose oil with food
- Vitamin K: 100 mcg per day
- If you have iron deficiency use Floradix iron: 2-4 capfuls per day

These nutrients may take up to two menstrual cycles to start reducing the symptoms of uterine fibroids. Many women achieve relief of symptoms and shrinkage of fibroids using only the nutrients above, along with the lifestyle recommendations mentioned below. Once you have uterine fibroids, the goal is to shrink them or keep them from growing until you reach menopause, at which time they will naturally shrink. Therefore, the nutrients mentioned above should be taken every day until after menopause.

Some women will need more aggressive relief so they do not become severely anemic. Bioidentical progesterone can be added in two ways. You can use the nutrients above for two months and see if the symptoms abate, and, if not, add bioidentical progesterone as recommended below. Or you can start to use bioidentical progesterone immediately, with the nutrients recommended above. The nutrients are to be taken until your periods abate at menopause.

Additional Bioidentical Hormone Cream Recommendation

In addition to the nutrient recommendations above, use a divided dose of bioidentical progesterone cream 40 mg (20 mg applied in the morning and 20 mg applied at night) between days 5 and 28. Or, if you have a 21-day cycle, then use progesterone cream from day 5 to day 21. If you have extremely heavy bleeding, then during two full cycles continue the progesterone through the menstrual cycle and every day. Do not take a break from the hormones for two months. If you are using nutrients, it takes approximately two cycles to see symptoms recede. Once the nutrients have a chance to start working, you can discontinue the progesterone during bleeding. You will know that your condition is improving because your periods will start to normalize, and, if you have pain, it will begin to diminish. Have an annual ultrasound after one year of this program to confirm the fibroids are shrinking or maintaining their size. Just to reiterate: the nutrients should be taken until after periods have stopped at menopause.

Vitamin K

The liver uses vitamin K, called the "Koagulation" vitamin, to make protein factors that are essential to form blood clots. Vitamin K is manufactured in the body by bacteria that live in the intestines. Babies are given injections of vitamin K at birth to prevent bleeding until their gut bacteria can produce vitamin K. However, some experts on vitamin K and blood clotting believe that babies should not be injected and instead should be kept safe from bumps and bangs and protected in a bassinet for the first few weeks of life.

Vitamin K regulates clotting in the blood, making it beneficial for excessive menstrual bleeding. It is necessary for activating bone protein in order to increase bone mineral density to offset osteoporosis. A more recent application of vitamin K has been as a supplement during cancer treatment. There is an unusual property in vitamin K that allows it to enhance anticoagulant therapy, which prevents tumors from metastasizing, even during chemotherapy. For women with flooding periods caused by uterine fibroids, vitamin K is a godsend. Vitamin K2 (menaquinone MK-7) is the preferred form. Until 2001 Vitamin K was not available for sale over the counter in Canada, but now it is readily available at health food stores, just as it is in the U.S.

Recommended dosage: 100 mcg per day with food for flooding periods. 200 mcg per day for bone health.

Endometriosis

The Endometriosis Association of North America states it is extremely rare for a woman in this day and age to ever need a hysterectomy for endometriosis, no matter how severe. Endometriosis is one of the most common, yet misunderstood, female diseases. Approximately 15 percent of women between the ages of 20 and 45 are affected with this painful and debilitating disorder. Symptoms can begin with the onset of menstruation and progressively increase with pending menopause. Dysmenorrhea (pain with menses), dyspareunia (pain with intercourse), and infertility may also be present. The pain some women experience can be devastating. Many women also experience pain when they have a full bladder or bowel. Some women experience no pain but may have fertility, ovarian, or menstrual problems. The symptoms are many and vary from woman to woman.

Seven Early Warning Symptoms of Endometriosis

1. menstrual cramps that increase in severity
2. intermenstrual pain, usually at mid-month
3. painful intercourse (dyspareunia)
4. infertility of unknown origin
5. bladder infection is suspected, but test results are negative
6. pelvic pain that is all-encompassing
7. history of ovarian cysts

Pelvic examinations by a highly skilled gynecologist may disclose nodules or lesions on the ovaries. Ultrasound tests will only show endometriosis if the ovaries are involved. Laparoscopy is the only diagnostic technique that can clearly determine if endometriosis is present. This examination, performed under general anesthetic, involves inserting a telescope containing a light through a small incision in the navel and another one or two small incisions along the bikini line for the instruments.

A laparoscopy is only as good as the surgeon who performs the exam. Removing all the endometriosis tissue requires a physician who is committed to biopsy and getting rid of all suspicious abnormalities. Lorna had endometriosis, and her surgeon was meticulous, eliminating all the endometriosis in one surgery.

Endometrial tissue can look like tiny blueberries or black spots; white, yellow, or reddish cysts; or vary from tiny bluish or dark brown blisters to large chocolate-colored cysts up to 20 centimeters in diameter. Only a biopsy can confirm which tissue is truly endometriosis.

It is not uncommon for endometrial cells to grow on the ovaries; the fallopian tubes; the pelvic ligaments; the outer surface of the uterus, bladder, the large intestine; or the covering of the abdominal cavity. Women are often misdiagnosed with irritable bowel syndrome, bladder infections, an attack of appendicitis, "just" PMS, or painful cramps.

New research points to a glitch in the immune system as the possible cause of this debilitating disorder. Dr. David Redwine, a world-renowned expert, believes that some women are born with abnormally located endometrial cells and that something goes awry with the immune system, causing the cells to become active. This theory has gained acceptance because endometrial cells and growths have been found in the nose, lungs, and other organs far from the uterus. Dr. Redwine has a website where further information on his technique can be found; visit www.endometriosissurgeon.com or phone 541-382-8622.

Endometriosis is worsened by estrogen replacement therapy, and estrogen dominance can worsen symptoms. Surgery to remove the majority of the endometriosis lesions, along with the following nutrient recommendations, is successful in putting endometriosis into permanent remission.

Non-drug Treatments for Endometriosis

All recommendations in the book should be combined with excellent nutrition and a good multivitamin with minerals. Reduce or eliminate environmental estrogens from your home and diet, particularly commercially raised meat and dairy products (known to be high in estrogen).

Recommended daily treatment:
- EstroSense: 2 capsules at breakfast and 2 capsules at dinner
- Vitex (Chaste Tree Berry): 2 to 4 capsules per day with food
- Borage oil or echium oil: 4,000 mg per day with food

Additional Bioidentical Hormone Cream Recommendations

In addition to the nutrient recommendations above, use bioidentical progesterone cream in a divided dose of 20 mg (10 mg applied in the morning and 10 mg at night) between days 5 to 28, or days 5 to 21 if you have a 21-day cycle. If you have very painful periods due to endometriosis, continue the progesterone through two full menstrual cycles without taking a break during your period. It takes approximately two to three cycles to see symptoms recede when using nutrients. Once the nutrients have had a chance to start working, you can discontinue the progesterone during bleeding. Continue to take the nutrients daily until menopause.

Ovarian Cysts and Polycystic Ovary Syndrome

These two conditions have similar treatments and have been included under one heading for this reason.

Ovarian cysts are very common and often exist without symptoms. In a normal cycle, several follicles develop every month, each containing an egg. Surges of luteinizing hormone and follicle-stimulating hormone help mature and release the egg, and progesterone is produced by the corpus luteum. If the egg is not fertilized, the cycle starts all over again. Sometimes, however, no egg is released. Then no progesterone is secreted, and more estrogen is released. The follicles mature into fluid-filled sacs or cysts that will grow larger every month until progesterone is secreted.

Fluid-filled cysts can appear in a very short time and disappear just as quickly. They can be found singly or in groups and be small or large (even as big as a lemon!). Often when cysts are a few centimeters in size, doctors will recommend surgery. However, if a diet and supplementation program is followed, those cysts will usually shrink and disappear.

The risk of cancer increases when ovarian cysts become solid. Ovarian cancer is rare, but it is difficult to diagnose and remission rates with conventional treatments are poor, so early diagnosis is essential. Sometimes a follicle is able to grow tissue or skin cells within the cyst. These types of cysts, called Dermoid cysts, will not dissipate and must be surgically removed.

Often ovarian cysts are not noticed until your doctor performs a pelvic examination or you have an ultrasound scan. This is why it is so important to go for your annual Pap test; your doctor will perform a pelvic exam at the same time. For those with symptoms, the most obvious one is pain, either tenderness to the touch or a constant sore or burning sensation in the lower abdomen, off to the right or left. Pain may occur during ovulation or intercourse. If a cyst erupts in the pelvic cavity, blood and/or fluid will discharge, possibly causing pain.

Ovarian cysts occur when there is a hormone imbalance. Estrogen dominance brought on by poor elimination of waste by the lymphatic system, colon, liver, and kidneys is a factor. Emotional or physical trauma, prolonged stress, and even heavy exercise can cause increased estrogen. A diet rich in meat, dairy products, and alcohol is also responsible for elevated estrogen. (See page 166 for foods that affect estrogen levels.) Cysts that occur after menopause should be looked at by a physician as there is a greater risk of them being cancerous. The risk of ovarian cancer is increased with the use of fertility drugs or birth control pills, or if you have never been pregnant.

Polycystic ovary syndrome (PCOS) is a disorder characterized by many fluid-filled cysts and excessively high levels of male hormones. In this disorder, the release of excess luteinizing hormone by the pituitary gland increases the production of male hormones that can cause acne, oily skin, and coarse hair growth on the face or chest. Ovaries are typically enlarged and contain multiple cysts, but some women with PCOS have no cysts present. Symptoms often become apparent in puberty when menstruation is to begin: irregular menstrual periods with copious bleeding may occur, or PCOS can cause a lack of periods altogether.

Affecting up to 10 percent of the North American population, PCOS is the most common hormone dysfunction among women in their reproductive years. Because eggs are often not released, fertility is a problem. If pregnancy does occur, it frequently ends with first trimester miscarriage or is associated with gestational diabetes. The condition seems to run in families, with 20 percent of mothers and 40 percent of sisters of those with PCOS also showing varying degrees of the syndrome.

With the approach of menopause, androgen production declines, leading to a more normal pattern of menstruation. If left untreated, PCOS can lead to cancer of the uterine lining. Women with PCOS are also at increased risk for developing Type 2 diabetes, cardiovascular disease, and hypertension.

Although historically considered to be a gynecological problem, research now shows that PCOS is associated with hyper-insulinemia (production of too much of the insulin hormone) and impaired glucose metabolism. Perhaps not surprisingly, then, more than 65 percent of women who suffer from PCOS are obese. Reports indicate that early pubarche (breast budding and pubic hair growth), also called precocious puberty (puberty in girls 7 to 11 years of age), is linked to ovarian hyper-androgenism and insulin resistance, suggesting another hormonal trigger. Doctors typically try to determine if a tumor is responsible for the production of male hormones. Thyroid and prolactin abnormalities should also be investigated as possible causes of amenorrhea (lack of period).

Non-drug Treatments for Ovarian Cysts and PCOS

All recommendations in the book should be combined with excellent nutrition and a good multivitamin with minerals. Reduce or eliminate environmental estrogens from your home and diet, particularly commercially raised meat and dairy products (known to be high in estrogen).

Recommended daily treatment:
- EstroSense: 2 capsules at breakfast and 2 capsules at dinner
- Vitex (Chaste Tree Berry): 2 to 4 capsules per day with food
- Borage oil or echium oil: 4,000 mg per day with food

Additional Recommendations for those with PCOS

Use PGX. PolyGlycopleX (PGX) is a unique supplement which was developed at the University of Toronto. It regulates insulin and blood sugar levels. PGX is available for purchase either in capsules, sprinkles, or as a meal replacement. The dosage is determined by the type chosen, for example, two scoops of meal replacement. PGX also aids the loss of excess weight, a contributing factor in PCOS.

Additional Bioidentical Hormone Recommendations

In addition to the nutrient recommendations above, if your saliva or blood hormone tests show you are low in progesterone, use 20 mg of bioidentical progesterone in a divided dose (10 mg applied in the morning and 10 mg applied at night) between days 5 and 28 or whenever your cycle ends; for some women, this is day 21.

Fibrocystic Breast Disease

With the fear of breast cancer so prominent today, breast lumps are a concern for many women. Fibrocystic breast disease (FBD), also called cystic mastitis, is a common, non-cancerous condition. It can be mildly uncomfortable to severely painful, especially when breasts become swollen. Fluid that has not been drained via the lymphatic system fills in small spaces within the breast. The fluid is then encapsulated by fibrous tissue and thickens like scar tissue. The cysts may swell before and during menstruation. Although FBD does not increase the risk of cancer, it may make detecting cancerous tumors difficult through breast self-exams.

Twenty to 40 percent of women who are peri-menopausal (between the ages of 35 and 50) experience FBD, with the symptoms generally disappearing after menopause. FBD is affected by the rise and fall of monthly female hormones. Symptoms include breast tenderness and swelling and a lumpy feeling to the breast.

It can be very distressing to feel these lumps. Monthly breast self-exams, thermography breast scans, and/or ultrasound can help lay your fears of breast cancer to rest. If a breast lump is discovered, have your physician assess it— most lumps are benign. Lumps that suddenly grow larger and do not change with your menstrual cycle; discharge from your nipple; severe, unrelenting breast pain; or puckered or dimpled skin on your breast should be reported to your physician immediately.

FBD occurs when you are exposed to too much estrogen, causing excess estrogens or an imbalance in estrogen-to-progesterone ratio in the body due to stress, estrogen replacement therapy, or exposure to xenoestrogens. Elevated cortisol, which further elevates estrogen, is another contributing factor to FBD. It is also seen in young women with irregular periods. Lumps may come and go, with symptoms often disappearing after the monthly menstrual period has passed and hormone levels return to normal. It is now considered a risk factor for or precursor to breast cancer, especially if you are having multiple mammo- grams with repeated exposure to radiation.

Heavy coffee consumption (more than two cups per day) has been linked to FBD because coffee increases estradiol levels. A diet high in "bad" fats has also been linked to the disorder. (See page 151 for more information.) As well, being overweight is a risk factor for FBD.

Non-drug Treatments for Fibrocystic Breasts

All recommendations should be combined with excellent nutrition and a good multivitamin with minerals. Reduce or eliminate environmental estrogens from your home and diet, particularly commercially raised meat and dairy products (known to be high in estrogen). Eliminate coffee or other caffeinated beverages like black tea, colas, and hot chocolate. (Green tea, because it contains L-thea- nine, known to modify the effects of caffeine, is the exception.)

Recommended daily treatment:
- EstroSense: 2 capsules at breakfast and 2 capsules at dinner
- Vitex (Chaste Tree Berry): 2 to 4 capsules per day with food
- Borage oil or echium oil: 4,000 mg per day with food

Additional Bioidentical Hormone Recommendations

In addition to the nutrient recommendations above, if your saliva or blood hor- mone tests show you are low in progesterone, use a divided daily dose of 40 mg of bioidentical progesterone, 20 mg applied in the morning and 20 mg applied at night for 14 days before your period begins. If you have a 28-day cycle, this will be day 14, and if you have a 21-day cycle, this will be day 11.

Lifestyle Recommendations for all Estrogen-dominant Conditions

Do not eat commercially raised dairy products. Dairy products contain arachidonic acid, which promotes the "bad" prostaglandins and leukotrienes that cause inflammation and pain. Dairy products also contain xenestrogens. Both Canada and the U.S. have approved estrogen and testosterone replacement therapy for cows and steers to enhance their commercial output and fatten them up. Only consume organic dairy products, and, even then, limit them if you have the conditions discussed above. All commercially produced beef products contain hormones, so limit your intake of red meat, and, when you do eat it, make sure it is organic and free range.

Excess estrogens must be eliminated. To reduce your consumption of estrogens from pesticide-laden foods, buy organically grown foods whenever possible.

Reduce the stress in your life. Working women with Type-A personalities are the most prone to estrogen-dominant conditions. Women who are constantly under stress from job, family pressures, and personal expectations are also at higher risk for estrogen-dominant conditions.

Get regular exercise. This helps keep hormones balanced. For those with endometriosis, fibroids, and ovarian cysts, it is essential to exercise to ensure that circulation in the pelvic area is restored. If you sit all day, your lower abdomen becomes congested.

A Warning about Hysterectomies

Unsuccessful conventional treatments for many of the common perimenopausal conditions we have cited put women at risk for a hysterectomy, and we feel it is important to present some information about them. *Over 90 percent* of hysterectomies are unnecessary. Yes, you read it correctly. Only 10 percent of hysterectomies are deemed medically necessary!

A report prepared by the Ontario Women's Health Council says that Canadian women are having hysterectomies too frequently as a first line of treatment for discretionary reasons—to supposedly improve a woman's quality of life—rather than to save her life. The report found that hysterectomy remains the most common procedure used to treat non-life-threatening conditions such as abnormal uterine bleeding (heavy periods), uterine fibroids, endometriosis, unexplained pelvic pain, and prolapsed uterus. And the same holds true for American women.

Just turning 40 years old in North America puts you at risk of losing your uterus. Women aged 40 to 44 years had a significantly higher rate of hysterectomy, at 11.7 per 1,000, than any other age group in the study. Fifty-two percent of all hysterectomies are performed on women younger than 44 years of age. With the population's aging baby boomers, hysterectomy rates are only going to climb. The highest hysterectomy rate, 16.8 per 1,000, is in African American women aged 40 to 44 years.

Abdominal hysterectomies were performed more frequently than vaginal hysterectomies in all races. Hysterectomy rates are more than twice as high in northern and rural areas than in metropolitan centers that have teaching hospitals. Over 55 percent of hysterectomies also involve the removal of both ovaries, which immediately throws a woman into surgical menopause.

Facts About Hysterectomy

- The word hysterectomy comes from the Greek word hystra, which means suffering caused by the uterus.
- Hysterectomy is the removal of the uterus.
- Oophorectomy is the removal of one or both ovaries.
- A complete hysterectomy is the removal of both the ovaries and the uterus.
- Supracervical hysterectomy leaves the cervix in place, which leaves the vagina longer with less discomfort during intercourse.
- Laparoscopic-assisted vaginal hysterectomy involves using a laparoscope to remove the uterus and/or ovaries.

Female Castration

Dr. Stanley West, M.D., author of the *Hysterectomy Hoax*, states that "removal of the ovaries is castration. A man would never consent to having his testicles removed unless he had cancer or some other life-threatening condition, yet women have their ovaries removed in record numbers simply because doctors are not telling them they will be castrated."

If physicians started to adopt the terminology of castration and disclosed the potential side effects of hysterectomy, most women would refuse to undergo the procedure and seek alternatives. It is important to understand how a hysterectomy may affect your overall health, your hormones, and especially your ability to have and enjoy sex afterwards.

Potential Side Effects of Hysterectomy

Although many women report that they feel better after a hysterectomy, others are not so lucky. Vaginal, abdominal, and laparoscopic hysterectomies are each performed with their own inherent risks. The reported side effects may include:

- **Adhesions**: Adhesions are bands of tough, fibrous, scar-like tissue that can occur during injury or surgery. These adhesions can interfere with normal functioning of an organ. Pelvic adhesions, where organs bind together, can occur on the bladder and bowel, especially if the woman has endometriosis. During a vaginal hysterectomy, the surgeon's ability to see these adhesions may be impaired. If this happens, a woman who thought she was going to have a vaginal hysterectomy may end up with an abdominal hysterectomy.
- **Bowel injury**: If the bowel is accidentally cut, infection can occur, or a fistula (an opening between the rectum and vagina that allows fecal material to enter the vagina) can develop. This can be repaired during surgery, if the surgeon is aware that a cut has been made.
- **Bladder injury**: Infection from a cut to the bladder can occur; or a fistula between the bladder and vagina can occur, allowing urine to leak into the vagina. Again, this can be repaired during a hysterectomy if the surgeon notes the problem. This does not always happen but many women report incontinence and bladder frequency issues after hysterectomy.
- **Ureter injury**: The ureter is next to the cervix; it is the tube connecting the kidney to the bladder. It can be easily bruised, nicked, or otherwise injured, causing urinary tract problems.
- **Sexual dysfunction**: Many women report never having another orgasm once they have had a hysterectomy due to important nerves being cut during the operation; others report sad feelings related to a perceived decrease or loss of their sexuality. The uterus and ovaries are a large part of what makes us female, and many women grieve the loss of their organs. (Back in the nineteenth century, hysterectomy was used as a treatment to stop such perceived sexual perversions as masturbation and promiscuity.)
- **Depression and Low Libido**: Estrogen acts to stimulate the release of endorphins from the hypothalamus. Removal of the ovaries (a major

estrogen source) in some women has a profound effect on hormones related to happiness, resulting in mood swings and depression. The ovaries are also a source of testosterone, which promotes higher energy, vitality, and a desire for sex.

- **Estrogen-deficiency symptoms**: Vaginal dryness, incontinence, painful intercourse, severe hot flashes, night sweats, joint pain, heart palpitations, anxiety, and depression are reported.
- **Shortened vagina**: A technique called Worrelling (named after Dr. Worrell) can be used to peel the vagina away from the cervix and maintain the length of the vagina. Without this technique, many women are left with a shortened vagina and painful intercourse. Even with this technique, women have painful intercourse.
- **Weight gain**: Many women report a large weight gain after hysterectomy.

Think Twice About Hysterectomy

Dr. Laura Berman, Ph.D., author of *The Passion Prescription* states that "any surgery performed for gynecological conditions can challenge a woman's sexual wellbeing. The medical field still does not know where all of the important nerves and blood vessels are situated in a woman's pelvis. As a result, many are inadvertently damaged during pelvic surgeries, which can pose a real problem for sexual response. Severed nerves and blood vessels compromise lubrication, sensation, and feelings of fullness in the genital area when you are aroused."

If you have to have a hysterectomy due to cancer or another medically necessary reason, ensure that your surgeon understands you want to maintain your sex life. For all other women, use the safe, effective alternatives to hysterectomy for conditions like endometriosis, uterine fibroids, heavy periods, prolapsed uterus, and others we have provided above.

Support the Adrenal Glands

As you read in Chapters 1 and 2, the adrenal glands are among the most important glands in the body. The adrenals secrete cortisol, which is essential for regulating many metabolic and immune functions (including glucose metabolism), releasing immune system hormones, and assisting cardiovascular functions, as well as regulating the body's use of proteins, carbohydrates, and fats. The key role of these small glands is to release hormones that guide the body's reaction to stressors, as well as releasing sex hormones. Extended periods of high levels of stress in life result in continually high levels of cortisol, which you now know not only exhausts the adrenal glands but also affects how the body manages other key hormones such as progesterone (see page 5). The continual production of cortisol can exhaust the adrenal glands, and exhausted adrenals fail to perform many of their vital jobs.

During the peri-menopausal years, as estrogen and progesterone production by the ovaries begins to decline, the adrenals are meant to increase their manufacture of these hormones to make up for the deficiency. Adrenals that have been exhausted by constant stress will not be able to respond to the extra demands of peri-menopause. Therefore, it is important to support the adrenals during high-stress adulthood. Take the adrenal stress test on page 218 to assess the health of your adrenals.

Herbs that assist the body in adapting to stress by supporting the adrenal glands are aptly called adaptogens. Adaptogens have a normalizing effect— regardless of the condition, they help the body maintain the constant internal state necessary for health and life itself. For example, if blood pressure is high, an adaptogen will help lower it; if it is low, the same adaptogen will help normalize it.

During menopause or surgical menopause the workload of the adrenal glands is increased. At this time, the adrenals must not only help you cope with life's ordinary strains but also with all the emotional and physical stresses that attend the menopausal transition. And as mentioned, the adrenals must begin replacing the sex hormones once produced by your ovaries. Because these adaptogens support adrenal function, they can be very important to wellbeing during menopause.

SIBERIAN GINSENG (Eleutherococcus senticosus)

Siberian ginseng is respected for its ability to support adrenal function and enhance immune function. Toxicity studies have demonstrated that it is virtually non-toxic. In Russia, Siberian ginseng is well known for its ability to increase stamina and endurance in athletes.

Siberian ginseng counteracts fatigue, provides immune support, improves mental abilities, and supports the body during periods of high physical exertion.

Recommended dosage: 100 mg, 1 to 3 times daily with food. Or simply take AdrenaSense, an adaptogenic formula containing Siberian ginseng, rhodiola, suma, ashwagandha, and schizandra. For optimal results take 1 to 2 AdrenaSense at 3:00 in the afternoon with a protein snack when you feel a drop in energy.

AdrenaSense, is an adaptogenic formula containing Siberian ginseng, rhodiola, ashwagandha, suma, and schizandra. For best results take it mid-afternoon with protein snack.

RHODIOLA (Rhodiola rosea)

Rhodiola is one of the newer adaptogens to North America, but it has been studied intensively for over 35 years in Russia. Russian researchers have observed that rhodiola increases resistance to a variety of chemical, biological, and physical stressors, as well offering anti-fatigue, anti-depressant, immune-enhancing, anti-cancer, and cardio-protective effects. It also improves the nervous system and mental function by increasing blood supply and protein synthesis. Rhodiola is beneficial in the treatment of insomnia, and enhances mental performance, reduces fatigue and hypertension, improves memory, and relieves depression.

Recommended dosage: 100 mg, 1 to 3 times daily with food. Or simply take AdrenaSense, an adaptogenic formula containing Siberian ginseng, rhodiola, suma, ashwagandha, and schizandra. For optimal results take 1 to 2 AdrenaSense at 3:00 in the afternoon with a protein snack when you feel a drop in energy.

ASHWAGANDHA (Withania somnifera)

Ashwagandha is referred to as Indian ginseng, and it has been used in Ayurvedic medicine, the traditional medical system of India, for more than 3,000 years. Historically, ashwagandha has been used as an aphrodisiac, liver tonic, and anti-inflammatory. While numerous studies have explored this herb's ability to improve stress tolerance, combat fatigue, improve memory problems, enhance immune function, and benefit inflammatory conditions such as arthritis, recent research has also examined its positive effect on those suffering from hormone imbalances and low thyroid function (see page 113 for more on ashwagandha and thyroid function). Remember: the adrenals and thyroid are directly linked. When the adrenals become exhausted, thyroid function is reduced. Ashwagandha is also an excellent remedy for nervous system complaints such as anxiety and insomnia.

In a double-blind clinical trial, ashwagandha was tested in over 100 patients aged 50 to 59 years. A significant improvement in hemoglobin, red blood cell count, hair melanin, and seated stature was reported. Serum cholesterol also decreased and nail calcium was improved. Erythrocyte sedimentation rate (ESR), which is a measure used to determine inflammation, decreased significantly. High ESR means more pain and inflammation in the body. Most importantly for your sex life, a 71.4 percent improvement in sexual performance was reported using ashwagandha.

Recommended dosage: 80 mg, 1 to 3 times daily with food. Or simply take AdrenaSense, an adaptogenic formula containing Siberian ginseng, rhodiola, suma, ashwagandha, and schizandra. For optimal results take 1 to 2 AdrenaSense at 3:00 in the afternoon with a protein snack when you feel a drop in energy.

SUMA (Pfaffia paniculata)

In Brazil, suma is also called *"para todo,"* a Portuguese phrase meaning "for everything." Traditionally, it is used as an energy and rejuvenation tonic, as well as a general cure-all for many types of disorders. Its active ingredients include the phytosterols, beta-sitosterol and stigmasterol, along with glycosides and saponins. Suma is particularly useful in aiding the adrenal glands in times of stress and in treating adrenal fatigue. Suma is an excellent herb for the cardiovascular system, central nervous system, reproductive system, digestive system, and the immune system. In Europe, suma is commonly used to treat fatigue, menopausal symptoms, impotence and other sexual difficulties, respiratory problems, blood sugar imbalances and diabetes, cancer, and diseases related to chronic immune deficiencies. Suma is a source of beta-ecdysterone, which is used widely to help athletes increase muscle mass and endurance.

A study published in the *Journal of Reproductive Development* in 2003 found that mice that had their water enriched with suma over a 30-day period had an increase in progesterone and testosterone. This may be the reason why people using suma report a return of sex drive.

Recommended dosage: 100 mg, 1 to 3 times daily with food. Or simply take AdrenaSense, an adaptogenic formula containing Siberian ginseng, rhodiola, suma, ashwagandha, and schizandra. For optimal results take 1 to 2 AdrenaSense at 3:00 in the afternoon with a protein snack when you feel a drop in energy.

SCHIZANDRA (Schizandra chinensis)

In traditional Chinese medicine, schizandra is commonly used as a general tonic herb to purify the blood and restore the liver. It counteracts the effects of stress and fatigue. Scientific studies show it has normalizing effects in cases of insomnia, gastrointestinal problems, and immune system disorders. Schizandra improves mental function and enhances physical and intellectual endurance.

Recommended dosage: 80 mg, 1 to 3 times daily with food. Or simply take AdrenaSense, an adaptogenic formula containing Siberian ginseng, rhodiola, suma, ashwagandha, and schizandra. For optimal results take 1 to 2 AdrenaSense at 3:00 in the afternoon with a protein snack when you feel a drop in energy.

> Remember that the adrenal and thyroid glands operate on a feedback system. When adrenal function becomes impaired, thyroid hormone output often becomes low. Because the two are so directly linked, problems with one may lead to dysfunction with the other.

Correct Low Thyroid

The thyroid gland, located at the front of your throat, sets the rate of your body's metabolism, which means it regulates nearly every cell in your body. This butterfly-shaped gland receives messages from the thyroid-stimulating hormone (TSH) secreted by the pituitary and secretes thyroxine (T4) and tri-iodothyronine (T3), which travel through your bloodstream and affect the rate that your body metabolizes fats, proteins, and carbohydrates for energy at many sites. In other words, thyroid hormones set the rate that you use food as fuel, rev up your fat-burning furnace, set your heart rate and temperature, and determine how quickly waste moves through your body for elimination (bowel movements), among dozens of other important functions in the body.

If your thyroid is not operating at peak performance, you will not be able to lose weight or you may have drastic increases in your weight over a short period of time; your hair may thin, including your eyebrows; your skin will wrinkle excessively and be dry; your sex drive will be gone; and you may experience menstrual problems or severe menopause symptoms. For an in-depth look at the thyroid gland, see page 6; for more detail on thyroid hormones, see page 28.

In addition to making diet and lifestyle changes outlined in Chapters 6 and 8, you can support your thyroid with nutritional supplements. The following recommendations are for those with symptoms of low thyroid and a thyroid stimulating hormone (TSH) level of 2.0 and higher, which is indicative of low thyroid. See page 51 for more information on testing thyroid function. We have seen people take the nutrients in ThyroSense and have their thyroid hormone levels normalize quickly without medications.

Or, if you are like many who are already taking thyroid medications but find, after a time, that your symptoms return, you may not be converting your T4 thyroid hormone to T3, and you will also benefit from the thyroid support nutrients listed below. These nutrient recommendations are not to be used in place of the thyroid hormone your doctor has prescribed, but in addition to it. These nutrients are extremely safe and will not cause your thyroid to become overactive because they are simply support.

Please note that the following treatment recommendations do not apply to hyperthyroid (over-active thyroid). This is a complicated condition that is best treated by an endocrinologist.

L-TYROSINE

L-Tyrosine is an essential amino acid that is necessary for the manufacture of the thyroid hormones T4 (thyroxine) and T3 (triiodothyronine). Dietary sources of L-tyrosine are mainly derived from animal and vegetable proteins. Vegetables and juices contain small amounts, and it is also found in fermented foods such as yogurt and miso. In addition to being involved in the manufacture of protein, L-tyrosine is a precursor for the synthesis of epinephrine and norepinephrine (produced by the adrenal glands), as well as dopamine, and the pigment melanin.

Recommended dosage: 500 mg per day with food at breakfast, or simply take 2 capsules of ThyroSense. (Those on thyroid medication should take it on an empty stomach first thing in the morning and then take 2 ThyroSense with breakfast.)

ThyroSense is a combination of L-tyrosine, ashwagandha, guggals, potassium iodide, and pantothenic acid.

ASHWAGANDHA

Ashwagandha (Indian ginseng) has traditionally been used in Ayurvedic medicine to support the thyroid gland. Animal studies show that it enhances thyroid function and produces a significant increase in T4 thyroid hormone. As noted, Ashwagandha also has a positive effect on the adrenal glands by improving response to stressful events. Ashwagandha contains the active ingredients flavonoids and withanolides. Research has focused on ashwagandha's anti-inflammatory action in arthritis, immune-enhancing actions, and restorative properties. It is also well known in India for its endocrine effects of enhancing sexual desire. We know that when the thyroid is low, sex drive disappears, so this action likely has more to do with enhancing T4 thyroid hormone.

Recommended dosage: 150 mg per day with food at breakfast, or simply take 2 capsules of ThyroSense. (Those on thyroid medication should take it on an empty stomach first thing in the morning and then take 2 ThyroSense with breakfast.)

GUGGALS

Guggals, also called Commiphora mukul extract, supports complete thyroid health while enhancing the conversion of T4 hormone to the more potent T3 hormone. Look for a formula that contains both ashwagandha and guggals as these two herbs have a synergistic effect on improving the conversion of T4 to T3 thyroid hormone. Ninety-five percent of all cases of low thyroid are due to impaired conversion of T4 into T3 in the tissues of the thyroid gland. This is very common in persons taking Synthroid or levothyroxine (T4 thyroid hormone), and this is the reason why we recommend taking these herbs with your T4 thyroid medication.

Recommended dosage: 100 mg per day with food at breakfast, or simply take 2 capsules of ThyroSense. (Those on thyroid medication should take it on an empty stomach first thing in the morning and then take 2 ThyroSense with breakfast.)

POTASSIUM IODIDE

Iodine is essential for the manufacture of thyroid hormones. Now that table salt is being eliminated from the diet due to fears of high blood pressure, North Americans often do not get enough potassium iodide to support proper thyroid health. Unlike Asian populations, North Americans eat very few sea vegetables, which are a major source of iodine. Potassium iodide was added to table salt in order to prevent low thyroid and goiter. When telling patients to avoid all salt, doctors forget that they require potassium iodide for a healthy thyroid gland. (On another note, it is not salt that is the culprit in high blood pressure, but the lack of potassium and magnesium in the diet, which balance the effects of sodium.) The adrenal glands also require sodium for optimal health.

Recommended dosage: 100 mcg per day with food at breakfast, or simply take 2 capsules of ThryoSense. (Those on thyroid medication should take it on an empty stomach first thing in the morning and then take 2 ThyroSense with breakfast.)

PANTOTHENIC ACID

Pantothenic acid supports the adrenal glands, increases energy, helps you handle stressful situations better, and reduces cellulite. Pantothenic acid is also a supporting nutrient for thyroid hormone manufacture.

Recommended dosage: 100 mg per day with food at breakfast, or simply take 2 capsules of ThyroSense. (Those on thyroid medication should take it on an empty stomach first thing in the morning and then take 2 ThyroSense with breakfast.)

Additional Support for Thyroid Function

Minerals such as copper, manganese, and selenium are also necessary for the proper manufacture of thyroid hormones. A deficiency in several nutrients can cause or contribute to hypothyroidism. Supplementing with a good multivitamin that includes the vitamins A, B2, B3, B6, C, D, and E, plus minerals, will ensure optimal health of your thyroid gland.

VITAMIN D

Vitamin D is essential for the manufacture of thyroid hormones. There are higher rates of low thyroid in the northern hemisphere than in the southern, due to lower exposure to sunlight. Sunlight on the skin is how the body manufactures vitamin D. Most Canadians and those living in the northern U.S. are vitamin D deficient all year round—not just in the winter. Now that North Americans have a fear of the sun and are covering up and wearing sunscreen, vitamin D deficiency is on the increase.

Increasing vitamin D levels inhibits the development and progression of breast cancer, according to the Imperial College of London. A study in the *Journal of Clinical Pathology* states that there is an ever-growing body of evidence linking vitamin D status with incidence and risk of various cancers, including breast, colorectal, and prostate.

This link between vitamin D intake and protection from cancer is not new. This information dates back to the 1940s when Frank Apperly demonstrated a link between latitude and deaths from cancer and suggested that sunlight gave "a relative cancer immunity," noting that circulating vitamin D levels are lower in patients with advanced breast cancer than in those with early breast cancer.

The authors of a study published in 2006 in the *Journal of Clinical Pathology*, recruited 279 women with invasive breast cancer. The disease was in its early stages in 204 women and advanced in the other 75. Measuring serum levels of 25-hydroxyvitamin D, the researchers reported that women with early stage disease had significantly higher levels of vitamin D (15 to 184 millimoles per litre) than the women in the advanced stages of the disease (16 to 146 millimoles per litre). It is not known whether the low levels of vitamin D among those with advanced disease are a cause or consequence of the cancer itself, but previous studies have reported that vitamin D sufficiency and exposure to sunlight may reduce the risk of developing breast cancer.

It is almost impossible to eat a diet rich in vitamin D without fortified foods or vitamin supplements because no food is naturally rich in vitamin D. Most vitamin D is made in the skin on exposure to sunlight. Have your blood tested for 25-hydroxyl vitamin D levels as a measure of vitamin D status. This test is covered by most insurers.

Recommended dosage: Everyone should take a minimum of 400 I.U. per day. If you have a family history of breast or colon cancer, you should use 1,000 I.U. vitamin D per day.

Thyroid Problems in the Transitional Years

It is common for women to have symptoms of low thyroid function during the transitional years from peri-menopause through menopause. If the situation is addressed at this point, further depletion of both thyroid and adrenal function can be prevented. Many of the symptoms women suffer at menopause are due to low thyroid and/or exhausted adrenals.

Unfortunately, most women are given synthetic estrogen for their complaints, which further shuts down the thyroid because high estrogen levels interfere with the thyroid hormones, particularly the utilization of T3, the more potent biologically active form of thyroid hormone. Weight gain and increased blood pressure are common side effects of the synthetic estrogens because when the estrogen blocks thyroid hormone the body's metabolic rate slows down, making it very difficult to lose weight. In addition, serum cholesterol or triglyceride levels may increase. When bioidentical estrogen is used in the correct form and optimal delivery method, and the dosages are monitored, weight gain from estrogen replacement therapy does not occur.

Depression and fatigue are the most common low thyroid symptoms in menopausal women. Often the prescription is anti-depressants or hormone replacement therapy or both, when thyroid hormones would be more appropriate. In 1993, Dr. Frank Tallis reported in the *British Journal of Psychiatry* that up to 14 percent of the patients referred to him for depression or some other emotional disorder turned out to have clinical hypothyroidism (underactive thyroid). Once the hypothyroidism was treated, the emotional cloud lifted. Hyla Cass, M.D., psychiatrist and author of *Natural Highs*, also states many women are incorrectly treated for a psychiatric condition when they actually have thyroid problems.

The correlation between low thyroid and the rise of emotional symptoms needs to be made to protect women from unnecessary drug side effects. The side effects of anti-depressant medications include low libido, vaginal dryness, weight gain, hot flashes, and more. Many of these are symptoms women are trying to treat during the transitional years.

Case Study: Lost My Hair—Mary

Mary is 39 years old, and she suffered for years with heavy periods caused by uterine fibroids. Her fibroids started to reduce in size (see page 95), and her periods normalized after following our recommendations on page 96 above. She used to have a thick head of hair, and she noticed her hair was thinning terribly on top, and the ends of her eyebrows were thinning as well.

Dr. Pettle and I recommended that Mary have thyroid hormone blood tests and a hemoglobin and ferritin blood test. She also had a saliva hormone test performed to look at her levels of estrogens and progesterone. Mary's thyroid stimulating hormone (TSH) test came back at a 5.5, which is borderline low thyroid, based on the current inadequate reference range (see page 51 for more information). Her hemoglobin was low, and her iron storage (ferritin) levels were poor as well. Mary's saliva hormone test came back indicating she had low progesterone and very high estrogens. She was suffering the effects of high levels of estrogens, which block the uptake of thyroid hormone. Her heavy periods had caused anemia, which worsens hair loss and makes monthly bleeding heavier.

Hair loss in women can be due to many factors, one being low thyroid. Low levels of iron in the blood, and, conversely, high levels of iron in the blood, a deficiency of zinc in the diet, autoimmune disease, and too much stress are also associated with hair loss.

We recommended that Mary take a complete multinutrient formula like FemmEssentials, which contains all the cofactors needed for strong, thick hair. It also contains the minerals and vitamin D that are necessary for the manufacture of thyroid hormones. FemmEssentials contains zinc citrate, needed for thick hair, and evening primrose and flaxseed oil for shiny hair, among other important nutrients. You can read more about the need for a good multinutrient formula in Appendix A.

Another excellent nutrient we wanted Mary to add is BioSil. BioSil has been clinically researched at the University of Brussels. It enhances collagen, not only in the hair, but also the nails, bones, and skin. Collagen, an essential part of hair, makes hair elastic so there is less breakage and less hair in the brush. BioSil has been found to improve hair thickness and strength within six weeks. Mary is also anemic and needs a good iron supplement. Floradix is a non-constipating iron; 2 capfuls per day are prescribed.

Mary is now taking low-dose thyroid hormone, along with 2 capsules of ThyroSense with breakfast. ThyroSense is added to her thyroid hormone regimen to ensure her thyroid medication is converting properly. We have also added bioidentical progesterone cream, 20 mg divided (10 mg applied in the morning and 10 mg applied at night), stopping during her menstrual cycle.

Our Gorgeous Hair Program

To correct low thyroid function and anemia, and restore gorgeous hair:

- FemmEssentials: 1 to 2 packets per day
- BioSil: 10 drops per day in juice or 2 capsules per day
- ThyroSense: 2 capsules with breakfast
- Floradix: 2 capfuls per day for diagnosed anemia. Iron is only given to those with iron deficiency diagnosed by blood tests.

Solve Insomnia

One of the worst conditions affecting women today is insomnia. It is a particularly challenging problem for women during the transitional years. Women who do not sleep well have a worsening of their hormone-related symptoms. Menopausal women suffering with insomnia will have more hot flashes and anxiety the following day, creating a vicious cycle of symptoms.

There are two types of insomnia: for some women, they cannot fall asleep easily; other women fall asleep easily but wake up several hours later and are unable to return to sleep. Night sweats can be a cause of insomnia; women often wake up due to damp bedding and night clothes. If this is the problem, the appropriate herbs mentioned on page 125 will help alleviate night sweats. Layer your bedding as well so you can cool down if necessary, and purchase a pair of "wick-away" long johns as your night clothes. Originally designed for skiers, they work fabulously for women suffering night sweats to keep the dampness away from the skin and absorbed instead of awakening the sleeper. If you have a loved one sharing your bed, get separate bed covers for your queen-sized bed. Make the bed up with twin sheets and blankets so that your loved one is not woken up every time you fling off the covers. He will be happier the next day. Sleep deprivation causes a severe drop in sex drive. Restoring deep, restful sleep goes a long way to enhancing sexy hormones.

Different types of insomnia require different recommendations. Melatonin is used for women who cannot fall asleep, whereas 5-HTP is used along with adrenal support herbs for women who wake up in the middle of the night and cannot return to sleep. Melatonin and 5-HTP can safely be taken together if you have both problems. Melatonin can be taken every night without concern that your body's own natural production will decline. It is a myth that you become dependent on this very safe hormone. Extensive research on melatonin's safety has been performed on children and adults.

MELATONIN

Melatonin, identified in 1958, is a hormone manufactured from serotonin, your "happy" hormone, and secreted by the pineal gland. The human body is governed by an internal clock that signals the release of many hormones that regulate various body functions. Melatonin is most well known for its ability to control sleep and wake cycles—it is secreted in darkness and suppressed by light. Melatonin is also used to treat jet lag—it resets your internal clock when you travel by air across several time zones. Children have much higher melatonin levels than adults do, and sadly, as we age, melatonin is dramatically reduced. Anti-aging specialists believe melatonin to be essential in slowing the aging process. Low levels of melatonin are also found in those individuals with sleep and depressive disorders.

Research has shown that melatonin:
- promotes restful sleep
- helps induce sleep
- reduces jet lag symptoms
- it protects against breast cancer and is anti-estrogenic
- protects against colorectal cancer
- when low blood levels are present, an increased risk of endometrial cancer occurs
- reduces harmful effects on the heart associated with insomnia or shift work
- protects against the effects of stress in those with diabetes and high blood pressure

Melatonin Protects Against Female Cancers

Exciting research shows that melatonin is important for much more than insomnia. A study published in *Neuroendocrinology* in 2003 found that melatonin has an anti-estrogenic effect on estrogen-receptor-positive breast cancer cells. Further research released in the *Journal of the National Cancer Institute* found that nurses who worked rotating night shifts three nights per month for fifteen years had a higher incidence of colorectal cancer. Earlier studies had confirmed that night shift workers had higher rates of breast cancer, but the colorectal study found melatonin also had an anti-cancer effect on intestinal cancers.

Another study reported in *Gynecologic and Obstetric Investigation* showed a significant correlation between melatonin deficiency and endometrial cancer. Unlike cervical cancer, there is no screening method for endometrial cancer (besides an invasive endometrial biopsy), which is the most common pelvic cancer in women. In this study, they looked at 138 women. Sixty-eight women were diagnosed with endometrial cancer, and 70 with abnormal bleeding. The researchers compared the blood melatonin levels of each group and found that there was a six-fold lower difference in melatonin levels in those with endometrial cancer. The researchers believe that melatonin levels may be an indicator of endometrial cancer and declining levels of melatonin may be a risk factor for developing the disease.

Melatonin has also been evaluated as a treatment to maintain normal

blood pressure in those with diabetes. It also protects the stomach mucosa from
acute gastric lesions caused by stress. For those people having difficulty weaning
themselves off sleeping pills (benzodiazepines), melatonin has been used effectively to help withdraw from these drugs without side effects.

B12 and Melatonin

Those who cannot get to sleep at night may need vitamin B12. Studies show
that B12 causes an earlier release of melatonin at night, which resets the sleep-
wake cycle. B12 acts directly on the pineal gland to provoke a faster release of
melatonin. Research has also shown that B12 helps you get to sleep more easily,
and it sensitizes you to morning light, which helps you wake up feeling refreshed.

Melatonin is best taken as a sublingual tablet put under your tongue and
allowed to dissolve. Do not chew or swallow it. Every person is different in
regards to dosage. Melatonin comes in 1 mg and 3 mg sublingual tablets. Take
it along with 1,500 mcg of sublingual B12. The tablets are usually peppermint
or berry flavored.

Recommended dosage: Get into bed and put one 1 mg or 3 mg tablet along
with one 1,500 mcg B12 under your tongue. If you do not achieve restful sleep
the first night, then the following night use two tablets of melatonin along with
1,500 mcg of B12. Most women can start with 3 mg at bedtime and go up to 9
mg. Remember, melatonin is very safe. If you take too much, you may feel
groggy the next day, which means you should reduce your dose. Melatonin can
be taken long term because you do not become dependent on it nor does your
body reduce its own melatonin production.

Do Not be Afraid of the Dark

Night lights and street lights streaming through your bedroom window at night
have been found to inhibit melatonin production while sleeping. Purchase
light-inhibiting drapes for your windows, turn off those night lights, and close
your bedroom door at night to shut out the light and enhance your body's own
melatonin levels.

5-HTP for Insomnia and Anxiety

If you fall asleep easily but wake up several hours later and lie wide awake for
hours, only to crash back to sleep early in the morning, this is often a sign of
adrenal exhaustion. See page 108 for the nutrients necessary to support the
adrenals, but one additional nutrient that has the ability to quickly deal with
insomnia and anxiety is 5-HTP.

5-HTP (5-hydroxytryptophan) is a metabolite of the amino acid tryptophan. Proteins in the food you eat provide amino acids, including tryptophan. Tryptophan is broken down by vitamins, enzymes, and other co-factors into 5-HTP, and 5-HTP is then turned into serotonin.

5-HTP
- stops carbohydrate cravings
- enhances serotonin, your "feel good" hormone
- improves mild depression
- reduces PMS symptoms
- aids restful sleep
- helps prevent anxiety
- during the years around menopause, it improves reactions to stress
- provides fibromyalgia relief
- reduces panic attacks
- aids weight loss

A healthy liver is essential to proper conversion of tryptophan to 5-HTP and then serotonin. Serotonin is the neurotransmitter that tells your brain that you are satisfied and do not need to eat more. Serotonin deficiency contributes to weight gain, depression, sleeplessness, anxiety, inflammation, and joint pain, among other symptoms. Low serotonin levels also lead to carbohydrate cravings (sugar cravings) and overeating. 5-HTP reduces appetite while it enhances your mood, and increases your energy levels.

5-HTP has also been extensively researched for the treatment of depression, anxiety, and insomnia and other sleep disorders. 5-HTP allows for natural sleep, without the drugged feeling in the morning which can occur in those taking prescription sedatives. 5-HTP's natural relief for depression and related problems also comes without the side effects of pharmaceutical alternatives.

Weight loss is another benefit of taking 5-HTP. One small but well-controlled trial used 600 mg a day of 5-HTP in 20 obese individuals allowed to eat their usual diet for the first 6 weeks and a prescribed diet for the following 7 to 12 weeks. Researchers found a significant weight loss in the 5-HTP group but not in the control group taking a placebo.

Look for 5-HTP that is pure and enteric-coated. Enteric coating ensures the 5-HTP is absorbed in the small intestine. Non-enteric-coated 5-HTP can cause nausea when taken in optimal doses. It is also important to take 5-HTP without vitamin B6 in the same tablet because some women have Technicolor dreams when taking high doses of vitamin B6. When you take 5-HTP in the dose required for restful sleep and anxiety relief, you will be taking too much B6 if your 5-HTP has B6. 5-HTP is extracted from the herb Griffonia. Poor quality 5-HTP extracts can also cause nausea. Hence the reason we recommend pure 5-HTP that is enteric-coated.

5-HTP is very safe, but if you are taking MAO inhibitors, SSRIs (Prozac, Luvox, Paxil, Effexor, Zoloft) and/or the tricyclic anti-depressants (Elavil, Tofranil, Pamelor), do not take 5-HTP without discussing it with your health-care provider. 5-HTP is used to help wean people off of SSRIs and other anti-depressants, but this should be done under the guidance of a physician.

Recommended dosage: Start with 50 mg at breakfast, 50 mg at dinner, and 50 mg at bedtime. You can go as high as 200 mg three times a day, but start with the lower dosage as it is often very effective at aiding sleep and reducing anxiety. It can be taken with melatonin and vitamin B12 at bedtime if you have trouble falling asleep and staying asleep. 5-HTP provides relief within two weeks, and it can be taken long-term with no side effects. HappySense is the name of the brand we recommend.

End Urinary Tract Infections (UTI)

Urinary tract infections affect 80 percent of women at least once in their life-times. According to pharmacist Sherry Torkos in her book *The Benefits of Berries*, while the burning, frequency, and urgency of UTIs are not an exclusively female burden, women constitute the overwhelming majority of those affected. Half the women over age 65 experience at least one infection per year.

The vast majority of UTIs are caused by bacteria (the most common is E. coli), which are commonly found in the vagina and/or colon and rectal area and are introduced through the urethra (the tube that carries urine out of the body). Women are more susceptible to infection than men because their urethra is shorter and situated closer to the anus, making it easier to transfer the bacteria from fecal material to the urethra.

Conditions that can increase vulnerability to UTIs are blockages in the urethra (due to either past infections or structural abnormalities), stress, pregnancy, food allergies, sexual intercourse, oral contraceptive use, diaphragms, diabetes, a weakened immune system, and hormonal imbalances brought on by menopause (particularly a deficiency in estriol). Herpes virus is also a factor because during an active outbreak, it may be so painful to urinate that the bladder is not fully emptied, thus allowing for infection. Waiting too long to pee also increases the risk of an infection. Candida overgrowth is also a contributing factor. Women with recurring vaginal infections experience more UTIs.

Sexual intercourse is the most common cause of UTIs in women aged 20 to 40. During intercourse bacteria may be pushed from the rectal area into the urethra. Position yourself on top and urinate immediately after intercourse to reduce your risk of developing an infection.

Antibiotic therapy is the most common treatment. Bacterial resistance, candida yeast overgrowth, irritable bowel, and stomach upset are some of the few side effects from antibiotic treatment. Antibiotics inhibit the CP450 enzyme system in the liver, causing a shift in the balance between good estrogens and the bad, cancer-causing metabolites. Furthermore, if you have recurring UTIs, antibiotics become less effective. Today many doctors and researchers are recommending that natural treatments using cranberry and probiotics be used before antibiotics are prescribed, if no fever or pain is present.

Whole Cranberry NOT Juice

Cranberries are an effective treatment for UTIs. The proanthocyanidins, also called tannins, in cranberry, prevent the E. coli bacteria from sticking to the bladder wall and halt the infection. Several studies using Cran-Max, an extremely potent form of whole cranberry, proved that it provided relief for UTIs. It takes 34 pounds of cranberries to produce one pound of Cran-Max— all the vital parts, including the fruit, seeds, skin, and juice, are used. Most cranberry products only use dehydrated juice. A new study published in the *Canadian Journal of Urology* involved 150 women between 21 and 72 years of age. These women were followed for one year, and those given Cran-Max had a 44 percent lower incidence of UTIs than the group getting the placebo.

Probiotics, which are friendly bacteria, are essential not only for preventing and treating yeast infections and enhancing healthy gut bacteria but also for protection against UTIs. *Bifidobacterium longum* (a special strain called BB536), found in Probiotic Essentials, has been extensively researched for the last 30 years where it has been proven to prevent and treat candida yeast infections and replenish the good bacteria after use of antibiotics. It also supports the immune system, lowers cholesterol levels and has been shown to reduce E. coli infection and prevent diarrhea and constipation. Probiotic Essentials is a strain of probiotic that is shelf-stable, so it does not require refrigeration, and it has the highest counts of friendly, good bacteria found in these types of supplements. (See the Appendix for details on Probiotic Essentials.)

Health Tips to Halt UTIs

- Drink plenty of water throughout the day. It is the cheapest substance to reduce pain and burning due to UTIs.
- Enhance your immune system by taking your multivitamin with minerals every day.
- Eat plain, probiotic-rich yogurt daily.
- Urinate when your body tells you. Don't wait—this increases the likelihood of infection.
- Wear cotton underwear.
- Use Natracare unbleached panty liners, pads, and tampons instead of the bleached type commonly sold.
- Position yourself on top during intercourse to reduce the amount of bacteria being pushed into the urethra.
- Urinate immediately after intercourse.
- Do not use douches.
- Do not use lubricants with harmful preservatives, parabens, or alcohols (see more on lubricants on page 208).

Additional Bioidentical Hormone Cream Recommendations

Use vaginal estriol, low-dose, short-term if recurring UTIs are due to estrogen deficiency. The recommended dosage for intra-vaginal estriol is 0.5 mg to 1 mg once daily for three weeks, with 0.5 mg to 1 mg once weekly for six months. Upon elimination of UTIs, you can discontinue use of estriol or use it 0.5 mg to 1 mg once every other week for another six months.

A Simple Operation Prevents Incontinence

Four extra stitches can help prevent a lifetime of bladder problems in women. Dr. Linda Brubker of Loyola University published a study in the *New England Journal of Medicine* (April 13, 2006), showing that a simple technique could solve years of problems in those having surgery for uterine prolapse, a painful condition that occurs when the uterus weakens and sags into the birth canal.

Frequent childbirth increases the chances of this happening. Hundreds of thousands of women in North America have repair surgery or many more have a hysterectomy to solve the problem of prolapse uterus. The operation can often lead to bladder problems, especially leakage. This study revealed that simply adding four permanent stitches, two on either side, from the vagina to the pelvic ligament to form a hammock, keeps the urinary control muscle stable. If you are having surgery, ask your surgeon to do this simple step. It can solve years of bladder leakage problems.

Restore Hormone Balance at Menopause

Menopause means one year with no menstrual period. The average age of menopause for North American women is around age 52, but some women go through natural menopause at age 35 and others at age 60. Menopause can also occur abruptly when a woman's ovaries and uterus are surgically removed during a hysterectomy. Other women may experience chemically induced menopause due to certain drug treatments. All these triggers for menopause can create similar symptoms. Do all women experience menopausal symptoms? No! Many women sail through menopause with no symptoms or just minor symptoms but, for those who do not, there are many solutions.

During natural menopause, the ovaries slow down their production of estrogens, and the adrenal glands must compensate by producing the precursor hormones DHEA and androstenedione, which can be converted to estrogen. If the adrenals are exhausted, symptoms of estrogen deficiency will appear. If you are not sure of the state of your adrenals, go to page 39 and complete the questionnaire, and then see page 228 for specific information on how to support the adrenals. Remember: healthy adrenals are the key to an effortless menopause.

Restoring hormone balance can be challenging for about 20 percent of women. It can be complicated to treat menopausal hormone problems even when blood and saliva testing is carefully evaluated and a detailed symptom questionnaire and history are assessed. It is not as simple as having a saliva test performed, discovering you are low in estrogen, and then supplementing estrogen. Although some women do very well with this approach, others will experience a myriad of new symptoms. That is why it is important to work with a healthcare professional to monitor your treatment so changes can be made to ensure you achieve vibrant health.

No one should feel tired, worn down, brain-fogged, or lacking vitality. Our goal is to have you feeling fantastic. And you should feel fabulous: you have no more periods to worry about and no more concerns about potential pregnancy. Menopause should be all about you. This is a time when you can focus on yourself. Eat right, exercise, and start new hobbies and activities that you did not have time for when your children were young or your career was in full swing.

Menopause symptoms such as hot flashes, night sweats, insomnia, and anxiety can be treated successfully with herbs and nutrients, exercise, and diet changes. Some women will experience complete relief with this approach while others may need low-dose, short-term bioidentical hormone treatment.

The herbs we recommend have been used for hundreds of years in traditional herbal medicine. They are extremely safe, well-tolerated, and, in comparison to synthetic estrogen replacement therapy, fairly inexpensive. You will note that several of the herbs should be taken in combination for more effective, faster relief of hot flashes, night sweats, mood swings, insomnia, and anxiety.

If you are currently using synthetic HRT and want to wean yourself off this medication, see page 144 for the guidelines for symptom-free withdrawal.

BLACK COHOSH (Cimicifuga racemosa)

Black cohosh is the most thoroughly studied herb in the treatment of menopausal symptoms and other female hormone imbalances, including amenorrhea, dysmenorrhea, sterility, threatened abortion, and severe after-birth pains. It has been found to enhance milk production. New research has found that black cohosh may also affect serotonin receptors, enhancing mood. Its effectiveness is due to the action of key compounds (isoflavones and triterpenes) on a number of the regulatory centers in the body, such as the hypothalamus and pituitary.

Black cohosh is thought to inhibit the pituitary release of luteinizing hormone (LH). Surges of LH are responsible for hot flashes. LH rises and dramatically increases until approximately three years after menopause, and levels often do not decline for two to three decades after menopause. In menopausal women, follicle-stimulating hormone (FSH) also elevates, peaking around two to three years after the cessation of monthly periods. Again, a decrease in FSH is not seen in many women until 20 to 30 years after menopause. Persistently high serum FSH-to-LH is used by many doctors to determine menopause status (see page 42 for why this is not a very good indicator). When FSH and LH surge, estradiol levels drop. Black cohosh inhibits LH without affecting follicle-stimulating hormone (FSH). FSH is responsible for stimulating estrogen, so maintaining normal FSH function is a good thing.

Furthermore, prolactin levels increase at menopause. Excess prolactin can, among other symptoms, trigger menstrual abnormalities (such as erratic periods of longer duration), male facial hair growth, and acne.

Black cohosh has been found to be very effective in the treatment of the following symptoms: hot flashes, profuse perspiration, headaches, heart palpitations, depression, PMS, dysmenorrhea (painful menstruation), sleep disturbances, vaginal atrophy or dryness, nervousness and irritability, and loss of concentration. A decline in symptoms usually starts within four to eight weeks. In all black cohosh research, the optimal reduction in hot flashes occurred by 12 weeks. For this reason, we recommend you take black cohosh with other herbs to maximize relief. Many women who have tried black cohosh did not take it long enough or at an optimal dosage to see results.

Safety Research Supports Black Cohosh

The German equivalent of the U.S. Food and Drug Administration and Health Canada list no contraindications or limitations for use of this herb in cancer patients where estrogen is contraindicated, such as breast cancer. Black cohosh is extremely well tolerated.

Several studies have focused on women with estrogen-receptor-positive breast cancer who were taking tamoxifen (an estrogen-blocking drug). These women were given double the dose of black cohosh for one year with excellent safety results and effectiveness in the reduction of menopause symptoms.

Research published in the *International Journal of Oncology* in 2003 finally put to rest the myth that black cohosh is estrogenic. Researchers stated black cohosh does *not* have estrogenic activity and does *not* promote breast cancer cell growth. If you hear otherwise, the person telling you this information has not read the latest research.

Over the last few years there has been outstanding research on black cohosh's safety and effectiveness. Unfortunately, pharmacists and medical doctors continue to provide out-dated information regarding this herb. Dr. Pettle and I continue to get questions regarding black cohosh's effect on the liver and whether it is estrogenic or not. A review of the safety and toxicity data published in 2005 in *Treatment Endocrinology* (and compiled at the Department of Pharmacy Practice, Center for Botanical Dietary Supplements Research, Program for Collaborative Research in the Pharmaceutical Sciences, College of Pharmacy, University of Illinois, Chicago) states:

> Since the publication of the results of the WHI that described the risks of hormone replacement therapy, many women are actively

seeking alternative treatments for post-menopausal symptoms. Black cohosh (*Cimicifuga racemosa*) is one such alternative that has been used in the U.S. for over 100 years. Review of the published clinical data suggests that *cimicifuga* may be useful for the treatment of menopausal symptoms, such as hot flashes, profuse sweating, insomnia, and anxiety… A few cases of hepatotoxicity have been reported, but a direct association with the ingestion of *cimicifuga* has not been demonstrated. The most recent data suggest that *cimicifuga* is not estrogenic.

When researchers looked at the cases of liver toxicity noted above, they found the women were taking NSAIDS, drinking alcohol, or had other liver-affecting conditions that created the liver enzyme elevation and therefore toxicity was not attributed to black cohosh.

Maturitas is one of the most respected medical journals, and in July 2006 an excellent article was published about what doctors should be prescribing for menopausal symptoms. The authors say,

Black cohosh appears to be one of the most effective botanicals for relief of vasomotor symptoms, while St. John's wort can improve mood disorders related to the menopausal transition. Many other botanicals have limited evidence to demonstrate safety and efficacy for relief of symptoms related to menopause. A growing body of evidence suggests that some botanicals and dietary supplements could result in improved clinical outcomes. Health care providers should discuss these issues with their patients, so they can assist them in managing these alternative therapies through an evidence-based approach.

Recommended dosage: 80 mg at breakfast and 80 mg at bedtime. Or simply take MenoSense, 2 capsules at breakfast and 2 at bedtime.

MenoSense contains black cohosh, dong quai, vitex, gamma oryzanol, and hesperidin in the doses recommended. MenoSense is readily available at all North American health food stores.

DONG QUAI (Angelica sinensis)

Dong quai has been used for centuries in other cultures as a blood builder or tonic. In traditional Chinese medicine, blood tonics are used to promote healthy reproductive function. Because blood tonics build the blood, they indirectly strengthen the heart energy complex, which controls the blood and houses the spirit. In traditional Chinese medicine, insomnia indicates an imbalance in the heart energy complex, and dong quai can be helpful in this case.

In menopausal women, this herb is particularly useful for promoting vaginal health and for easing hot flashes. In menstruating women, dong quai has proven its worth in treating infertility and painful periods. Scientific investigation has shown that dong quai has both a balancing effect on estrogen activity and a tonic effect on the uterus. Furthermore, one of the active ingredients in dong quai stimulates the corpus luteum in the ovary to secrete progesterone, so this herb has a progesterone action as well.

As the Asian herbal tradition suggests, dong quai has beneficial effects on the cardiovascular system, such as decreasing blood pressure and preventing atherosclerotic plaque formation. Dong quai has potent anti-tumor effects. It is also a very effective immune system regulator. It should be used in combination with other herbs.

Recommended dosage: 200 mg at breakfast and 200 mg at bedtime. Or simply take MenoSense, 2 capsules at breakfast and 2 at bedtime.

VITEX

Vitex, also called chaste tree berry, was discussed earlier (see page 91) and is a progesterone-enhancing herb. It contains no hormones, has no direct hormonal activity, and is not estrogenic. Its main active ingredients are aucubine and agnusides, which work on the pituitary gland to stimulate the production of luteinizing hormone (LH), which in turn increases progesterone. The LH increases the level of progesterone (as in the luteal phase of the menstrual cycle), thereby shifting the ratio of estrogen-to-progesterone in favor of progesterone. The increase in progesterone created by Vitex is thus achieved indirectly; the plant does not have direct hormonal action.

Most importantly for menopausal women, Vitex inhibits excessive production of prolactin, which causes male facial hair growth. Excess prolactin is also found in polycystic ovary syndrome, and in women who are infertile. Prolactin levels have also been found to be elevated in women with low thyroid.

Recommended dosage: 160 mg at breakfast and 160 mg at bedtime daily. Or simply take MenoSense, 2 capsules at breakfast and 2 at bedtime.

HESPERIDIN

Hesperidin, like many other flavonoids, improves vascular integrity, lessening excessive capillary permeability, which is a primary factor in hot flashes. Hot flashes are associated with vasodilation of the capillaries. When combined with vitamin C, it was found that hot flashes were relieved in 53 percent of patients and reduced in 34 percent of those treated. Leg cramps, nosebleeds, and easy bruising also declined.

Recommended dosage: 150 mg at breakfast and 150 mg at bedtime daily. Or simply take MenoSense, 2 capsules at breakfast and 2 at bedtime. Additionally take with at least 1,000 mg vitamin C.

GAMMA-ORYZANOL (ferulic acid)

Gamma-oryzanol is found in grains and is isolated from rice bran oil. It is effective in alleviating menopausal symptoms, including hot flashes. Gamma-oryzanol also lowers elevated triglyceride and cholesterol levels.

Recommended dosage: 150 mg with breakfast and 150 mg at bedtime daily. Or simply take MenoSense, 2 capsules at breakfast and 2 at bedtime.

SAGE (Salvia officinalis)

Garden sage is very effective for treating menopause symptoms, particularly night sweats and hot flashes. It is tranquilizing and acts as an excellent anxiety remedy. Garden sage also has strong antioxidant properties and improves digestion and assimilation. When digestion is improved, symptoms and illnesses improve.

Recommended dosage: Drink sage tea throughout the day instead of coffee. For excessive sweating, let tea steep until it is strong.

You will note that we have not included estrogenic herbs like red clover or soy isoflavones. The research is contradictory on these two supplements. At the time of publication, red clover had not been subjected to enough research. Soy studies have been conflicting, with one study showing positive protective effects on breast cancer and others showing breast cancer proliferation. One of the reasons for this is the type of soy used in the studies compared to the type of soy eaten in Asian cultures. We do not recommend soy unless it is fermented. Asian diets do not contain the regular GMO soy that is found in North America nor do they contain soy beans or soy milk. Fermented soy is a completely different food than regular soy. Read more about fermented soy and its healing benefits on page 158.

Case Study: Hot Flash Hell

Margaret's hot flashes were so bad she said that when she is buried, the gravestone will read "Died from hot flashes—Stay back! Fire below!" and her gravesite will be steaming. Margaret was 56 years old and about 30 pounds overweight. Her periods had stopped four years before she came to see Dr. Pettle, and she had been battling symptoms since. Dr. Pettle took a full case history and ordered thyroid tests and saliva hormone testing. Margaret had hot flashes and night sweats that were severe—up to 20 a day and as many at night. Margaret had not slept in weeks due to the night sweats, and she had developed severe memory problems and urinary incontinence. One of her daughters had moved back home due to divorce and brought her three children with her. Margaret's job as an accountant was full of deadlines, and she was exhausted. She is also allergic to peanuts. Her saliva hormone test results were as follows:

estradiol	1.0 pg/ml	low
progesterone	45 pg/ml	normal
testosterone	2.8 pg/ml	low
cortisol AM	18 ng/ml	high
DHEAS	3.5 ng/ml	low
thyroid	TSH 6.0	low

Margaret has low thyroid and low estrogen, which cause her severe hot flashes, night sweats, incontinence, and memory problems.

Although her progesterone is normal for post-menopause, progesterone is a precursor to both testosterone and estradiol and both are low, so compounded, micronized progesterone, 100 mg at bedtime every night, was prescribed to help balance all hormones and help her sleep. Oral progesterone causes sleepiness, hence the reason for taking it at bedtime. Margaret was also prescribed MenoSense, two capsules at breakfast and two at bedtime.

She was advised to reduce the stress in her life and help her daughter find a new place to live. High cortisol in the long term can burn out the adrenal glands, creating more hormone imbalance, so stress reduction is paramount. Daily weight-bearing exercise of 10 minutes will help increase testosterone and decrease cortisol. Margaret also had to eat an exceptionally healthy diet with protein at every meal and take a good multivitamin with minerals. Vaginal estriol of 0.5 mg once daily for three weeks, with 0.5 mg weekly for six months, was prescribed to clear up the incontinence. Margaret was also prescribed thyroid hormone and will be monitored until the correct dosage is achieved. Low thyroid is common in those with high cortisol as the adrenals and thyroid are directly linked (see page 7). Once optimal thyroid hormone levels are achieved, Margaret will have an easy time losing the weight.

Anti-Depressants Are Not for Hot Flashes

Without synthetic HRT to prescribe, some physicians are now writing scripts for anti-depressant medications to ease menopausal symptoms. In Canada, the Canadian Medical Association Journal is questioning the dramatic increase in these prescriptions since the WHI estrogen-and-progestin study was halted. See the following graph showing the spike. This spike has been seen in the U.S. as well. Are doctors now treating menopause as a psychiatric disorder? Maybe or maybe not, but physicians are opening another Pandora's Box of side effects with this approach.

According to several studies, including a landmark Canadian study, certain kinds of anti-depressants can double the risk of developing breast cancer. These drugs include paroxetine (sold under the brand name Paxil), amoxapine (Asendin), clomipramine (Anafranil), desipramine (Norpramin), and trimipramine (Surmontil and Rhotrimine). It is one thing to take anti-depressant medication when you are medically depressed, but another to use it to treat hot flashes and night sweats. Other side effects from anti-depressant medication include sexual dysfunction; a 7 to 10 lb (3 to 4 kg) weight gain; increased sweating, particularly at night; sleep disturbances; and urinary problems. Some women report 20 to 30 lb (8 to 12 kg) weight gains in a very short period after starting anti-depressant medication.

Strangely enough, these side effects are also some of the symptoms of menopause that women are seeking relief from. Do not trade your menopause symptoms for anti-depressant side effects. Read about 5-HTP (see page 120) and St. John's wort (see page 135) before filling that prescription. It can be more challenging to get off anti-depressants than it is to stop synthetic HRT. There is not one reason why women should take synthetic HRT or anti-depressant medication to treat hot flashes and night sweats when there are so many effective natural options that promote vibrant health.

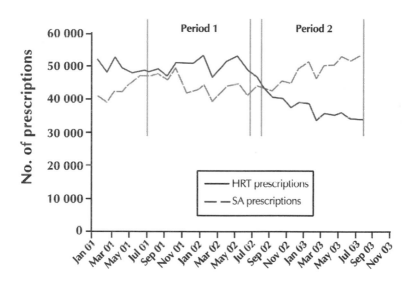

Total estimated prescriptions dispensed in Ontario for hormone replacement therapy (HRT: oral and transdermal estrogen monotherapy and estrogen-progesterone combination therapy) and serotonergic anti-depressants (SAs: citalopram, fluoxetine, sertraline, fluvoxamine, paroxetine, venlafaxine, nefazadone and trazadone) to women 45-65 years old, from January 2001 to June 2003. Source: McIntyre, R. S. et al. CMAJ 2005;172:57-59

Case Study: Thinning, Dry Vagina

Sarah is 62, active, beautiful, and fit. She sailed through the menopause transition with minimal hot flashes and night sweats. Sarah takes EstroSense, two capsules every day, to help reduce her risk of breast cancer. She wanted to "do" menopause naturally with no hormones. She has been suffering with extreme vaginal dryness, bleeding during intercourse caused by thinning of the vagina, and urinary leakage when she exercises, which she never had before. Sarah eats very well and supplements her diet with vitamins and minerals and fatty acids, along with bone nutrients. Her saliva hormone test revealed the following:

estradiol pg/ml	1.2 pg/ml	low
progesterone pg/ml	68 pg/ml	normal
testosterone pg/ml	26 pg/ml	normal

Based on Sarah's symptoms and her saliva hormone test, she is low in estrogen. Vaginal estriol of 0.5 mg morning and night every day for three weeks, with 0.5 mg morning and night once weekly for six months, should clear up the vaginal dryness, atrophy, and incontinence. Sarah is worried about the effects of estrogen, but, as we discussed in Chapter 4, vaginal estriol at this dose has not been shown to increase or thicken the uterine lining nor is it dealt with by the liver. The dosage recommended is also low and for the short term. Since Sarah is taking EstroSense along with her estriol, this ensures the healthy detoxification of estrogen from her body and protects her breasts, cervix, and ovaries.

Sarah should also use a vaginal lubricant like LOVE, which contains no parabens, alcohols, or any substance that would interfere with the estriol (see page 208 for more information). Lubricants are used during intercourse but also throughout the day to ensure adequate lubrication. LOVE will not stain panties nor leave any residue. It is identical to the body's lubrication and available at health food stores. Do not use lubricants containing parabens, dangerous preservatives, or alcohols.

Lift Depression

Depression is a very real condition during the peri-menopause to menopause transition. In this section we would like to highlight St. John's wort as it has excellent research for the treatment of depression when used with black cohosh.

ST. JOHN'S WORT (HYPERICUM PERFORATUM)

St. John's wort is one of the most popular and well-researched herbal remedies for mild to moderate depression. It is also used to relieve anxiety and to treat sleep disturbances. St. John's wort also relieves menstrual cramps, PMS, and menopausal symptoms; promotes wound healing; and enhances the immune system to fight viral infections. In numerous studies, St. John's wort has been effective in reducing symptoms of depression in those with mild to moderate but not severe depression. When compared with tricyclic anti-depressants, including imipramine, amitriptyline, doxepin, desipramine, and nortriptyline, St. John's wort is equally effective and has fewer side effects. Research has also shown this to be true for anti-depressants known as selective serotonin reuptake inhibitors (SSRIs), including fluoxetine and sertraline.

St. John's wort and black cohosh are the solution for many women suffering with low mood or low to moderate depression at menopause. In a study published in *Advances in Therapy* in 1999, 111 women were given St. John's wort at a dose of 900 mg daily for twelve weeks. The women were between 43 and 65 years old and had peri-menopausal symptoms. The incidence and severity of typical psychological symptoms were recorded at the beginning and after 5, 8, and 12 weeks of treatment. Dramatic improvement in psychological symptoms was observed in 79 percent of the women treated with St. John's wort. Peri- and post-menopausal symptoms were reduced dramatically or disappeared altogether in 76 percent of participants. Most importantly, sexual desire also improved after treatment with St. John's wort extract.

Another study published in *Obstetrics and Gynecology* in 2006 looked at the combination of black cohosh and St. John's wort. In this double-blind, randomized, placebo-control study, 301 women experiencing hot flashes, night sweats, and other post-menopausal complaints with psychological symptoms were treated with St. John's wort extract and black cohosh for 16 weeks. The combination of black cohosh and St. John's wort was found to be far superior to a placebo in alleviating climacteric complaints, including the related psychological component.

Prolonged high-dose (over 1,800 mg per day) consumption of St John's wort may cause the skin to become photosensitive to the sun, especially in individuals who are already sensitive to sunlight. Therefore, persons taking high doses of St. John's wort should avoid excessive exposure to sunlight, tanning lights, or UV sources.

Because of its MAO-inhibition type of activity, it may decrease the effects of other MAOIs (Monoamine oxidase inhibitors). Secondly, St. John's Wort may cause serotonin syndrome (a rare condition that occurs when you combine drugs that enhance serotonin with herbs or nutrients that naturally increase serotonin). These drugs include: selective serotonin reuptake inhibitors (SSRI) and tricyclic anti-depressants.

Recommended dosage: 300 mg 3 times daily with food. Do not exceed the recommended daily dose. Look for St. John's wort that is standardized to 0.3 percent hypericin. Women with mild to moderate depression and menopausal symptoms should take 2 MenoSense at breakfast and 2 MenoSense at bedtime along with 300 mg of St. John's wort 3 times a day.

Boost a Low Libido

We explained earlier that the brain is the master conductor of your hormones. The pituitary is directed by the hypothalamus to secrete sexy hormones. The front part of the pituitary secretes LH and FSH, which control ovulation and the production of estrogen and progesterone. The pituitary also produces prolactin, the hormone that not only stimulates lactation but also interacts with thyroid, cortisol, and DHEA hormones, to name a few. Excessive prolactin levels cause a decline in testosterone, a decrease in libido, and are associated with sexual dysfunction. High prolactin also decreases the action of DHEA on DHEA receptors, and low levels of DHEA are associated with a decline in libido. Low thyroid also causes excessive prolactin secretion. This is one reason why low sex drive or no sex drive is a side effect of low thyroid.

When prolactin levels get higher, the number of days between periods shortens and then periods become irregular in length. Prolactin increases during the menopausal years, which is another reason why as some women age, they lose their desire for sex.

The brain's neurotransmitters dopamine, norepinephrine, and serotonin also affect sexual function. Dopamine levels drop as women age, and some of the decline in sexual function is a result of aging. Levels of the brain's dopamine play an indirect role in stimulating the production of testosterone because it inhibits testosterone-suppressing prolactin. Dopamine inhibits prolactin so when dopamine is suppressed, prolactin goes up and testosterone drops. It is amazing any of us have a sex drive with all these hormones interacting with one another.

Drugs and Libido

In addition to the hormone havoc brought on by synthetic hormones, sexual health, in particular desire, can be affected by many medications.

Drug manufacturers should be cognizant of the quality of a patient's sex life when developing new medications. The list of drugs that adversely affect sexual functioning is enormous. If you had a healthy sex drive, and it has declined since starting a new drug, low libido could be a side effect. Your medicine cabinet could be the culprit.

Many drugs interfere with one or all phases of sexual response: desire, excitement and climax. Pain relievers can stop orgasm; sedatives reduce libido; anti-anxiety or anti-depressants delay orgasm; blood pressure medications cause vaginal dryness and inhibit orgasm. Alcohol, not thought of as a drug, causes delayed orgasm. All of these drugs decrease desire.

Birth control pills inhibit testosterone and disrupt sex-hormone-binding globulin. As we mentioned earlier the Pill can kill your sex drive and it may not return. See page xx-xxi for more information.

The following drugs predominantly decrease desire and inhibit orgasm in women.

High blood pressure medications (antihypertensives)	Reserpine, Methyldopa, Propanolol, RAldactone, Timolol, Clonidine
Depression medications	Anti-depressants, Prozac, Wellbutrin, Imipramine, Paxil, Zoloft
Anti-anxiety medications	Xanax, Valium, Compazine, Fluphenazine, Lithium
Over-the-counter medications	Tagamet, Benadryl, Zantac, Codeine, Nizoral (treats yeast infections)
Prescription hormones	Ethinyl estradiol (birth control pill)

Many of the natural herbs and nutrients we recommend for low libido and sexual difficulties have an effect on the hypothalamus, the pituitary, and the neurotransmitters and hormones secreted by these glands. We chose these ingredients because of their safety and effectiveness. You may ask why we are not just recommending testosterone. That is because not all sexual difficulties are related to a deficiency in testosterone. Also, many people do not want to take a hormone and prefer to use a natural remedy that gets to the root of the imbalance.

There is a tremendous sexist bias in the area of female sexual health research. As a result many of the herbs, nutrients and amino acids we recommend are not researched for their effects in women's bodies even though they have an effect on key systems that are involved in sexual desire, frequency and intensity of orgasm, vaginal lubrication, personal enjoyment, and emotional satisfaction.

Despite knowing that 48 percent of North American women have no sex drive, investigators have totally ignored research in this area. We feel this is appalling. Combining the fact that women have no sex drive with men using the "little blue pill" in record numbers is a recipe for relationship disaster. We have personally had great success with the following supplements when it comes to reviving women's sex drives. Remember: a nutrient will not repair a poor relationship—in other words, you still have to like your partner.

L-ARGININE

Arginine is an essential amino acid. ("Essential" means your body cannot make it, and in this case, you have to obtain it from foods like meat, chicken, turkey, other fowl, nuts, and dairy products.) In supplement form, it is known as "L-arginine." In women, L-arginine increases staying power. Both men and women report that L-arginine increases their libido (desire for sex).

L-arginine is the main source of the primary molecule nitric oxide (NO), which is responsible for sexual arousal in women. Your body's NO plays a role in keeping your blood pressure normal; regulates immune function; kills cancer cells and microorganisms; and helps control muscle activity, balance, and coordination. Dietary arginine is the primary source of NO. Without arginine, there is no NO and no sexual arousal. In research on women, L-arginine in supplement form has been reported to increase the intensity of sensation during sex. That is because NO stimulates blood flow to the genitals to lead up to orgasm.

Female rat studies show that NO release initiates a chain of events that begins with the release of luteinizing hormone (LH). When this hormone is secreted by the female rat, male rats are attracted. In other rat studies, the female rats were deprived of L-arginine. This deprivation of L-arginine resulted in slow sexual development and less sexual activity. In women we know that L-arginine enhances NO and promotes the secretion of LH, thereby increasing testosterone and the desire for sex. Some researchers believe that L-arginine, with its cascade of hormone events, causes secretion of pheromones that make women more attractive to men.

Recommended dosage: Women can take 1,000 mg of L-arginine per day with meals. (If you have herpes, L-arginine may cause an outbreak in some people.) We find that women need to take prosexual nutrients such as Sex Essentials every day to improve sexual pleasure. Women should take 3 capsules per day with food.

> Sex Essentials contains a combination of L-arginine, Tribulus terrestris, Ginkgo biloba, eurycoma longifolia, choline bitartrate, and pantothenic acid (vitamin B5).

TRIBULUS TERRESTRIS

Tribulus terrestris, also known as the puncture vine, has been used as a prosexual herb for thousands of years. Its active ingredient is protodioscin. The Chinese used it as a cure for impotence. Tribulus terrestris works as an adaptogen, which means it has a general effect of bringing a variety of hormones and other biochemicals into balance. Tribulus terrestris raises testosterone levels when they are low. There also appears to be no downside to taking Tribulus terrestris. Based on long-term studies, you can take it continuously for years without any negative effects on hormone balance and, in addition to improving your sex drive, it will also improve your overall health.

Tribulus terrestris works in a special way. You learned about luteinizing hormone (LH) in Chapter 2. One of luteinizing hormone's many functions is to command the production of testosterone. As you age, follicle stimulating hormone (FSH) increases in huge amounts, peaking a few years after menopause and staying high for several decades thereafter. The ratio of FSH to luteinizing hormone increases, and LH does not have the same ability to increase testosterone. Tribulus terrestris helps to naturally boost the levels of luteinizing hormone to FSH, which then helps produce more testosterone. Tribulus terrestris is both a libido enhancer (and has been proven in multiple clinical trials in this regard) and has an ability to increase testosterone.

Clinical trials using Tribulus terrestris were performed at the First Obstetrical and Gynecological Hospital in Sofia, Bulgaria, on 150 women with abnormal ovulation associated with hormone imbalances (dysovulatory syndrome). Those with fertility problems and peri-menopausal and menopausal symptoms were included in one group. Women who had had a complete hysterectomy were included in a separate group. All the women were given Tribulus terrestris with a high percentage of the active ingredient protodioscin. They compared these two groups to another group of women that received estrogens and testosterone only, with no Tribulus terrestris.

The results of the study showed:
- normalization of ovulation (24 of 36 women in one group had normalized ovulation)
- improved fertility
- a reduction in peri-menopausal and post-menopausal symptoms (complete or almost complete disappearance of hot flashes, missing sex drive, sweats, insomnia in 49 of 50 treated women)
- a longer menstrual cycle (which is known to protect women from the effects of excess estrogen)

Tribulus terrestris was also compared to a group receiving a combination of estrogen and testosterone. Tribulus terrestris was found to provide better results in women in regards to increasing libido than the hormone therapy alone. The estrogen/testosterone therapy has the adverse effect of weight gain and male facial hair growth, whereas taking Tribulus terrestris does not. In addition, one in-vitro study performed in Shanghai (published in Chinese) found that Tribulus terrestris inhibited breast cancer cell lines.

Recommended dosage: Take 150 mg per day. Or keep it simple and take Sex Essentials, 3 capsules per day with food.

GINKGO BILOBA

Ginkgo biloba has been used in several clinical trials in women with low libido. One trial found that women on anti-depressant medications, which can cause sexual dysfunction (including low libido), had their libido improve and orgasms return. Another study, published in *Advances in Therapy* in 2000, found that study participants using a combination of Ginkgo biloba and Muira puama (another herb) reported having significant increases in sexual desire, had intercourse more often, had more sexual fantasies, and were able to reach orgasm.

Other research studies have shown Ginkgo biloba to be a major aid in improving blood flow to small blood vessels. Enhancing blood flow to the genitals heightens sexual sensations. Research has also shown that Ginkgo biloba significantly increases mental acuity and memory—and sexual desire starts in the brain. Look for Ginkgo biloba extract that is standardized to 24 percent ginkgo flavonglycosides and six percent Terpene lactones.

Recommended dosage: 150 mg per day. Or keep it simple and take Sex Essentials, 3 capsules daily with food.

EURYCOMA LONGIFOLIA (The "Blue Pill" for women)

Eurycoma longifolia, also known as Malaysian Ginseng, is the missing ingredient in helping women's libido. This potent herb brings the zest back in your sex life and aids vaginal dryness. Published research has been performed in male mice and men. We have yet to see a published research study in women or in female mice. The Malaysian government is currently investigating the traditional use of Eurycoma longifolia for libido enhancement in women.

Testimonials from women using Eurycoma longifolia have reported that they are finally having orgasms again, and that the orgasms they are having are longer and more intense. Women have reported to us that they are waking up in the middle of the night with strong orgasms. The combination of Eurycoma longifolia, L-arginine, vitamin B5, choline, and Gingko biloba has been on the market in Canada and the U.S. for over two years. Women have sent letters and emails telling us that this combination has changed their sex lives. It has them thinking about sex again. The added benefit of increased vaginal lubrication has them more comfortable while they are doing it as well.

Recommended dosage: 150 mg per day, with food. Or keep it simple and take Sex Essentials, 3 capsules daily with food.

CHOLINE BITARTRATE

For women, the neurotransmitter called acetylcholine (ACh), which sends sexual messages to the nerves, is also a very important part of sexual function. Too little ACh and sexual activity goes down; increase ACh levels and sexual activity goes up. ACh is involved in the build-up toward orgasm and the urethral and vaginal contractions that occur during orgasm, as well as the subjective perception of orgasm intensity and duration. Female rat studies have shown that when ACh is increased, female rats seek out male rats and are receptive to them.

Choline bitartrate, along with pantothenic acid (vitamin B5), helps to enhance acetylcholine, thereby enhancing orgasm.

Recommended dosage: 75 mg per day, with food. Or keep it simple and take Sex Essentials, 3 capsules daily with food.

PANTOTHENIC ACID

Pantothenic acid, also known as vitamin B5, is part of the B group of vitamins. Along with choline bitartrate, pantothenic acid enhances acetylcholine, the neurotransmitter that sends sexual messages to the nerves. Secondly, vitamin B5 is involved in the Krebs cycle, which is responsible for the energy supply for all living cells. Vitamin B5 increases endurance, so you will have better staying power.

Recommended dosage: 75 mg per day, or keep it simple and take Sex Essentials, 3 capsules daily with food.

Case Study: No Sex Drive

Angie is 45 years old and peri-menopausal. She has been using over-the-counter progesterone daily for the last two years. She did not tell her doctor and has never been tested to ensure her hormones are not becoming unbalanced due to the progesterone she is using. Over the last year Angie's sex drive has disappeared. She misses the intimacy with her husband, and she is afraid he is getting frustrated enough to leave her. She cannot understand what is happening because she still desires her husband, but she cannot get excited or lubricated. Angie also reported that even if she does proceed despite the lack of desire, she cannot have an orgasm. This is a very common problem among women today. Angie's problem can be understood from her saliva hormone test results, which were taken on day 20 of her normal menstrual cycle.

estradiol	4.5 pg/ml	normal
progesterone	19,000 pg/ml	high
testosterone	26 pg/ml	normal

A normal progesterone range for a peri-menopausal woman with regular periods is between 25 and 250 pg/ml. Angie's over-the-counter progesterone, taken daily with no break, has caused her to become progesterone-dominant. Side effects of this condition include having no sex drive and an inability to achieve orgasm. Upon discussion with Angie, we found she had stopped measuring the dose, which was supposed to be 1/4 teaspoon morning and night. She was just dipping her finger in the cream and applying what was approximately 10 times the prescribed amount. Even though her testosterone levels were normal, the extremely high progesterone was reducing her sex drive. This is a case where if there was no saliva hormone testing, her physician may just have prescribed testosterone, which would not have solved the problem.

Angie started to measure the progesterone cream and use it every other day, stopping from day 1 to day 14 of her cycle. Within a few months, her progesterone levels normalized and her sex drive was restored. Angie also took Sex Essentials, 3 capsules per day with food, to enhance her sex drive naturally.

Maca for Mice and Men

Maca is a traditional food, formerly grown almost exclusively in the cold climate of the Andes with poor soil. It was so valuable as a food source that it was traded as currency. Today it is also grown outside the Andes, but it may have very different constituents when grown in warm climates. Traditional maca contains about 60 percent carbohydrates, 10 percent protein, and 8 percent fiber. It also contains a variety of minerals, fatty acids, and polysaccharides. Researchers have concluded that a whole food is very different from an extract of that food, or when an isolated, active ingredient is selected. The food in its whole form may have very different action standardized in the body than the sum of its parts. This has been found to be true with maca.

Maca has been researched in men in small trials, where it has been shown to enhance sperm quality and motility as well as libido. The majority of the research, however, has been performed on mice and rats. No research has been performed to date on women, although there are a multitude of claims for everything from fertility enhancement and menopausal symptom relief to breast enhancement. Let us look at the animal studies where maca has been evaluated in ovariectomized mice or rats (i.e., their ovaries have been removed).

Research published in *Reproductive Biology and Endocrinology* in 2005 looked at the effects of maca on several fertility parameters of female mice of reproductive age. There was an improvement in all fertility parameters studied. This study showed the uterus was increased in size, which occurs when estrogen is increased—not a good thing for women with uterine fibroids, endometriosis, or a thick uterine lining. The scientists believe the increase in uterine size is why maca may have been used by traditional healers to increase fertility. Many studies use ovariectomized rats or mice because these animals have low to no estrogen present, so they are a good study for how foods, herbs, or drugs may affect estrogen levels. This study suggests an increase in estrogen affecting the uterus.

One study in *Cell Biology and Toxicology* in 2006 looked at rat hepatocytes (liver cells) and human breast cancer MCF-7 cells. These researchers found that maca extracts exhibit estrogenic activity. A study published in the *Journal of Ethnopharmacology* in 2006 looked at maca in post-menopausal osteoporosis in ovariectomized rats. The scientists found that maca was effective in the prevention of estrogen-deficient bone loss. Maca has not been researched in women and, at the time of publication, we would only recommend maca for men and mice, adding a caution for women until studies are done to determine how it affects estrogens or estrogen metabolites in women. For men, research has shown it does not increase testosterone or affect other sex hormones, but maca does improve the action of sperm and libido.

Symptom-Free Withdrawal from Synthetic Hormones

If you are currently on synthetic hormones, it is time to wean yourself off them. If you eat a healthy diet rich in vegetables and good sources of protein and exercise every day, you will have an easier time weaning yourself off synthetic hormones. Women who have been on synthetic hormones for decades may find it takes many months to do this, while others may be able to come off quite easily. We have provided a few scenarios for coming off your hormones as examples. Some women may want to switch over to bioidentical hormones, while other women will want to stop hormone therapy and use herbs and nutrients instead.

Case History: From Synthetic Hormones to Nutrients

Lisa, who is 72, has been taking Premarin for over 30 years, after having a complete hysterectomy. After the WHI estrogen-and-progestins study results were published, Lisa decided it was time to get off those hormones. Although she is well past menopause, her body is dependent on the synthetic hormones. Lisa does not want to switch to bioidentical hormones; she wants to come off hormones entirely.

In order to stop hormone therapy without nasty menopause symptoms, it is necessary for Lisa to wean herself off the drug slowly. It is important that all post-menopausal women who stop taking synthetic estrogens ensure they are using an excellent bone supplement containing a minimum of at least calcium citrate, magnesium citrate, vitamins D and K, and ipriflavone. Research has shown women are at higher risk of fracture at this time

Weaning Off Oral Estrogens

Ask your physician for consecutively lower and lower dose prescriptions for estrogen to make the weaning process easier. MenoSense dosage is 2 capsules at breakfast and 2 at bedtime to provide 24-hour support.

Weeks 1 and 2	1 day HRT	1 day MenoSense
Weeks 3 and 4	1 day HRT	2 days MenoSense
Weeks 5 and 6	1 day HRT	3 days MenoSense
Weeks 7 and 8	0 to 1 day HRT	MenoSense every day

If you are using the patch Estrogen HRT:

The longer you wear the patch, the weaker it becomes. You can also ask your physician for a lower-dose patch as well.

Weeks 1 and 2	apply and wear for 5 days	alternate MenoSense
Weeks 3 and 4	apply and wear for 7 days	alternate MenoSense
Weeks 5 and 6	apply and wear for 10 days	MenoSense daily
Weeks 7 and 8	apply and wear for 14 days	MenoSense daily
Week 9	do not wear	MenoSense daily

If you cannot sleep or develop anxiety, follow the recommendations for sleep and anxiety disorders on page 120.

Every woman is different. Some women will be able to wean off HRT over an eight-week period; other women may take 18 months. The goal is to wean off symptom-free, so go slower than suggested above if you have to.

Case Study: From Synthetic to Bioidentical Hormones

Sandy is 59 and has been taking Premarin (synthetic estrogens) and Provera (synthetic progestins) for nine years. She wants to switch to bioidentical hormones. Sandy has an intact uterus and ovaries. Saliva hormone test results showed she was very high in estradiol for a woman using estrogens and low in progesterone. Remember: synthetic progestins are not recognized by the body as progesterone, so a low progesterone test result makes sense. Sandy gained 35 pounds within one year of starting synthetic hormones, and her breasts are painful. These are both symptoms of estrogen dominance.

Sandy's program had her stop taking Provera, replacing it with bioidentical progesterone cream, 20 mg applied morning and night for 25 days with a five-day break each month. Because she is showing signs of estrogen dominance, Sandy will follow the directions on page 144 to wean off Premarin and switch to MenoSense morning and night as recommended above. Sandy will do well on this program, if she weans off Premarin slowly. If she starts to have estrogen-deficiency symptoms like vaginal dryness, she will use vaginal estriol 0.5 mg once daily for three weeks and 0.5 mg once weekly for six months. Sandy should also take an excellent bone supplement along with Biosil, eat an excellent diet and exercise regularly.

Monthly breast self-exams are important for all women, but especially for women who have taken Premarin and Provera. The WHI estrogen-and-progestin study showed that women taking this combination of hormones had a 26 percent increase in invasive breast cancer. Thermography should also be performed, and EstroSense, 2 capsules at breakfast, added to reduce her risk of any negative effects from nine years of taking synthetic hormones.

Now that you have balanced your hormones and increased your vitality, we can give you some tips on how to use all that energy. Next you'll discover how diet and exercise can improve not only your health but your sex drive. And you will also find tips on how to love yourself, and more.

6

Sexy Hormone Diet
Part One:
Maintaining Hormone Balance

Food is the most important factor to consider when working toward balancing hormones and achieving maximum vitality. Now that you have learned about your body chemistry, tested your hormone levels, added key nutritional supplements and perhaps added bioidentical hormone therapy, we will teach you how to use food to keep your hormones stable by improving your overall health. This chapter will tell you how to give your body the nutritional building blocks it needs to accomplish its day-to-day tasks of energy production, growth, and repair. In the following chapter, we will give you nutrition tips to not only maintain hormone balance but also to boost your sexy hormones.

Make no mistake—food has a powerful effect on hormones. Food can make you feel content and satisfied; it can make you feel happy or sexy. It can also make you feel bloated and grumpy. Some foods contain ingredients that act exactly like or increase the body's production of progesterone or estrogen or testosterone, while others can inhibit hormone action. When it comes to sexy hormones, food can either enhance those hormones or suppress them. The ancients were correct when they said that food is our medicine. Food aids thousands of actions and reactions. On the flip side, processed foods can disrupt healthy body processes, including the ones that make us ready for love.

Nutritionists and dietitians advise us that we can get adequate nutritional requirements from the foods we eat. "Adequate" nutrition is just not good enough anymore—especially for women suffering hormone imbalance. People often resist changes in diet until a health crisis forces them to rethink nutritional choices. "Diet" is simply a four-letter word for the food you eat every day. But if that diet is high in refined carbohydrates, devoid of good fats, or lacking in protein, it will create hormone havoc. Dr. Pettle and I are constantly surprised that the women we care for are confused as to what a carbohydrate is, or that they are avoiding all dietary fat, or that they basically eat no protein. Excellent nutrition is the foundation on which you add nutritional supplements and possibly hormone therapies. Without super nutrition in the form of high-quality foods, you cannot feel vibrant, let alone have an abundance of sexy hormones. Eat the following foods for health and vitality.

Carbohydrates

Carbohydrates supply your body with energy. All carbohydrates, with the exception of fiber, are converted into glucose, a major source of fuel for your body. Found mostly in plant foods and, to a lesser extent in milk and milk products, carbohydrates are divided into two groups: complex carbohydrates, made up of hundreds of sugar molecules linked together; and simple carbohydrates, usually made up of no more than three sugar molecules.

Carbohydrates are divided between two types because their different structures have a big impact on how the body uses them. Simple carbohydrates, made up of just a few sugar molecules, are quickly used by the body. Complex carbohydrates, also known as "good carbohydrates," are starches made up of many sugar molecules, and they require some effort on the part of the digestive system. It takes longer for complex carbohydrates to be broken down and have the glucose (and other nutrients) gradually released into the bloodstream and distributed throughout the body. Complex carbohydrates can be further categorized as high-fiber and low-fiber carbohydrates. High-fiber complex carbohydrates are the better choice.

Refining foods can change a good carbohydrate to one that is less nutritious—for example, grains are stripped of their hulls and other fibrous parts and finely ground to become flours that no longer nutritionally resemble the original food. In other cases, the pulp is removed from fruits to create pure juices devoid of fiber and high in fructose. As a result, these foods behave more like a simple carbohydrate, moving through the digestive system faster, with glucose hitting the bloodstream soon after consumption. When this occurs, the body has to quickly supply a high level of insulin, the hormone that acts as the body's traffic cop for blood sugar, in order to deal with the influx. Insulin is also a hormone that negatively affects levels of testosterone, sex-hormone-binding globulin—and your sex drive. That is a big impact on your sexy hormones from a spike in your blood sugar.

Even worse, a side effect of the refining process is that the parts of the plant that are stripped away are also the parts that contain most of the vitamins and minerals in the food. Not only do these foods boost blood sugar—they are almost always devoid of key building blocks that the body needs.

Simple carbohydrates are most often identified by their sweet taste. Simple carbohydrates include fructose (fruit sugar), sucrose (table sugar), and lactose (milk sugar). Products that are primarily simple carbohydrates are fruit juices without pulp, baked goods made with white flour (such as cookies, cakes, and crackers), white pastas and breads, and any sugar-laden food (such as gooey desserts or candies). You can identify these not only by their taste but by checking the ingredient lists on the labels. If sugars such as fructose, sucrose, or maltose are in the top five ingredients, you are holding a potentially dangerous blood-sugar booster. These foods should be avoided or limited in your sexy hormone diet.

Complex carbohydrates include fiber and starches, which are found in all vegetables, legumes, beans, nuts, seeds, and whole, unrefined grains. Complex carbohydrates like cruciferous vegetables (broccoli, Brussels sprouts, cauliflower, cabbage, and kale) have the ability to balance estrogens. In addition, cruciferous vegetables stop your estrogens from converting into toxic estrogen metabolites like 16 alpha-hydroxyestrone. They also ensure that when your liver metabolizes estrogens for excretion, the estrogens are removed from your body safely. Cruciferous vegetables are stars at hormone balancing and protecting you from hormone-related cancers. The fiber found in flaxseeds and legumes acts as a vehicle for excess hormones and toxins that are being eliminated. Lignans, which you will read about later, have a potent, positive hormone effect. These are the types of high-fiber complex carbohydrates you want to eat more of.

You will note we have not mentioned fruits to this point. Fruits, although a complex carbohydrate, contain high amounts of naturally occurring fructose. Some fruits are low in fiber, bananas for example, so our recommendation is to eat no more than one serving of fruit a day and ensure it is a high-fiber fruit like berries. Do not drink the juice, which is devoid of the pulp.

Craving those Refined Carbohydrates

If instead of heading for the complex carbs, you find yourself craving refined carbohydrates like baked goods or other sugar-laden foods, you likely need to enhance your levels of serotonin, which is your happy hormone (read about 5-HTP to enhance serotonin on page 120). When you eat an abundance of refined carbohydrates, your serotonin level does go up, but it plummets just as fast because the refined carbohydrates are processed so quickly. This will make you crave more and lock you into a vicious cycle of craving, sugar highs and lows, weight gain, and depression over your perceived lack of willpower.

Shortly you will read that protein and healthy fats provide a better source for boosting your serotonin levels. If you eliminate all white pasta, white rice, white flour, and white sugar from your diet, you will have more energy and will be able to maintain a healthy weight and kick-start your hormones. These refined foods drag you down physically and emotionally. So pack your sexy hormone diet with lots of dark-colored vegetables instead of high-sugar snacks.

No Fake Sweeteners

If those natural sugars like fructose are bad news, what about artificial sweeteners? Dr. Pettle and I recommend that you avoid synthetic sugar substitutes like aspartame (NutraSweet) and sucralose.

Aspartame is more sinful than sugar. It is a synthetic substance made up of phenylalanine, aspartic acid, and methanol (wood alcohol). Canada's Health Protection Branch regulates methanol, which is a potent neurotoxin, and has banned the food supplement phenylalanine for safety reasons, yet allows aspartame to be sold freely. Opponents of aspartame say there are links between aspartame and memory problems, seizure disorders, birth defects, headaches, and brain tumors. Although no long-term studies have proven these side effects, there are better, natural choices available.

Sucralose is a chlorinated sucrose derivative with no long-term, human-based research on its effects. A 1992 abstract published in *Science Health Abstracts* reported that large doses of sucralose shrank the thymus glands of rats by up to 40 percent. Because the thymus is so important to a healthy immune system, the Center for Science in the Public Interest, a non-profit watchdog group, requested that further studies be performed before sucralose was released in the U.S. This recommendation was ignored, and sucralose, sold under the name Splenda, is available as a sweetener in North America today. Hundreds of animal studies have been performed using sucralose, some of which show the following hazards:

- enlarged liver and kidneys
- atrophy of lymph follicles in the spleen and thymus
- reduced growth rate
- decreased red blood cell count
- hyperplasia of the pelvis
- extension of the pregnancy period
- aborted pregnancy
- decreased fetal body weights and placental weights
- diarrhea

Safe Natural Sweeteners

There are two safe, natural sweeteners available that we recommend: stevia and xylitol. Stevia is 300 times sweeter than sugar, has no calories, and is safe for people with diabetes. Stevia leaves have been used as herbal teas by patients with diabetes in Asian countries and have been used as a sweetener in South America for centuries. In a study published in 1993, no side effects were noted in people with diabetes who used stevia for years. Two other research studies published in 1981 and 1986 found that stevia extract can actually improve blood sugar levels.

The sweet secret of stevia lies in a complex molecule called stevioside, which is a glycoside composed of glucose, sophorose, and steviol. It is this complex molecule and a number of other related compounds that account for *Stevia reubaudiana's* extraordinary sweetness. Stevia is available in health food stores and a growing number of drug and grocery stores in powder form for cooking and baking, and in drop and tablet form for use in coffee and tea.

Xylitol, another natural sweetener, was discovered in 1891 by German chemist Emil Fischer. It occurs naturally in fruits and vegetables. Xylitol has one-third fewer calories than white sugar and reduces the development of dental cavities. Xylitol is sold as a white, crystalline powder for use as a sweetener for foods and beverages. It is also used as an ingredient in chewing gum to improve dental health.

Dietary Fats

Western society has become terrified of eating any fat. Yet, like carbohydrates, there are good and bad fats. Good fats not only contain healthy, hormone-promoting components; they also enhance overall health. In the push to help everyone keep their weight down, consumers have been trained to search food packaging for the words "no fat" or "low fat" without being trained to distinguish fat that is good from fat that is not. Furthermore, when manufacturers remove fats from foods, they often put sugar in its place. As you now know, sugars, or even worse, fake sugars, disrupt your body's hormone chemistry.

Foods containing fat make you feel satisfied, and good fats are essential for healthy brain function. Fat is also the most concentrated source of energy your body will receive.

Without the right fats in your diet, your hair will fall out, your thyroid gland will not function well, depression and low mood will set in, your sex drive can die, and you will crave those refined carbohydrates that cause weight gain and worsen the cycle of hormone dysfunction. The right fats will help your hormones. Think about giving your body good fats from foods like nuts and seeds and their oils, rather than those from poor sources such as margarines, processed oils, shortenings, lards, and foods containing trans fatty acids (those cancer-causing, heart-disease-promoting fats labeled as hydrogenated or partially hydrogenated). You don't fuel your car with dirty gasoline, yet every day you pollute your body with these toxic fats, which contribute to health problems.

Good fats found in nuts and seeds and their cold-pressed, organic oils such as flaxseed, hemp, evening primrose, echium, and borage are the precursors to many hormones. Fish and their oils also play a role in hormone formation.

Saturated Fats

Saturated fats are semi-solid at room temperature and are found in animal products, such as red meat (beef, veal), pork, lamb, and lard, and dairy products like milk, cheese, and butter, as well as in some processed foods. They are generally considered "bad" fats because they are associated with increased risk of heart disease, cancer, hormone problems, inflammation, and more. Many of the foods that contain saturated fats are good sources of protein. Our recommendation is to eat these foods in moderation and always choose the sources that are organically raised and free-range.

However, not all saturated fats are created equal. Good saturated fats— found in butter and coconut oil—do not clog arteries, nor do they cause heart disease. Rather, they are easily digested and a good source of fuel for energy.

The Truth about Coconut Oil

Coconut oil has been wrongly branded as a nutritional evil for too long. In the 1960s, data collected from research was misinterpreted, concluding that coconut oil raised levels of LDL blood cholesterol (the "bad" cholesterol). In fact, it was the omission of essential fatty acids (EFAs) in the experimental diet that caused the observed cholesterol problems, not the inclusion of the coconut oil.

Coconut oil is a short-chain fat that is easily digested and used by the body. Subject groups studied more recently in the South Pacific for their regular use of coconut oil exhibited low incidences of coronary artery disease and low serum cholesterol levels. Little or no change is evident in serum cholesterol levels when an EFA-rich diet contains coconut oil (or butter). Coconut oil also supports healthy thyroid function. Coconut oil is naturally saturated, so it does not need to go through hydrogenation to stabilize it. It will become harder when it is exposed to lower temperatures. Other benefits of coconut oil are that it is slightly lower in calories than most other fats and oils, and you do not need to use as much coconut oil as you would other oils when cooking or baking. Coconut oil is a rich source of medium-chain triglycerides. New research shows coconut oil also enhances metabolism, aiding weight loss. Purchase virgin, cold-pressed, organic coconut oil. It is delicious.

Butter is Better

The great debate over whether butter is better than margarine is still going on, and it is a travesty that butter continues to be demonized. Fat and oil experts, including Mary Enig, author of *Know Your Fats*, and Udo Erasmus, author of *Fats That Heal, Fats That Kill*, also believe that butter is an important fat and one that should not be replaced by hydrogenated fats like margarine.

Butter contains many healthful components, including lecithin, which aids the body in breaking down dietary cholesterol. It is also a rich source of vitamin A, which is necessary for the healthy functioning of the adrenal and thyroid glands. The vitamins A and E and the mineral selenium in butter serve as important antioxidants in protecting against free radical damage that can destroy tissues and weaken artery walls. Butter from cows that have been allowed to graze on grass has high amounts of conjugated linoleic acid, an important fat for weight loss and metabolism.

If you look at the fat component of butter, it is made from cream and contains a wide range of short- and medium-chain fatty acids, as well as monounsaturated and some polyunsaturated fatty acids. The dangers of butter's saturated fat components have been blown out of proportion. If used in moderation (like all good things), butter is an excellent fat to have in your diet. It can even be improved upon by adding an essential fatty acid component, if you use the recipe below.

Better Butter Recipe

1 lb	butter	.5 kg
1 cup	high-quality essential-fatty-acid-rich oil	250 mL
	(such as VegaOmega, flaxseed oil, Udo's oil,	
	or any other organic, cold-pressed oil)	

Cut butter into eight pieces. Put butter and oil into the food processor, and blend until smooth. Spoon into covered container and refrigerate. Not only will you have better butter, but it will remain soft even though refrigerated. Makes 2 cups (500 mL).

Trans Fatty Acids

The fats that are so bad they are downright dangerous are trans fatty acids. These fats are abundant in restaurant fried (fast) food, junk food, packaged baked goods, and processed foods. These fats are bad because they have been processed in order to stabilize them (so the foods will last longer). The processing, called hydrogenation or partial hydrogenation, changes the chemical structure of the fat, making a liquid into a solid that is more shelf-stable. The quest to prolong the shelf life of foods has led to the development of a more poisonous form of fatty acid, called trans fatty acids, the deadliest of all fats.

Although government health departments are reviewing the acceptable level of trans fatty acids allowed in foods, currently no laws have been agreed upon and manufacturers' withdrawal of trans fatty acids is voluntary. Trans fatty acids are found in all fast foods that have been cooked in oils that contain trans fatty acids, including potato chips, French fries, baby biscuits, breakfast cereals, cookies, microwave popcorn, and some margarines, to name just a few. All the oils used in commercially produced salad dressings—except extra virgin olive oil—also contain trans fatty acids as a result of the high-heat process used to make these oils shelf-stable.

In North America there is a push to eliminate trans fatty acids from foods. In the fall of 2006 New York City banned trans fatty acids from restaurant food. (You will now even see French fries being touted as trans fatty acid free—be aware that even though there are no trans fatty acids, French fries are still an unhealthy food because they contain acrylamides and other bad fats as a result of high-heat frying.) Eliminate all foods that contain trans fatty acids.

Unsaturated Fats: Not Just Good, but Fabulous

Unsaturated fats are categorized as omega-3 (richest sources are fish, flaxseed, and echium seed), omega-6 (see below), and omega-9 (found in flaxseed, olives, pistachios, pumpkin seeds, hazelnuts, and coconut). The omega-3s and omega-6s are polyunsaturated and are called essential fatty acids (EFAs) because the body cannot make them. You must consume them in order to get your supply. The omega-9s are monounsaturated and non-essential because your body can make them from other fatty acids.

Essential fatty acids contain their own hormones, called eicosanoids, which are the precursors of some of your sexy hormones. These special hormones act as the intracellular communications control center, balancing virtually every system in the body, including, but not limited to, inflammation, blood clotting, and blood vessel dilation.

Good Omega-6 Oils, Bad Omega-6 Oils

Omega-6 oils are divided further into good omega-6 oils and bad omega-6 oils. Conflicting information abounds on the benefits of omega-6 oils, mainly because of poorly designed studies that do not make a distinction between the types of omega-6 oils. Omega-6 oils include soy, safflower, sunflower, corn, flax, hemp, pumpkin, peanut, canola, borage, echium, evening primrose, and, to a lesser extent, olive oil.

The good omega-6 oils contain gamma linolenic acid (GLA). The richest sources of GLA are evening primrose oil (8 to 10 percent GLA), echium oil (12 to 18 percent GLA), and borage oil (20 to 24 percent GLA). Hemp oil contains minimal GLA (2 to 4 percent). The bad omega-6 oils are made from corn, canola, peanut, and include refined safflower and sunflower oils; they do not contain GLA. Peanut, safflower, and sunflower oils are predominantly highly refined. (Safflower and sunflower oils are available cold-pressed and organic but should still be used in moderation as they contain no GLA.)

Research has confirmed that GLA-containing evening primrose and borage oils have positive effects in breast cancer treatment; they enhance lubrication in those with Sjögren's syndrome; help relieve PMS symptoms, breast pain, skin conditions (including eczema), and attention-deficit hyperactivity disorder in children; improve cardiovascular health and mental health; and the list goes on. GLA is a well-researched, safe fatty acid.

Borage oil (and the related echium oil) contains more GLA than evening primrose oil per milligram, so people can take less to get the same effect.

A British study published in 2000 observed women who had locally advanced metastatic breast cancer (when cancer cells have spread out from the primary tumor). They found that women with breast cancer who were taking tamoxifen (a common drug for estrogen-receptor-positive breast cancer) and received GLA from borage oil demonstrated faster clinical response than those taking amoxifen alone. Study participants received 3 grams of GLA (approximately 12,000 mg of borage oil). The researchers concluded that GLA was a useful adjunct to primary tamoxifen treatment with no serious side effects: "our Phase II study suggests high-dose oral GLA to be a valuable new agent in the treatment of hormone-sensitive breast cancer."

Echium Oil: Better than Fish Oil

Echium oil is a "new kid" on the shelves. Echium oil is derived from the seeds of the species *Echium plantagineum*, a member of the *Boraginacea* family of plants that includes the borage plant. Echium oil is rich in stearidonic acid, a precursor to eicosapentaenoic acid (EPA). Up until now, EPA has been provided mainly from fish oil and, to a lesser extent, flaxseed oil. Flaxseed oil provides less than 10 percent EPA conversion in a healthy person. Echium, on the other hand, provides 30 percent EPA. Echium also contains high levels of GLA, similar to those levels found in borage oil. There is a huge demand for EPA for vegetarians and for those people who are concerned about the impact the fish farms (the main source of fish oil) have on the environment. Also, fish oils have to be heavily processed to remove the impurities, PCBs, and other toxic substances like mercury. A daily dosage of echium oil is anywhere from 250 mg to 1.5 grams per day, with food.

Vegetarian DHA

DHA (docosahexaenoic acid) is one of the two important fatty acids in fish oils (the other is EPA, eicosapentaenoic acid, mentioned above). Docosahexaenoic acid (DHA) is an omega-3 fatty acid. It is found in cold-water fatty fish and in fish oil supplements, along with eicosapentaenoic acid (EPA). For vegetarians or those concerned about fish oil contaminants or the environmental impact of fish farms, algae is a vegetarian source of DHA. DHA is essential for the proper functioning of the adult brain, and for the development of the nervous system and visual abilities during the first six months of life. DHA research has shown it reduces the risk of heart disease. DHA can be obtained from fish in the diet or from food supplements. Daily dosage is 200 mg per day with food.

VegaOmega is a new vegetarian fatty acid supplement containing echium and DHA and provides the equivalent EPA and DHA found in fish oil. We believe this fatty acid supplement to be better than fish oil because it also contains high amounts of GLA.

Every woman reading this book should include GLA-containing oil as part of her sexy hormone diet to improve overall hormone balance, protect her breasts, and aid vaginal lubrication.

Dietary Fats: Do's and Don'ts

- Do not eat margarine, even if the package says it is non-hydrogenated
- Do not fry foods
- Avoid canola oil because it is genetically modified rapeseed. Canola is found in salad dressings and spreads, so please read labels
- Avoid peanut oil because it is heavily refined. Instead: Use virgin coconut butter in place of lard and shortening

- Use extra-virgin olive oil for salad dressings, low heat sautéing, and dipping bread. (Do not purchase light olive oil; it has been processed to remove the good fats.)
- For low-heat sautéing, use healthy oils, including extra virgin olive oil, sesame oil, or coconut butter
- For salad dressings, use cold-pressed oils from organic flaxseed, hempseed, walnuts, extra-virgin olives, pumpkin seed, or macadamia nuts
- For baking, use cold-pressed organic sunflower oil, butter, or coconut butter
- Make better butter from the recipe on page 153

Dietary Protein:
A Building Block for Hormones

The importance of dietary protein for optimal hormone health cannot be overstated. Your body requires 20 amino acids to facilitate the production of protein for the repair of your cells and tissues. Protein is also required for the manufacture of CP-450, a protective enzyme that acts as a protector of the body and decreases the risk of breast cancer. Of the 20 amino acids, 12 are synthesized by your liver and the remaining eight must be obtained from your food—these are called essential. The richest sources of amino acids are legumes, fresh fish, free-range poultry and eggs, free-range red meat, nuts, seeds, fermented soy, whey protein, and fermented organic dairy products. Many conditions are related to inadequate consumption of dietary protein, especially:

- breast cancer
- depression due to a lack of serotonin
- fragile, soft nails
- heart problems
- hormone dysfunction
- hypoglycemia
- accelerated aging
- lack of sex drive
- lack of muscle tone, including sagging chin

- osteoporosis
- poor wound healing
- poor digestion
- thinning hair
- weak immune system
- wrinkled skin

Two groups of proteins are found in your diet: complete proteins—including meat, fish, poultry, cheese, eggs, milk, tofu, fermented soy and whey protein powders—contain all of the essential amino acids. The second group, comprised of incomplete proteins that do not contain all the essential amino acids, include grains, legumes, and leafy green vegetables. Eat protein at every meal. Your plate should have 40 percent protein, with the balance of the plate filled with lots of dark-colored vegetables and good fats.

Why Fermented Soy?

You may be unfamiliar with the term "fermented soy." There are two types of soy: fermented and non-fermented. Fermented soy includes miso, tempeh, soy sauce, fermented soy powders, and fermented soy yogurt. Traditional Asian diets contain mainly fermented soy foods, not isolated soy protein, soy milk, or whole soybeans. In addition, most non-fermented soy products are genetically modified, unless the label clearly states that the soy is certified organic.

Before the days of refrigeration and canning, fermenting foods was a preservation method devised for foods to be stored for longer periods of time. Fermentation also enhances the digestibility of the food and the bioavailability of the nutrients found in the food. In Asian countries, the popular diet consists of sea vegetables rich in iodine, sea foods, meat, poultry, and plenty of vegetables, with fermented soy products used as a condiment. Fermented soy is a healing food. Other fermented foods that are healing include yogurt (fermented milk), sauerkraut (fermented cabbage), and olives.

Non-fermented soybeans contain enzyme inhibitors that can block protein absorption and therefore inhibit the production of the protein-derived hormones. Non-fermented soybeans also contain hemagglutin, which is known to decrease the ability of red blood cells to properly absorb oxygen and distribute it through the body. Non-fermented soy beans are also highly goitrogenic, meaning they inhibit the uptake of thyroid hormone. And non-fermented soy products contain phytic acid, which latches onto (or chelates) certain nutrients, including iron, to inhibit their absorption.

When soybeans are naturally fermented, as found in tempeh, miso, and fermented soy powder, they become a very different food than unfermented soy. The fermentation process deactivates hemagglutinin and enhances protein absorption. Soy is cooked and then mixed with probiotics or a starter of "good" bacteria and then left to ferment over time. Tofu, although not fermented, goes through a process whereby anti-nutrients (like hemaggluten and phytic acid) are removed. The fermentation process also breaks down phytic acid, so nutrients are absorbed. Fermented soy powders also provide safer forms (alglycone forms) of the isoflavones genistein and daizein.

Isoflavones are sold as individual ingredients in health food stores for women in the transitional years for menopausal symptoms. There is negative research showing that soy isoflavones may stimulate estrogen-receptor cells in breast tissue. When soy is fermented, the activity of the isoflavones is reduced by two-thirds, and the isoflavones become safer forms of the original molecule. The late Dr. John R. Lee, M.D., father of natural progesterone, recommended choosing fermented soy foods in moderation, along with a varied diet rich in vitamins, minerals, and other essential nutrients. The fermentation process also creates probiotics—helpful bacteria the body needs to increase the quantity, availability, digestibility, and assimilation of nutrients in the body. The fermentation process actually removes nearly all of the negative side effects of soy and converts it into a powerful health food. We love fermented soy but would still caution women with estrogen-receptor-positive breast cancer to avoid all soy products.

Replace your morning Coffee with a Protein Power Shake

Excess consumption of caffeine can lead to a magnesium deficiency characterized by heart palpitations, twitchy eyelids, high blood pressure, anxiety, sleep disturbances, poor response to stress, osteoporosis, restless leg syndrome, urinary tract infections, and fibroid breast cysts, to name a few problems. And coffee (not caffeine but coffee) is estrogenic. Caffeine has a strong presence in North American drinking habits, and not just in your morning latte. Soda pop, tea, chocolate, over-the-counter medications such as Excedrin and Midol, and even decaffeinated coffee have caffeine. Caffeine causes the body to excrete magnesium, which a serious side effect, given that North Americans already tend to have magnesium-deficient diets. The table below gives you some idea of the caffeine content of popular beverages, compared to medication designed to keep you awake. Note that the beverages' caffeine content is for a 6 oz/175 ml cup. If you are in the habit of pouring or buying jumbo servings, multiply the numbers accordingly.

Caffeine Countdown
(per 6 oz/175 ml cup)

pill (No-Doz, Vivarin)	100–200 mg
drip coffee	103 mg
cappuccino	75 mg
instant coffee	57 mg
black tea	36 mg
analgesics (Excedrin, Anacin)	35–65 mg
soft drinks	26–34 mg
iced tea, instant	30 mg
green tea	30 mg
chocolate	18 mg
decaf coffee	2 mg
herbal tea	0 mg

Protein shakes are refreshing, provide quick energy, and are a wonderful alternative to caffeine-laden beverages.

PROTEIN POWER SHAKE

1 cup	plain, acidophilus, organic yogurt
2 scoops	of your favorite protein powder from whey, fermented soy, rice, pea, or hemp protein
1 tbsp	VegaOmega oil (vegetarian EPA and DHA)
1/2 cup	fresh fruit, mango, papaya, berries, or banana
1 cup	water
3	ice cubes

Combine all ingredients in a blender, and blend until smooth. Drink immediately.

Dietary Protein Requirements

Some people have greater dietary protein requirements than others. If you are very active, exercise strenuously, or do heavy labor, or if you are pregnant, you will need more protein than a couch potato.

When choosing your dietary protein sources, opt for free-range poultry and eggs and wild fish over farm-grown fish to avoid contamination from antibiotics and growth hormones. In Canada and the U.S., hormones are used to fatten up cattle. Hormones, including estradiol, progestins, testosterone, zeranol, melengestrol acetate, and trenbolone acetate, are approved for use in the beef industry. The Canadian Animal Health Institute's *Fact Sheet*, entitled "Hormones: A Safe, Effective Production Tool for the Canadian Beef Industry," states that: "Although there are cost benefits associated with the use of hormones in beef production, never has there been any compromise in regards to human health. To ensure the safety of all new drugs, Health Canada's Food and Drugs Act makes it law for all veterinary drugs used in food production processes to pass stringent tests and regulations set by the Veterinary Drugs Directorate."

In this fact sheet, the Institute reports that "using hormones is a matter of limiting inputs while increasing outputs." In other words, make more money by increasing the size of the animal without having to spend a lot of money or time doing it. They "spin doctor" the hormone issue by saying that four ounces of cabbage has more estrogen than six ounces of hormone-treated beef. Cabbage is an anti-estrogen—blocking the negative effects of estrogen and aiding the elimination of toxic estrogens—not an estrogen. (See page 161 for more information on the benefits of cabbage.)

If you are sedentary and weigh approximately 130 pounds, you will need 45 grams of protein per day. You can get this protein from sources like the ones listed on the following page.

Sources of Food Protein

	Protein (grams)
Dairy and eggs	
Cheddar cheese, 1 oz./28 g	7
cottage cheese (2%), 1/2 cup	16
egg, 1 medium	6
milk, skim, 1 cup	8
mozzarella, part skim, 1 oz./28 g	8
ricotta, part skim, 1/2 cup	10
yogurt, low-fat, plain, 1 cup	12
Meat and fish (4 oz.)	
chicken, light meat, roasted, no skin	31
ground beef, extra-lean, broiled	33
sirloin steak, choice cut, trimmed, broiled	35
tuna, canned, in water	33
turkey breast, roasted, no skin	24
Grains	
oatmeal, 1 cup cooked	6
rice, brown, 1 cup cooked	5
whole grain spaghetti, 1 cup cooked	6
whole wheat bread, 2 slices	6
Legumes and nuts	
almonds, 1 oz./28 g	6
cashews, dry roasted, 1 oz./28 g	4
lentils, 1/2 cup cooked	8
lima beans, 1/2 cup cooked	8
peanut butter, 2 tbsp	10
red kidney beans, 1/2 cup canned	8
soybeans, 1/2 cup cooked	10
tofu, 4 oz./113 g	9

Dietary Support for the Adrenals and Thyroid Function

A diet based on good sources of carbohydrates, fats, and protein is key to supporting healthy adrenals and thyroid function. Use the following tips to reinforce your food choices and ensure optimum health.

- Eat high-quality free-range, organic or wild protein. Your plate at lunch and dinner should contain a piece of protein and lots of green vegetables.
- Breakfast should be predominantly protein, such as boiled or poached free-range eggs, a protein shake, yogurt with protein powder added, or a chicken breast.
- Avoid refined foods at breakfast, including breads (especially those made with refined flours) and refined breakfast cereals, and concentrated carbohydrates such as instant oatmeal and fruit juices.
- Eat foods rich in the mineral iodine. The thyroid needs iodine to make thyroid hormones. Iodine-rich foods include beef, lamb, and beef liver (hormone-free); eggs; raw nuts and seeds; seafoods (such as clams, oysters, sardines, and other saltwater fish); sea vegetables (such as wakame, hijiki, kelp, nori, arame, and dulse); and fresh fruits and vegetables, especially green peppers, lettuce, and pineapple. Raisins contain iodine as well.
- Avoid all regular soy foods as they contain goitrogens, which cause a decrease in the absorption of iodine. Fermented organic soy foods are fine (including tempeh, miso, soy sauce, and fermented soy yogurt and powders).
- Use only pure, cold-pressed organic oils, including flaxseed, extra virgin olive oil, echium, borage, and sesame.
- Avoid all artificial sweeteners, including sucralose and aspartame. Use only natural sweeteners like xylitol and stevia.
- Exercise daily for 20 minutes, if possible. Exercise is particularly important for those with low thyroid as it stimulates the thyroid gland and increases metabolism.

Now you have the basics of a health-enhancing diet, setting the stage for the add-ons that will enhance your sexy hormones.
- Eat plenty of complex carbohydrates in the form of dark-colored vegetables; choose good fats, and clean sources of free-range or organic proteins.
- Do not consume artificial sweeteners. Use stevia or xylitol instead of sugar and artificial sweeteners.

7

Sexy Hormone Diet Part Two: Boosting Sexy Hormones

Throughout history, cultures around the world have been convinced of the power of foods, particularly when it comes to enhancing sex drives. Modern interest in the subject is not new, but now research on food-based nutrients and how they affect sexual enhancement is catching up with traditional theories and practices.

John Harvey Kellogg, M.D., founder of the "Snap, Crackle, and Profitable" Kellogg breakfast cereal corporation, believed that food could be so sexually stimulating that people suffering from "sexual excesses" should avoid all stimulating foods such as spices, pepper, ginger, mustard, cinnamon, cloves, all condiments, pickles, "flesh" foods in any but moderate quantities, chocolate, coffee, and tea. Kellogg had no science to prove his recommendations, but today researchers know many of the foods purported to be sexual enhancers by him back in the 1800s do exactly that—enhance sexual arousal, stamina, and satisfaction.

To keep budding libidos under control, Dr. Kellogg recommended a bland diet to delay puberty in the children of his day. That diet consisted of oatmeal, wheat flour, boiled vegetables, and ripened fruit. These foods, he stated, were "wholly free from injurious properties" and "the immense evils of self-pollution" (masturbation). No flesh foods, chocolate, or oysters for these kids. You, on the other hand, are free to nourish yourself for maximum desire and pleasure.

Chocolate: The Love Drug

Researchers have been unlocking the secrets of your chocolate desires. They now know chocolate has some very powerful ingredients that affect neurotransmitters, the chemical messengers in the brain. The natural love drug chocolate contains high levels of tryptophan, the precursor to serotonin (meaning your body uses tryptophan to make serotonin), the happy hormone that positively affects your emotions and body sensations. As a result, chocolate makes you feel elated or happy, and your mood elevates.

Chocolate's aphrodisiac qualities can be attributed to another neuro-chemical —phenylethylamine, also known as chocolate amphetamine. By elevating your levels of phenylethylamine, you can promote feelings of attraction and excitement. Phenylethylamine works by stimulating the brain's pleasure centers and reaches peak levels during orgasm. Although chocolate contains only small amounts of tryptophan and phenylethylamine, the combination of the two, plus other neurochemicals present in chocolate, may be the reason for chocolate's sensual effects.

When you eat chocolate, your body releases endorphins, also called opiate peptides. Endorphins are responsible for the "high" produced by strenuous exercise. And endorphins produce the sensation of sexual arousal. No wonder chocolate makes people feel sexy!

Chocolate connoisseurs know that one square of dark chocolate contains more phenols than a glass of red wine. Phenols are antioxidants that help keep bad fats from clogging up arteries. Chocolate contains around 300 known chemicals, including stimulants such as caffeine, although 1 ounce (28 g) of dark chocolate contains only 30 mg of caffeine—equivalent to one-third of a cup of coffee. Caffeine provides the stimulant effect and, when combined with the hormones and neurotransmitters in chocolate, can be quite pleasurable. Cocoa and chocolate fats include substances that are chemically related to the brain lipids anandamide ("ananda" means bliss). Anandamide does indeed give you that blissful feeling. How chocolate feels in your mouth, with its sweet taste and smooth, melting texture, also enhances sensory perceptions.

When choosing chocolate, reach for the darker variety at 70 percent cocoa or more. This is the chocolate that is packed with all the sexy hormone enhancing goodies. Remember, despite all the good things in chocolate, it should be eaten in moderation because of the high caloric content.

Testosterone-boosting Foods

Nothing boosts testosterone like regular exercise, but there are also foods, particularly flesh foods (as Dr. Kellogg called them), that are known to enhance testosterone. Foods that are referred to as aphrodisiacs have ingredients, like the mineral zinc, that work to enhance testosterone.

In women, zinc deficiency can lead to such problems as impaired synthesis and secretion of follicle-stimulating hormone (FSH) and luteinizing hormone (LH), both of which figure in the menstrual cycle, abnormal ovarian development, and recurring miscarriage. Women must have adequate amounts of LH because LH promotes the manufacture of testosterone; low levels will inhibit desire. Zinc is important for normal sexy hormone function.

Oysters have long been touted as sexual enhancers. They contain high levels of zinc and have been shown to increase testosterone in men. Research on the effects of oysters in women has not been performed. Actually, research on women and testosterone is sadly lacking.

Red meat is also a testosterone-enhancing food. Most animal foods like wild game, poultry, lamb, and pork enhance testosterone. Goose and duck contain the highest levels of testosterone. Remember to buy wild, free-range, organic animal foods whenever possible. Vegetarians should add baked beans and nuts to their diets because those foods have been shown to enhance testosterone.

Foods for Testosterone
- free-range red meat, wild game
- goose and duck
- oysters
- baked beans
- nuts

Estrogen and Foods:
The Great, The Good, and The Ugly

Estrogens have a tangled relationship with food. Some foods and herbs block estrogens, that is, they keep estrogen molecules from fitting into estrogen receptors on cells. Some foods enhance the action of estrogen, making it stronger. Some foods contain high levels of estrogens and should be avoided or eaten in moderation. Some foods keep estrogens at healthy levels by aiding the liver in detoxifying excess estrogens, while some foods contain progesterone that helps to balance out estrogens. Other foods stop estrogen-related cancers from forming.

You learned in the Prologue that you also get a good dose of xenoestrogens from the environment, contributing to your toxic load and estrogen-dominant conditions. Many foods are so powerful they can detoxify estrogens and halt the conversion of 2-hydroxyestrone to 16 alpha-hydroxyestrone (the bad estrogen metabolite involved in cancer). These foods are the super protectors of the body and should be eaten often.

Phytoestrogens

Phytoestrogens (*phyto* means plant) are naturally occurring plant estrogens. Plants can produce chemicals that mimic estrogen, block estrogens, or reduce or detoxify estrogens. However, only a limited number of plant-based foods have the ability to mimic estrogen or fit into estrogen receptors. Some phytoestrogens have no estrogenic action and are estrogen-blocking.

This is why the term "phytoestrogen" is confusing to women who have been told to avoid them because they are possibly cancer-promoting. Making matters more confusing, the phytoestrogen activity of a plant depends on the plant's stage of growth, the season it is harvested, where the plant is grown, and the nutrient content of the soil in which the plant grows.

Sprouted seedlings contain the highest amount of phytoestrogens. For example, broccoli sprouts contain high levels of estrogen-blocking or estrogen-balancing compounds, particularly indoles and sulforaphane. Broccoli, Brussels sprouts, cauliflower, cabbage, and kale are also high in indoles and other chemicals that help detoxify excess estrogens and keep your body's own estrogens in their healthy form. Lignans (which are phytoestrogenic) found in flaxseeds and cranberry can help block the action of estrogen and balance the estrogen-to-progesterone ratio. Fermented soy foods contain estrogens, and these can fit into estrogen receptors, enhancing total estrogens in the body.

We have broken the foods and herbs into categories so you can see which foods help regulate estrogens, which foods protect you from estrogen's negative effects, and which foods should be avoided or limited because they contain estrogen. We have also included the foods that are progesterone-enhancing because estrogen and progesterone have a direct feedback mechanism—if one goes up the other is reduced and vice versa.

The Great: Super Estrogen and Testosterone Regulators

Flavonoids and indoles are super regulators of estrogen and testosterone. Flavonoids are a group of plant chemicals that includes flavones, isoflavones, isoflavonones, catechins, and chalcones, among dozens of others. Flavonoids are found in high concentration in fruits, vegetables, nuts, and grains. Flavonoids are anti-inflammatory, antioxidant, antiviral, and anti-cancer. Most importantly, they either increase the function of sexy hormones and their receptors by fitting into the receptor or decrease its action by blocking the receptor. Indoles, primarily found in cruciferous vegetables, are powerful regulators of hormones. We discuss them at length below. There are many foods that contain indoles and flavones, but the super regulators with excellent research include:

- apigenine: passiflora and chamomile
- chrysin: passiflora and to lesser extent bee propolis
- galangin: bee propolis
- indole-3-carbinol: cruciferous vegetables

The ability of flavones to balance estrogens and enhance testosterone has been evaluated in many studies. Some of the most potent estrogen-inhibiting flavones are found in passiflora, chamomile, and bee propolis. These flavones work on the aromatase enzyme, which is found in the liver and is responsible for the conversion of the male hormones (androgens) androstenedione and testosterone into estrogens. We know that inhibiting the aromatase enzyme ensures that less estrogen is produced by tissues, thereby maintaining healthy testosterone levels. As men age, aromatase activity increases, converting precious testosterone into estrogen. Researchers believe this is the reason for male menopause (also called andropause), enlarged prostate, and prostate cancer. Both male and female body builders often use aromatase-inhibiting flavones to increase lean muscle mass and lower body fat. In women, aromatase, especially in fat cells, produces estrogens. The more fat cells you have, the more estrogen you produce. Aromatase inhibitors are being studied in women for the development of estrogen-blocking treatments for estrogen-receptor-positive breast cancer. Powerful drugs like Arimidex and Femara inhibit aromatase and are now the first choice in many breast cancer treatment procedures. Male body builders are so aware of the estrogen connection that many use the drug Arimidex to stop the conversion of testosterone to estrogen.

Wild Yam is Estrogenic, NOT Progestogenic

Wild yam, known as dioscorea, has been and is still eaten in Mexico, China, and Africa as a staple food. Wild yam's fame began in the 1940s when Russell Marker took Mexican wild yam and produced progesterone from diosgenin, one of its active ingredients. (Diosgenin was also used to make the hormones found in the Pill until cheaper synthetics were produced.) In 1970, the Mexican government nationalized the yam industry. Mexico still remains the principal grower, but India, South Africa, and parts of Asia also supply the drug industry with wild yam. Over 100,000 tons have to be harvested every year to provide the over 700 tons of the saponin diosgenin used by the drug companies. Hydrocortisone was also originally derived from yam's constituents.

One very important point that most people overlook is that wild yam is actually estrogenic, not progestogenic. (Dioscorea-containing herbal products are currently being sold as progesterone precursors. Manufacturers claim that dioscorea can be converted into progesterone upon consumption.) Research published in the *Journal of the American College of Nutrition* in 2005 evaluated what happens to women's sex hormones, urinary estrogen metabolites, lipids, and antioxidants when wild yam (dioscorea) is eaten. Twenty-four post-menopausal women were asked to eat 39 g of wild yam per day for 30 days. Twenty-two women completed the study. After yam ingestion, there were significant increases in serum concentrations of estrone (increased 26 percent), sex-hormone-binding globulin (increased 9.5 percent), and near-significant increase in estradiol (27 percent). No significant changes were observed in serum concentrations of dehydroepiandrosterone sulfate, progesterone, androstenedione, testosterone, follicle-stimulating hormone, or luteinizing hormone. Most important, urinary concentrations of the toxic metabolite of estrogen, 16 alpha-hydroxyestrone, decreased significantly–it was down 37 percent. Plasma cholesterol concentration also decreased significantly (5.9 percent). This study, like others, shows that wild yam increases estrogens but, more important, decreases toxic 16 alpha-hydroxyestrone. It does not have an effect on other hormones, only estrogens.

If you are taking wild yam supplements, they will not convert to progesterone but will provide an increase in estrogens, which may or may not be a positive. Regular yams that can be purchased in North American grocery stores are not the same as wild yam.

See page 72 for more on wild yam creams.

Some of the other super hormone-regulating flavones include naringenin (found in grapefruit) and quercitin (found in most fruits and vegetables, especially citrus fruits, black tea, onions, red apples). There are hundreds of flavones; many have not been researched yet.

Foods that Balance Estrogens

These foods have been found to keep 2-hydroxyestrone levels in a healthy range while stopping the conversion to bad estrogens (16 alpha-hydroxyestrone). These foods are also high in fiber to aid elimination of excess and/or bad estrogens. These foods have weak estrogenic action and will not promote breast cancer or worsen estrogen-dominant conditions. Eat these foods often:

- alfalfa sprouts (rich in vitamin K)
- apples
- berries (blueberry, cranberry, bilberry, blackberry, raspberry, pomegranate)
- borage, echium, evening primrose oils
- carrots
- dried beans, lentils, chickpeas
- extra virgin olive oil
- grapefruit
- mung beans
- non-genetically modified, organic, fermented soy products (tempeh, miso, soy sauce, fermented soy powders)
- pears
- rice bran
- sesame seeds, flaxseeds (they contain lignans)
- wheat germ, barley
- whole grain rice and oats
- wild yam

The Great: Veggies that Inhibit Bad Estrogens

All vegetables contain plant chemicals that are effective in balancing hormones, but the cruciferous vegetables—members of the Brassica family, such as cabbage, Brussels sprouts, broccoli, cauliflower, radish, turnips, kale, kohlrabi, and collard greens—are the super powerhouses that contain indole glucosinates, called indoles for short, that help detoxify excess estrogens, halt the conversion of estrogens into dangerous metabolites, block the action of estrogens, and balance the estrogen-to-progesterone ratio.

Indoles affect estrogen levels in three key ways. First, they reduce the amount of unhealthy estrogen metabolites like 16 alpha-hydroxyestrone and 4-hydroxyestrone, while regulating the amount of healthy estrogen in the body. Second, indoles speed the removal of excess estrogens and estrogen metabolites from the body. And third, indoles can increase the activity of enzymes that detoxify the body of cancer-causing toxins. Indoles have been heavily researched in the area of cancer prevention and treatment. Cruciferous vegetables are rich in Indole-3-carbinol, which is further broken down in the gut by enzymes into di-indolylmethane (pronounced *die-in-do-lyl-meth-ane* or simply DIM).

Broccoli also contains sulforaphane, which was presented on page 90. Along with its estrogen-protective effect, sulforaphane also stimulates certain enzymes that deactivate cancer cells, allowing them to be digested and eliminated from the body. Cancer cells are often not recognized by the immune system as foreign invaders, and as a result they are allowed to "set up house." Sulforaphane turns on specific immune cells so they recognize cancer cells as invaders and destroy them. For those who have heard that broccoli is bad for your thyroid, you would have to eat 10 cups of broccoli per day, every day, to have a negative effect on thyroid.

Broccoli sprouts have over 10 times the sulforaphane as mature broccoli spears. Consumption of broccoli sprouts is also effective at inhibiting *Helicobacter pylori* (the bacteria responsible for stomach ulcers and, potentially, stomach cancer). Sprouting cruciferous vegetables is one way to get the maximum benefit from the plants. Do not buy grocery store, ready-to-eat sprouts, as they have high bacteria counts and have been linked to salmonella poisoning. Sprout your own at home in a jar on the kitchen windowsill.

D-glucarate, another powerful hormone balancer (see page 85), is made in the intestines from all fruits and vegetables you have consumed. It is a super detoxifier of estrogens and dangerous estrogen metabolites like 16 alpha-hydroxy-estrone. It keeps your liver's detoxification system working well. Remember, your liver is the key organ in processing and packaging your hormones.

Your sexy hormone diet should be packed with organic fruits and vegetables. Sulforaphane, D-glucarate, DIM, and Indole-3-carbinol are all available in nutritional supplements in higher doses for hormone balancing. EstroSense, described on page 83, contains all these super good-estrogen-balancing ingredients.

Foods that Inhibit Bad Estrogens

Eat plenty of these foods every day to improve your estrogen-to-progesterone ratio. They are also cancer-preventing.

- broccoli
- Brussels sprouts
- buckwheat
- cabbage
- cauliflower
- figs
- flaxseeds (ground)
- green beans
- green tea, chamomile tea
- kale
- kohlrabi
- melons
- squash

Note: If you have heard that cruciferous vegetables block the uptake of thyroid hormone, please note you would have to eat several cups of broccoli, Brussels sprouts, cauliflower, cabbage, and/or kale every day for months to have them negatively affect your thyroid or inhibit thyroid hormone. These vegetables are super regulators of your hormone levels and should be eaten daily.

Foods that Enhance the Action of Progesterone

Progesterone is decreased in those exposed to excessive estrogen. Consume these foods to protect your progesterone.

- dong quai (herb)
- nutmeg
- turmeric (containing curcumin)

The Good: Lignans Promote Healthy Estrogen Levels

Ground flaxseed: look no further for the perfect food to enhance overall health, balance hormones, and protect you from diseases like breast cancer. Flaxseed is bursting with lignans. Other flaxseed components, such as fiber and the essential omega-3, also lower breast-cancer risk and protect you from the dangerous effects of estrogen. This ancient grain is the newest superfood. In the last decade, studies have shown that adding ground flaxseed to your diet can prevent and slow the progression of breast cancer.

Lignan content is highest in flaxseed, with lignan content of cranberries coming a close second. Many fruits and vegetables, such as strawberries, apricots, broccoli, cabbage, Brussels sprouts, and kale, contain lignans to a lesser extent. Some lignans are also formed by bacteria in your intestines. When plant lignans are eaten, they are metabolized by intestinal bacteria into two forms of lignans: enterodiol and enterolactone. Enterodiol can also be converted to enterolactone by intestinal bacteria. Enterolactone levels measured in serum and urine reflect the activity of intestinal bacteria in addition to the dietary intake of plant lignans. Lignans are eventually excreted in the urine. A high urinary lignan excretion corresponds with a high dietary intake of lignan-rich foods, while a low urinary excretion of lignans is associated with an increased risk of certain cancers. People at high risk of breast, prostate, and colon cancer have been found to have a urinary excretion of lignans that is significantly lower than those without cancer and those who eat vegetarian diets.

Flaxseed has a lignan concentration of 75 to 800 times that of other plant foods. Studies have indicated that a semi-vegetarian diet rich in fruits and vegetables high in lignans balances estrogens and enhances the action of the immune system. Lignans help by reducing the total estrogens and bad estrogens, balancing overall estrogen levels, thus reducing the risk of breast cancer and other estrogen-dominant conditions.

Lignans Reduce Estrogen Exposure

Flaxseed lignans exert physiological effects, such as increasing menstrual cycle length, which has also been associated with lower breast-cancer risk. A study conducted by the Department of Obstetrics-Gynecology at the University of Rochester confirmed the relationship between consuming flax-based lignans and length of menstrual cycle. The researchers evaluated the effect of the ingestion of flaxseed powder (a concentrated source of lignans), which is known to produce high concentrations of urinary lignans. The number of days from ovulation until menstruation increased in women consuming flaxseed powder. Longer cycles correspond with less exposure to the body's estrogen production. This is significant as high levels of estrogen promote breast and ovarian cancer.

The potent anti-cancer effects of lignans, especially in hormone-sensitive cancers like breast cancer, are acknowledged and accepted by the scientific community. An impressive number of studies have shown that flaxseed lignans are very potent anti-cancer agents because of their ability to block the action of too much estrogen and eliminate excess cancer-causing estrogen metabolites produced in the body. We believe ground flaxseed, with its high lignan content, is essential for the prevention and treatment of estrogen-related conditions.

In a 2002 study, researchers from the Department of Nutritional Sciences at the University of Toronto examined the effect of ground flaxseed or soy supplementation on urinary excretion of estrogen in a well-controlled study. Post-menopausal women were randomized into three groups. One group supplemented their diet with a muffin containing 25 grams of ground flaxseed; another group with regular soy; and the third group received a muffin with no supplementation (placebo). Urine samples were collected, and after 16 weeks, results data showed that ground flaxseed, not soy or the control, significantly increased urinary estrogen excretion. The researchers confirmed that ground flaxseed supplementation has a more powerful action at normalizing estrogen metabolism than regular soy and therefore may be more cancer-protective. We believe that ground flaxseed is the best choice for women with positive-estrogen-receptor breast cancer.

Flaxseed Slows Breast Cancer Cell Growth Rate

For women who already have breast cancer, ground flaxseed supplementation can slow its progression. Researchers at the University of Toronto, Princess Margaret Hospital, and The University Health Network studied a group of 39 women with newly diagnosed breast cancer tumors. Each day the women received either a muffin that contained 25 grams of ground flaxseed or a muffin that contained no ground flaxseed. The researchers found that women who received the ground flaxseed muffins experienced slower tumor growth.

This research is significant because it suggests that consumption of ground flaxseed in the diet may reduce the risk of developing breast cancer as well as slowing the progression of the disease. This research confirms population data that suggests people who consume ground flaxseed have lower breast cancer risks.

In a related study, the same researchers who did the earlier studies also examined the role of ground flaxseed in cyclical mastalgia (a syndrome of breast pain, swelling, and lumpiness) that recurs in each menstrual cycle. This syndrome has been associated with an increased breast cancer risk. The researchers found that a daily muffin with 25 grams of ground flaxseed was effective in relieving symptoms of cyclical mastalgia, without significant side effects. The researchers believe that the benefits are the result of the anti-estrogenic effects of the lignans found in ground flaxseed.

Researchers feel that one of the reasons lignans may be so beneficial for fighting breast cancer is because the lignan structure is very similar to anti-cancer compounds such as tamoxifen, which have anti-estrogenic properties. Lignans are able to displace excess estrogen by fitting into estrogen receptors. Some lignans have also been found to improve immune function; in addition, they have antiviral, antibacterial, and anti-fungal properties.

Flaxseed should be consumed daily. It should be ground fresh and added to your protein shake (whole flaxseeds act like a laxative when not ground). Cranberries are also a rich source of lignans. You could combine ground flaxseed and chopped or pureed whole cranberries (not the forms dried and sprayed with glucose) in your protein shake for a super lignan combination.

The Good: Pomegranate to Fight Estrogen Dominance

The pomegranate is a berry. The fruit is described as a many-seeded berry that is surrounded by a juicy, fleshy outer layer. Interestingly, the French word for pomegranate is "grenade." Pomegranate seeds possess anti-inflammatory properties; they inhibit cyclooxygenase and lipoxygenase enzymes, which are responsible for inflammation.

The Laboratories of Food Engineering and Biotechnology, Technion-Israel Institute of Technology, Haifa, showed that pomegranate juice has heart-protective, immune-enhancing properties similar to those of green tea, and significantly greater than those of red wine.

Pomegranate seeds have been used in Middle Eastern countries to treat menopausal and hormone concerns since written records have been kept. In human studies, pomegranate has been shown to lower the risk of heart disease; new studies show it may also have a role in preventing and treating estrogen-related cancers. Pomegranate contains compounds like punicalagin, antioxidants, flavonoids, punicic acid, and coumestrol. But it is the only plant currently known to contain estrone. Estrone in the human body is converted from estradiol in the liver and other hormones like progesterone and androgens. Estrone is often the main source of estrogen in post-menopausal women or women who have had their ovaries removed. Pomegranate's medicinal ingredients alter the way estrogen receptor cells respond to the body's own estrogen, which is important for North American women who are so overloaded with estrogen from the environment and endogenous estrogen. Pomegranate, a good phytoestrogen, blocks the activity of aromatase, the enzyme that makes estrogen from androgens. In the Petri dish, pomegranate reduced the activity of 17-beta-estradiol, making it a "safer" estrogen. Estradiol-17b is the estrogen of concern in 50 percent of breast cancers. There is no human research showing that pomegranate works the same way in women, but its ability to inhibit the activity of aromatase is very encouraging. According to other research, pomegranate juice is effective in lowering bad (LDL) cholesterol and increasing the good (HDL) cholesterol. Drink a glass of pomegranate juice every day for its heart benefits. It could be that a few ounces of pomegranate juice will keep bad estrogens at bay too.

The Ugly: Flavones that Enhance Aromatase

Isoflavones found in regular (unfermented) soy increase the production of aromatase and therefore increase levels of estrogens. Regular soy also negatively affects thyroid hormone uptake. Regular soy is a true phytoestrogen because it fits into estrogen receptors; therefore it is a strong estrogen and should be completely avoided. Bad omega-6 oils, including corn, canola, safflower, and soy oil, also enhance aromatase activity, stimulating the production of estrogen. These foods should not be eaten.

Forskolin, derived from *coleus forskolii*, is used in some weight-loss and fitness products to promote fat loss. This is one supplement you should avoid. Forskolin is another potent substance that stimulates aromatase, thus increasing estrogen. Although there is interesting research involving the use of forskolin in eye drops for treating glaucoma, oral preparations should be approached with caution if you have breast cancer or are at risk of breast cancer.

The Ugly: Alcohol Raises Bad Estrogens

It has been known for over a decade that drinking alcohol increases estrogen levels in women. This is the reason why alcohol consumption increases the risk of breast cancer. You do not have to be a big drinker—just three glasses of wine a week can increase your risk. A study in *The Journal of the American Medical Association* shows that the increases in estrogen and breast cancer risk are much higher when drinking even small amounts of alcohol while taking estrogen therapy. The study found that when post-menopausal women taking oral estradiol drank the equivalent of just half a glass of wine, the levels of estrogen circulating in their blood nearly doubled. After a drink comparable to three glasses of wine, estrogen surged more than threefold. Another study by the same researchers found that estrogen levels rose in women who drank while using the estradiol skin patch, although the increase was just 40 percent. Previous studies in men have found that alcoholic men have seriously elevated levels of estrogen. Enjoy the occasional drink, but realize if it is an everyday occurrence, it will increase estrogen to dangerous levels and negatively disrupt your balance of sexy hormones.

The Ugly Estrogenic Foods

Avoid these foods altogether or limit their intake. These foods contain either estrogen, fit into estrogen receptors, or enhance the action of aromatase, and therefore promote the production of estrogen.

- soy beans
- tofu
- soy beverages
- soy oil
- coffee (drink only organic if you like coffee)
- cotton seed oil (often found in sardines or other canned fish)
- corn oil
- hops in beer (both alcoholic and non-alcoholic)
- red clover in supplement
- commercial chicken, pork and beef
- commercial dairy products
- farmed fish
- alcohol

Quick Food Guide for Sexy Hormones

- Eat lots of foods that help block excess estrogen and stop your healthy estrogens from converting into cancer-causing estrogens.
- Increase your consumption of cruciferous vegetables (broccoli, cauliflower, Brussels sprouts, kale, cabbage or broccoli sprouts). Steam or cook them to absorb more of the indole-3-carbinol. Broccoli sprouts rich in sulforaphane and indoles should be eaten raw.
- Choose organic as often as possible; pesticides are estrogenic and cancer-causing.
- Research has shown that you need to consume a higher concentration of the anti-estrogen and aromatase-inhibiting foods than those foods that are estrogenic to keep hormones balanced.

- Eat plenty of omega-3 fatty acids from ground flaxseed, hempseeds, or wild fatty fish, including salmon, mackerel, and tuna. Include fish, or echium or flaxseed oils too.
- Do not eat omega-6 oils derived from soy, canola, or safflower. (They do not contain GLA.) Do not eat margarine, even if it is trans fatty acid free.
- Eat omega-9 fatty acids, including olive oil and nuts that are neutral in estrogenic action.
- Minimize the amount of meat or dairy products you consume, unless they are organic or free-range and hormone-free.
- Minimize alcohol intake. Alcohol increases levels of estrogen.

8

Get Physical:
Exercise Your Sexy Hormones

The human body was made to move, yet less than 25 percent of North American adults exercise on a regular basis. Instead, most people spend their non-working time performing sedentary tasks like surfing the Internet, playing video games, and watching television. (And most of our working hours are filled with sedentary tasks as well.) This lack of exercise leads to insulin resistance, hormone dysfunction, and inevitable weight gain.

Exercise enhances mood. The same feel-good hormones unleashed by dark chocolate—endorphins—are secreted by the brain during exercise. Endorphins resemble opiates in that they produce a natural pain-killing effect and an increased sense of well-being. These feel-good hormones help you handle stress successfully. As an endorphin generator, exercise is so powerful that its mood-elevating effect can last for several hours.

Regular exercise also reduces your risk of heart attack and stroke, builds strong bones, and aids weight loss. And it boosts your sexy hormones and supercharges your sex drive. Women who walk, swim, bike, dance, or perform other aerobic activities have higher levels of good cholesterol, improved estrogen-to-progesterone ratios and enhanced testosterone, and reduce their risk of breast cancer.

Soothing Hormone Havoc with Exercise

There are several important hormones affected by exercise, including estrogen, testosterone, growth hormone, endorphins, and thyroid hormone. Exercise aids menopausal symptoms by enhancing key hormones. Women who walked briskly 30 minutes per day were able to cut their incidence of hot flashes in half.

In one study, women were asked to swing their arms while they walked and keep up the pace. Researchers know that even 10 minutes of aerobic exercise can enhance the levels of good estrogen and testosterone in post-menopausal women. Think about exercise as a hormone enhancer.

Estrogens

Estrogen levels normalize when women exercise. The estrogens/exercise connection has also been evaluated in women who are at risk of breast cancer. Research has shown that women who exercise three to four times a week for 30 minutes or more have a reduced risk of breast cancer. Exercise reduces the overall size of fat cells, and it inhibits the action of aromatase—both of which are protective against breast cancer. As you now know, all hormones have an effect on other hormones, so the added benefit of exercise, which normalizes high cortisol and improves the action of insulin, is a positive effect on estrogens.

Women athletes who exercise excessively often lose their menstrual cycle due to serious reductions in estrogen with little to no changes in progesterone. Dr. Pettle and I are not suggesting this amount of exercise; putting women into a hypoestrogenic state has its own set of side effects, including osteoporosis.

Testosterone

The best way to enhance testosterone is to exercise. This hormone of desire is essential for maintaining muscle tone, stamina, and strength. Testosterone starts to naturally decline in women over the age of forty who do not exercise regularly. This is about the time you notice that slow slide in muscle tone, with your breasts racing to meet your waist. Testosterone increases your metabolism— the speed at which your body burns food as fuel—so you burn fat faster. Testosterone also makes women feel sexy and strong. Blood levels of testosterone increase with just 20 minutes of exercise and remain elevated for up to three hours after.

Growth Hormone

Growth hormone stimulates the manufacture of protein. Protein, as you learned in Chapter 6, is important for the strength of your bones and is involved in the repair and regeneration of all body cells, organs, and tissues. Growth hormone is elevated during exercise and increases your body's use of glucose and fat for fuel. This means that growth hormone maintains normal blood sugar levels and reduces body fat. This is important for female hormones because fat cells are a source of excess estrogens; reducing fat cells goes a long way to balancing hormone levels. Also, excess blood sugar elevates estrogen and cortisol levels and reduces testosterone, so by exercising you can keep your cortisol and estrogen levels healthy. Growth hormone helps you make more muscle, and muscle helps burn fat and improve the way you look and feel about yourself.

Endorphins

Endorphins are those "feel good" hormones secreted by your pituitary gland to reduce anxiety and pain, decrease your appetite, and create a feeling of euphoria. You have most likely heard of "runner's high." This high is caused by an increase in endorphins during intense exercise. If you exercise for more than 30 minutes, your blood levels of endorphins increase more than five times the level found at rest. You do not have to be a marathon runner to experience an increase in endorphins; women who performed a combination of weight and aerobic exercise (bike riding) had an increase in endorphins. And the longer you exercise, the more endorphins you produce and the longer they stay in your system.

Thyroid Hormone

Thyroxine (T4), produced by the thyroid gland, is increased by almost 35 percent during exercise. The longer you exercise, the longer your thyroxine levels will stay high after exercise. And if you incorporate regular exercise into your day, your thyroid responds by keeping thyroxine levels stable even when you are not exercising. Thyroid hormones set the metabolism in most cells. By increasing thyroxine, you increase your energy production and elevate your mood. You can read more about how essential thyroid hormones are to overall health in Chapter 1.

Do not hesitate to incorporate some type of activity into your weekly routine. You do not have to visit a gym; buy yourself some weights and use them, or skip rope, dance, swim, walk, and, of course, have sex. You will feel more like having sex because your sexy hormones will be renewed and your body image will have improved, too. Sex is not just for the young; it is also for the young at heart.

Move It or Lose It

Your muscles are the key to your exercise program. The adage "Move it or lose it" is so true when it comes to your muscles. As you age, your muscles atrophy or shrink if they are not used. As noted, the more muscles you have, the more body fat you burn. Muscles contain "tiny engines" (called mitochondria) that produce the energy that keeps you moving. Those engines need plenty of fuel, which they get from your fat stores. By simply adding 5 lbs (2 kg) of nice, lean muscle, you could burn an additional 250 calories a day or 25 lbs (11.5 kg) of fat a year. And that muscle will help you burn calories even while you are sleeping or sitting in your chair.

Having sex is definitely one of the more enjoyable ways to burn calories. Leslee Welch's *Sex Facts: A Handbook for the Carnally Curious* states that 100 calories are burned during intercourse. The calorie expenditure during sex differs due to duration, intensity, effort, frequency, and position, but the overall consensus is 100 calories are burned during one encounter.

What else can you be doing while you burn those fat calories? These are the calories expended by a 125-lb (57-kg) woman doing 10 minutes of the following activities:

Activity	Calories expended
cross-country skiing	98
cycling	42
dancing	35
downhill skiing	80
house painting	29
making beds	32
running	90
shoveling snow	65
swimming (front crawl)	40
tennis	56
walking (a leisurely stroll, perhaps to take out the trash)	29
walking (briskly)	52
weeding	49

(*Source:* John Foreyt, Baylor College of Medicine's Behavior Medicine Research Center; Kelly D. Brownell, Ph.D., Yale University; and Thomas A. Wadden, Ph.D., University of Pennsylvania School of Medicine)

You will notice that none of those activities need to involve spandex tights and someone yelling at you from the front of a gym.

Just like muscles, bones adhere to the "use it or lose it" rule; they diminish in size and strength with reduced exercise. Weight-bearing exercise like walking will help increase your bone mass. Even if you already have osteoporosis, you can regenerate bone with weight-bearing exercise. It is the most effective tool in rebuilding bone.

In addition, exercise should be called the fountain of youth. Now that you are taking nutritional supplements every day and eating a healthy diet, you will notice that your skin is glowing and firmer, your hair is thicker, and you have more energy. Add 10 minutes of exercise per day, and your muscles will become stronger, your back will be straighter, and you will have a spring in your step, just like when you were younger. Mental clarity, more strength and stamina, normal blood sugar, reversal of pre-diabetes and diabetes, and improved cardiovascular health will not only improve your overall health but ensure that you live longer too.

The Healthy Exercise Program

Follow the 10-minute weight-bearing exercise program every morning. Many women are worried that exercising with weights will build big, bulging muscles, and they will end up looking like Arnold Schwarzenegger. They will not, and neither will you. It takes years of dedication, a serious weight-lifting program, and diet changes to look like Arnold. You want sexy, beautiful arms that do not have that jiggling, hanging skin between your armpit and elbow. You want a chin line that is not sagging toward your breasts. Exercise, combined with a healthy diet, will stop your thighs from slapping together, diminish your cellulite, and firm up your breasts and stomach. We know from research investigating women's body image and body esteem that exercising will also improve your body esteem, and your sex drive will increase when you are feeling better about yourself.

We want you to follow the 10-minute exercise program every morning to rev up your metabolic rate, which aids calorie burning throughout the day. When you exercise, your levels of cortisol (the stress hormone) naturally rise for several hours before they level off. This is why you should avoid evening exercise, if possible; high night-time cortisol levels can disrupt your sleep. (If you have a lot of weight to lose, read Lorna's book *The Body Sense Natural Diet: Six Weeks to a Slimmer, Healthier You.*)

Effortless Exercise

You can no longer avoid exercise with the excuse that you have a busy life. Exercise can be effortless and easily incorporated into your lifestyle.

Start by going to a fitness store or the fitness section of your local department store and purchasing soft, wrap-around Velcro weights for your wrists and ankles. They can be found in 1- to 5-lb (0.5- to 2-kg) sizes. If you have not exercised in a while, start with the 1- or 2-lb (0.5- or 10-kg) size and work your way up to 5 lbs (2 kg). The beauty of Velcro weights is that when you are walking, doing housework, or gardening, you can wear them. They increase the amount of fat you burn and help build nice, strong muscles effortlessly. That is what you want—effortless muscle gain and fat loss. When Lorna gets ready in the morning, she straps them on. When you watch television, you can lift your arms up and down throughout the program and tone those upper arms. The more slowly you do the lift, the better your workout. No more sagging skin on the backs of your arms—all while watching television.

Rebounding for Stability and Cellulite Reduction

A rebounder is a small, circular mini-trampoline that is another inexpensive tool you can use to get fit. It usually stands about 8 inches (20.5 cm) off the floor and is about 36 inches (91.5 cm) in diameter. It fits perfectly under your bed or in the back of your closet when not in use. Ten minutes of rebounding is equivalent to 30 minutes of walking. Some models also come with stability bars, so you can hold onto the bar while you bounce—you can use it even if you feel you have poor balance.

The best thing about rebounding is that you will also stimulate your lymphatic system, which is the drainage and filtration system that also produces infection-fighting cells. Your lymphatic system does not have a pump to move the fluid (lymph) that performs cellular cleansing. You must exercise (or deep breathe) to promote movement of lymph through this system of vessels and tubes. One added benefit of a healthy lymphatic system is cellulite reduction. Cellulite, that orange-peel-like skin, forms when fluid distorts the cells in and around your fat, creating dimples in your skin. Women, because they have more body fat, develop it more often than men.

Rebounding also improves your stability, which is essential to ensure you do not fall or feel unstable as you age. Strap on your Velcro weights while you use the rebounder, and get added weight-loss benefits. Rebounding also benefits your cardiovascular system. Rebounders are available at fitness stores and most department stores. Rebound during your favorite television show. No more guilt about watching television because you are now multitasking. Your children will love it too.

The Sexy Hormone 42-Day Program that Gets Results: Fitness Fun in 10 Minutes a Day

For this program, you need to buy yourself a set of dumbbell weights. These are widely available. Usually they come in three different sizes. For women, start with the 3-, 5-, and 8-lb (1.5-, 2-, and 3.5-kg) sizes. Do not start with weights that are too heavy, or you may injure yourself or give up due to difficulty. To choose the correct weight for your ability, pick a weight you can lift at least 10 times without stopping. Pick up the dumbbell, bend your arm at the elbow, and then slowly lift the weight up toward your shoulder. Do this 10 times. If you can do this easily, then you need a heavier weight. If you have a very hard time doing this 10 times, then you need a lighter weight. For the heavier weight, add 2 or 3 lbs (1 or 1.5 kg) and for the lighter weight, delete 2 or 3 lbs (1 or 1.5 kg), and then you will have the right mix of weights to get started.

You may also wish to use a thin mat or a folded blanket to lie on during some of the floor exercises. You should do a bit of warm-up before you begin.

- Stretch your arms to the ceiling. Breathe deeply. Then reach to the floor. Breathe deeply. Repeat 6 times.
- Jog in place for 30-60 seconds.
- Lie on your belly. Place your hands comfortably beneath your shoulders so you can push your chest off the floor and stretch your upper body toward the ceiling. This is not a push up, but more like a yoga position to stretch your upper body muscles and elongate your back.
- Drink water to ensure you are well hydrated before you begin, and remember to drink more water between the two sets of exercises. Dehydration can make you feel weak and dizzy.

The goal is to eventually do three sets of each exercise with successively heavier weights. Do the first set with the lightest weight and work toward the heaviest weight for the last set. Depending on your level of fitness, you may be able to do this easily. Other people will be able to do only a few repetitions with the lightest weight. Whatever your fitness level, build on your previous success. If on Day 1 you can lift the lightest weight only three times, then on Day 2 try to lift it four times. Then move on to a heavier weight and so on, until you finally reach the goal of three sets of 10 repetitions using successively heavier weights. The fact that you are trying is success. And remember, no matter what your age or fitness level, you will be able to do these exercises. So just have fun.

For the next 42 days, you will do 10 minutes of exercises each morning, five days a week, to a stronger, sexier, fitter you. You will be surprised how quickly your body will respond by becoming more toned and shapely.

Week 1, Day 1

Shapely Arms

Choose the lightest weight. Hold a dumbbell in each hand. Stand with your feet shoulder-width apart, with your arms at your sides. Breathe in a couple of deep breaths, then exhale and curl both arms to a 90-degree angle. Make sure your elbows are at your sides and not bending outward. Hold for two seconds. Inhale as you lower the weight. If you are pushing your stomach out and bending backward to compensate for the weight, the weight is too heavy. Make sure you are standing straight and strong. Exhale and repeat 10 times. Do not pause between curls. Next, pick up the medium weight, and repeat 10 curls. Then choose the heaviest weight, and repeat 10 curls. If you find that you cannot complete the last set of 10 curls, then use the medium weight for both the second and third set of repetitions. It is best to do the required 30 curls even if you have to use the lightest weight initially. This exercise also makes your neck muscles tighten up, so your chin stops sagging.

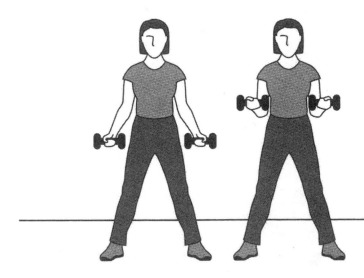

Arms without Wings

This is the exercise that makes the backs of your arms beautiful while also toning your abdominal muscles. Lie on the floor with your knees bent and the soles of your feet flat on the floor. Hold the lightest dumbbell beside your ears with your elbows pointing up to the ceiling. Exhale as you raise the weight from your ears toward the ceiling. Your arms should be straight up now. Hold for two seconds and inhale as you lower the weight. Repeat 10 times. Do not pause between curls. Next, choose the medium weight and repeat 10 curls. Then pick up the heaviest weight and repeat 10 curls. To really get the benefit of this exercise, hold your abdominal muscles tight and push your lower back into the floor after you inhale. Focus on your breathing. If you can't complete all three sets with successively heavier weights, just use the lowest weight at the beginning and within a couple of weeks you will be able to progress to the heaviest weight.

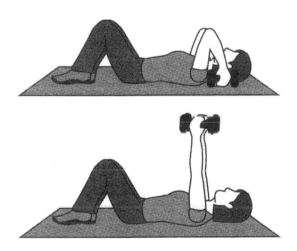

Week 1, Day 2

Sexy Calves

Stand tall with your feet shoulder-width apart. Hold the lightest dumbbell in your hands with your arms at your side. Keep your shoulders back but relaxed, not pulled up toward your ears. Exhale as you raise your heels. You should now be up on the balls of your feet, but not so high that you end up on your tiptoes. Hold for two seconds. Inhale as you slowly lower your heels. Repeat for 10 lifts. Next, pick up your medium weight and repeat. Then choose the heaviest weight, and repeat for 10 more lifts. Beautiful calves are the end result of this exercise. Once this exercise becomes effortless, instead of moving to heavier weights, use Velcro weights on your ankles while holding the dumbbells for increased results.

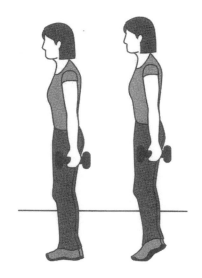

Tight Thighs and Cellulite Reducer

This is a favorite exercise because it gets the fastest results. Stand with your feet slightly wider apart than your shoulders, with your arms at your sides. Keep your back straight. Exhale as you squat down to about 90 degrees with your butt out as if you were going to sit down. Your knees should be in line with your toes if you are doing this exercise correctly. Hold for one or two seconds. Inhale as you straighten up. This is called a squat. Do 10 squats, then rest for a count of 10. Repeat 10 more squats. Soon you will be able to do an additional 10 squats, for a full 30 squats. This exercise sculpts great legs and helps tighten the skin on your upper thighs and butt to reduce cellulite. Once you get very good at this exercise, add the Velcro weights to your wrists.

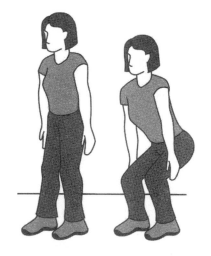

Week 1, Day 3

Chest and Breast Press

Lie on your back with your knees bent and the soles of your feet flat on the floor. Hold your lightest dumbbells in each hand. Stretch your arms out from your body along the floor like a cross, then bend your arms at the elbows toward the ceiling. Exhale as you push the weight up toward the ceiling, straightening your arms. Hold for a count of two, and inhale as you bring the weight back to the starting position. Repeat for 10 presses. Then change to your medium weight, and repeat for 10 presses. Finally, choose your heaviest weight and repeat. This exercise makes for strong arms and builds chest muscles. It tightens sagging breasts in women.

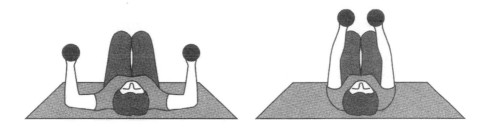

Tight Abdomen

We all want tight abdominals. You may be able to do only a few of these exercises at the beginning, which is fine. Start slowly and add a few more repetitions every time you do this exercise, but try to do as many as you can, up to 10 in each set.

Lie on your back with your knees bent and the soles of your feet flat on the floor. Cross your arms over your chest. Exhale as you curl up toward your knees. If you can raise yourself only a few inches off the floor, do not worry—it will get easier. Make sure your lower back is not arched upward. Repeat as many times as you can. Remember, the more you do this exercise, the tighter your abdominal muscles will become and the sooner the inches will fall off. You can do it!

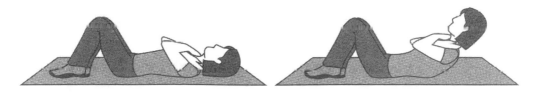

Week 1, Day 4

Butt Lift

Kneel on all fours on a rug or mat. You should have your hands and feet positioned so you feel steady. While keeping your head up off the mat, exhale and raise your right leg until your thigh is even with your back, then push your foot toward the ceiling. Hold for one second and inhale as you return your knee to the original position. Do 10 repetitions for the right leg, and then repeat for the left leg. This exercise gives you the greatest butt lift. As you get better at this exercise, increase the number of repetitions to 15 per leg and then 20 per leg.

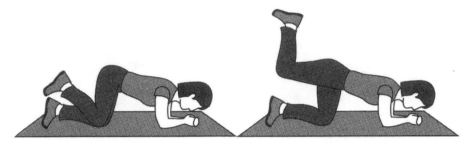

Even Better Butt Lift

Pick a sturdy chair that will not move or tip, and lie on the floor on your back with the chair at your feet. Place your palms flat on the floor with your arms at your sides. Lift your legs and put your heels firmly on the chair. Exhale as you contract the backs of your thighs and lift your butt toward the ceiling. Hold for two seconds. Inhale as you slowly lower your body back to the starting position. Do 10 repetitions. Stop, rest for 10 seconds, do 10 more repetitions, and then the last 10 repetitions. Once you feel strong doing 10 repetitions, add another five, and so on.

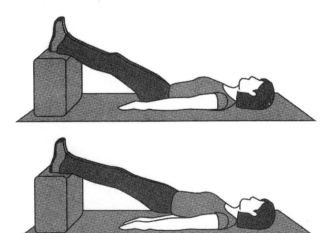

Week 1, Day 5

Shoulder Lift

Stand with your feet shoulder-width apart, your back straight, and your arms at your sides. Grip your lightest dumbbell in each hand, then raise your extended arms level with your shoulders; turn your palms toward the ceiling. Then turn your palms down, and hold for one second. Inhale as you lower the weight. Repeat 10 times. Choose your medium weight and repeat 10 times. Finally, complete 10 more repetitions with your heaviest weight. If you push out your stomach and arch your back, you are using too heavy a weight. Either use a lighter weight or reduce the number of repetitions.

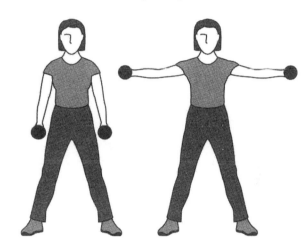

No More Back Fat

Put your lightest weights on either side of an armless chair, and sit down. Lean forward and down; pick up a dumbbell in each hand. Still in that position, exhale as you lift the dumbbells, pointing your elbows toward the ceiling. Stop the lift when your hands are at the height of your thighs. Hold for two seconds, and inhale as you lower your arms. Repeat 10 times. Next, use your medium weights and repeat 10 times. Finally, choose the heaviest weight and repeat. This exercise gets rid of the back flab that women accumulate around their bra strap, while making stronger back muscles.

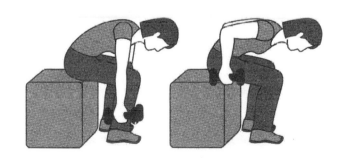

Week 1, Day 6 and Day 7

Go for a walk in the park, bicycle with your kids, swim, golf, play tennis, garden, or go dancing. Do anything that requires you to move your body. Add some exercise variety today and tomorrow. You have done fabulously and should be proud of yourself. Even after five days most people feel stronger and want to exercise. It is so easy to fit 10 minutes of exercise into your day. If you miss a day because you slept through your alarm, just remember to do your exercises the next day. You will succeed with this program because it is easy.

Week 2, Day 1

Arms and Shoulders

Sit in an armless chair. Make sure the chair has a straight back and is hard. Tighten your stomach muscles when you do this exercise and keep your back straight. Pick up your lightest weight. Raise your arms out from your sides until they are even with your shoulders. Then, bend your elbows into a 90-degree angle from your shoulders (make each arm an L-shape), then push the weight toward the ceiling while exhaling. Hold for two seconds, then inhale as you lower the weight to shoulder height. Do 10 repetitions if possible. This is a challenging exercise, so start with as many repetitions as you can do, building up to 10 in a set. Then, as you get stronger, do a second set of repetitions with your medium weight, and eventually a third set with the heaviest weight. Your shoulders will get that lovely curve, your breasts will lift, and your arms will be strong.

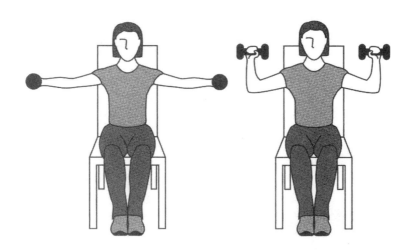

Shapely Arms

Stand with your feet comfortably apart. Hold a dumbbell in
each hand, your arms at your
sides with your elbows slightly
bent forward. Then lift the
weight so your elbows bend into
an L-shape. Hold for two seconds. Remember to exhale as
you raise the weight and inhale
as you return to the starting position. Do 10 repetitions and then
repeat with the medium weight.
Do a final set of 10 repetitions
with the heaviest weight.

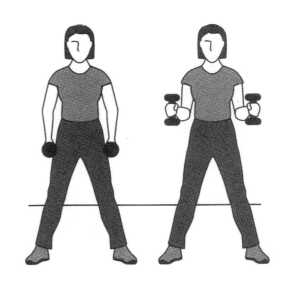

Week 2, Day 2

Slim Thighs

Stand straight with your hands at your sides. Then step forward with your right leg and
bend your knee in a 90-degree angle (L-shape). Keep your knee above your foot. The
knee should not extend past your foot. Hold this position for two seconds. Inhale as
you return to the original position. You may be able to do only a few of these to begin
with. That is fine. The key is to do this exercise with strength and precision and not

wobble, so if you can do only
two lunges with strength, then
do only two. Work up to 10 repetitions for each leg. This exercise makes the top of your
thighs nice and shapely, and
your butt muscles will tighten
along with your abdominal
muscles. This exercise is not
performed with weights, but
you could eventually do it holding your dumbbells or with
Velcro weights.

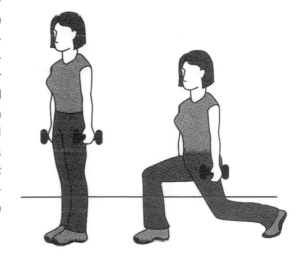

Inner Thigh

Lie on your side, using your lower arm with your elbow bent as a pillow to support your head, and your top arm with your elbow bent as a brace to keep your upper body from toppling forward. Align your legs with your body. Inhale and then exhale and raise your leg up toward the ceiling. Hold for two seconds. Initially you may not be able to lift it very high, but as you get stronger you will be able to lift it above shoulder height. Do 10 repetitions. Repeat on your other side with the other leg. This exercise firms your thighs and stops them from rubbing together. Once you get good at this exercise, add your Velcro ankle weights.

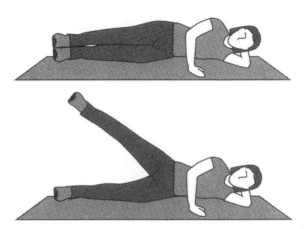

Week 2, Day 3

Back and Arms

Sit in an armless chair. Keep your back straight, and hold one dumbbell with both hands in front of you. Hold it firmly but comfortably. Exhale, and lift the dumbbell straight over your head; your arms should be on either side of your ears. Then inhale, and bend your arms back at the elbow so the dumbbell drops back level with the top of your head. Your elbows should be bent at a 90-degree angle. Hold for two seconds. It is easiest when you keep your elbows closer to your head, but do not squeeze your head. Exhale, and then bring the dumbbell back up above your head. Repeat 10 times. Move to the medium weight and repeat. Once you are strong, you will be able to complete three sets with small, medium, and heavy weights. If you don't feel confident using the weight above your head, do this exercise with your Velcro weights strapped on your wrists.

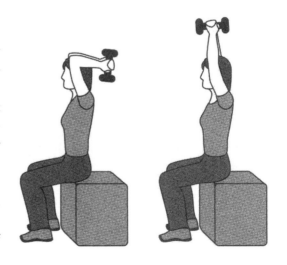

Shoulders, Arms, and Back

Stand with your back straight, your knees comfortably bent, and your feet about shoulder-width apart. Pick up the lightest weights. Let your arms hang straight down in front of your thighs and hold your dumbbells with palms turned in toward your thighs. Keeping your elbow slightly bent, raise the right dumbbell to eye level while exhaling. Now inhale and slowly lower the right dumbbell back to your thigh. Repeat with the left arm. Do 10 repetitions with each arm. Then switch to the medium weights, and repeat 10 times for each arm. Eventually you will be able to do another 10 with the heaviest weights.

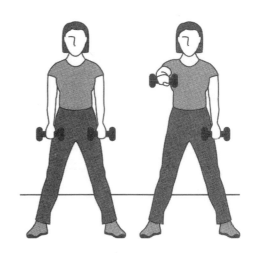

Week 2, Day 4

Great Legs

Stand with your back against the wall, your feet shoulder-width apart, and your hands on your thighs. Exhale as you slowly slide down the wall until you are in a sitting position. Hold this position for two seconds. Inhale and return to the upright position. Repeat this exercise 10 times. If you want to make this exercise more challenging, add Velcro weights to your wrists.

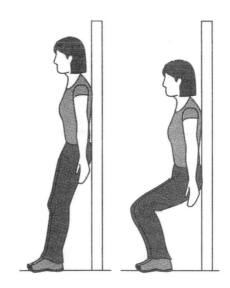

Better Butt

Stand with your feet comfortably apart and with your hands on your thighs. Squeeze your butt muscles and lower yourself into a sitting position. Hold for the count of two. Exhale and return to the upright position. Repeat this exercise 10 times. Rest and repeat 10 times. Then rest and repeat another 10 times. Initially many people will be able to do only one set. As you get stronger, you will be able to complete the full three sets. When you get really good at this exercise, add Velcro weights strapped to your wrists or hold dumbbells in your hands.

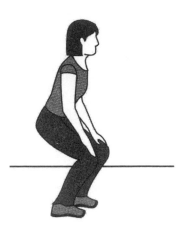

Week 2, Day 5

Long, Lean Leg Muscles

Stand tall with your feet comfortably apart, your arms at your sides. Place a chair beside you to use as a balance. Lift your right leg until you have your knee bent at a 90-degree angle. Straighten your leg in front of you, and hold it for two seconds. Do this exercise 10 times, and then repeat on the other leg 10 times. Repeat for a total of three sets on each leg. This exercise is designed to give you core balance. Once you become strong, add Velcro weights to your ankles, and watch those leg muscles become lean and beautiful.

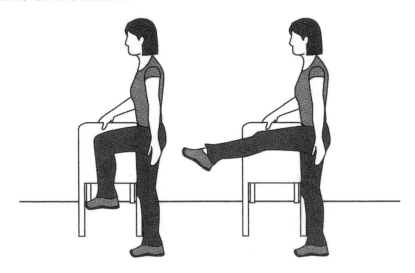

Flat Lower Abdominals

Get into a kneeling position with your hands placed firmly on the floor. Make sure your hips are over your knees and your shoulders are directly above your hands. Keep your back and tummy muscles in a relaxed position. Let your tummy sag down. Then gently use your stomach muscles to pull your belly button into your lower spine. Hold the position for 10 seconds. Then relax. Repeat this exercise 10 times. This quickly fixes sagging lower abdominals.

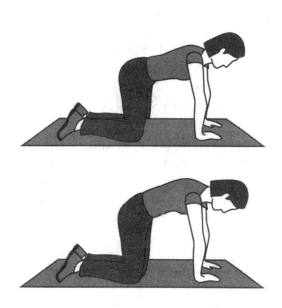

Week 2, Day 6 and Day 7

Have fun and spend time being active with your family. You have just finished two weeks of amazing exercises, and I am sure by now your muscles are getting stronger. You should be proud of yourself. Accelerate the process by walking, riding your bike, gardening, and doing other physical activities.

Repeat these exercises in this order for the next four weeks, and watch the inches melt off your body and your muscles start showing. Your body will respond quickly to these exercises, your skin will become clearer, and you will be able to breathe better. This 10-minute exercise program is so easy to do and provides such fast results you will want to continue it every day for the rest of your life. But the best part is feeling strong and fit and in control of your body.

Fitness has to be fun, or you will not do it. Ask yourself when you stopped exercising. Was it because you had a baby? Or did you stop when you started working overtime at your job? There is always a reason. Ask yourself why, and then tell yourself you will not let anything get in the way of attaining a flat stomach, better balance, and strong muscles. You'll love seeing those rolls around your abdomen and the jiggling skin between your armpit and elbow disappear. You'll start wearing short sleeves again and choosing pants that do not have an elastic waistband. People will remark on how fabulous you look. They'll want to know your secret. And your sex life will improve, too, because you feel great about your new body.

You are never too old or too unfit to begin an exercise program; in fact, increasing age and lack of fitness are all the more reason to start. Study after study has come to the same conclusion: inactivity promotes illness, and the right exercise for the condition can work wonders in reversing or delaying that illness. Activity encourages the flow of oxygen and other nutrients and enhances mood.

9

The Anatomy of Great Sex

Beyond improving your general muscle tone and bone strength, exercise is an important contributor to healthy hormone levels. And sex is an important contributor to your overall fitness. Here are some more reasons to do your basic fitness routine, and some tips on improving your chances of getting some satisfaction.

Sex is Good Exercise

Research performed back in 1983 and published in the *Journal of the American Medical Association* found that women who had sex more than 3 times per month had less thinning of the vaginal wall and significantly higher levels of androgens, including androstenedione and testosterone, along with luteinizing hormone, than women who had sex less than 10 times per year. Sex also strengthens the vaginal wall, which is important in preventing urinary and uterine prolapse and also ensures you do not suffer tears, pain, or dryness due to excessive thinning. Having a stronger vaginal wall will also give you more intense orgasms. Interaction between the chemicals in male ejaculate and a woman's hormones also has a beneficial effect on the vagina and female sex hormones.

Kegel for Your Sex Muscles

Beyond having sex, you can exercise your vaginal muscles too. The pelvic floor exercise popularized by Dr. Arnold Kegel is not new. It has been used by the Taoists of China and the Yogis of India and is still practiced today for health, longevity, and sexual gratification. Kegel exercises should be performed daily to develop strong vaginal muscles, prevent prolapsed uterus and bladder by strengthening muscles, and eliminate urinary incontinence and urinary frequency. They will also improve the intensity and duration of your orgasms. If you sneeze or laugh, and urine leaks out, you need to Kegel. (You may also need estriol: see page 71 for more information.)

You can Kegel anytime. Start Kegeling by squeezing the muscles of your vagina and urethra, then relax, then squeeze the muscles again, and relax. Kegel often. Do it while you are at work, when driving in your car, or waiting in a line-up. It is similar to the action you use to stop and start a urine stream or prevent gas from escaping. You can purchase an exerciser called the Energie Kegel to make the exercise more effective. Dr. Sue Johansen of the *Talk Sex* television show recommends this little device. This Kegel exerciser can be purchased online at www.natural-contours.com. (You will also find wonderful small, effective vibrators at this site.)

Exploring Your Sexual Anatomy

Too much focus is put on the "dys" in dysfunctional sex drive. Dr. Pettle and I have no desire to contribute to that. If you think you have never had an orgasm and you would like to experience one, it may simply be that you have not found what works for you. We can help you with some simple suggestions. At different times of your life, you will experience different desires and drives due to hormones being out of balance, stress, medications, and more. Do you think you are dysfunctional when it comes to sex? It is likely you are not. This section is about the physical, functional side of sex.

According to the *Journal of the American Medical Association* between 22 and 28 percent of women in all different age categories have never had an orgasm. However, when women are taught how their female genitalia function, they are able to experience this type of pleasure. So let's understand the beautiful female anatomy. All the structures we are discussing can provide great pleasure from sexual stimulation.

We have provided a basic diagram of what the female genitalia look like, but there are hundreds of variations. Take a mirror and get to know your genitals. Not only is this important for your sexual health, but you can also observe if you have any bumps, moles, or growths that should be evaluated. One woman told us that she did not want her husband to look at her "down there" because she was deformed. She thought because she had very long labia minora that she was not normal. We explained that Mother Nature does not provide "one size fits all" when it comes to physical assets and that some women have long labia minora, while other women have labia minora that look like small, flat testicles. Some women have a large clitoral hood, while others have a small one. All are normal.

Sexual Anatomy on the Outside: The Mound of Venus

Venus, the Roman goddess of love and beauty (her Greek counterpart is the goddess Aphrodite), has lent her name to the external female sexual anatomy. The "Mound of Venus" is a lovely term for the most beautiful and sacred parts of the female body. It is sad that so many women have never looked at their genitalia. It is equally sad that many women have been told this part of their body is not beautiful. The fact that women can bear children and nourish them tells the world how wonderful the female body is, and that wonder includes female genitalia.

The term "vulva" includes the mons pubis, the clitoris, the labia majora, the labia minora, the perineum, the urethra, and the anus. Some women have pubic hair from the anus to the mons pubis to their thighs. Others have very little.

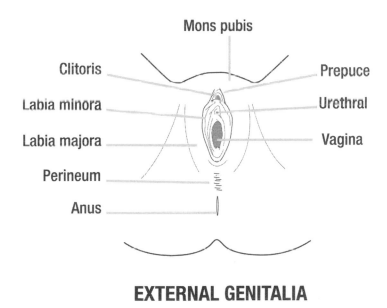

Mons pubis

Clitoris

Prepuce

Labia minora

Urethral

Labia majora

Vagina

Perineum

Anus

EXTERNAL GENITALIA

The **mons pubis**, also called mons venus, is the soft mound of fatty flesh over the female pubic bone. During puberty, the mons pubis becomes covered with hair. This area is rich in nerves and can be a source of sexual arousal and pleasure when stimulated or pressure is applied.

The **clitoris** is a very sensitive organ that contains a high concentration of nerve endings. It is covered by the clitoral hood (**prepuce**) and is at the top of the labia, just above the **urethra** (where urine is released). The clitoris has a small head called the glans. The glans has been called the small penis. The only function of the clitoris is to provide you with pleasure.

The clitoris is an extensive organ. You can only see the small head, which is about the size of a pea, but Helen O'Connell, an Australian urologist, showed that the clitoris is actually quite large and extends back into the pelvis. The clitoris engorges with blood upon arousal. A healthy vascular system is just as important for women as it is for men when it comes to ensuring adequate blood flow so an orgasm is possible. Many women have to have clitoral stimulation to achieve orgasm. Orgasms can be clitoral or vaginal. Surveys of women tend to show clitoral orgasms are more common.

The labia are composed of the **labia majora** or the outer lips and the **labia minora** or the inner lips. Pubic hair can grow on the outer lips but not on the inner lips. During arousal the labia darken in color and become engorged with blood. Thinning of both labia can occur as a result of low levels of testosterone and estrogens. In severe cases, the labia majora and minora shrink and fuse together, creating a very painful condition. Aging, menopause, and hormones out of balance can also change the labia.

The **perineum** is the hairless area between the vagina and anus. It is composed of an internal network of muscles. Women who have had children may have had the perineum cut (called an episiotomy) to make a larger opening for the baby's head during delivery or the perineum could have torn during childbirth. Some women lose sensation in this area after an episiotomy; others do not. Many women find stroking or pressure on this area quite pleasurable.

Sexual Anatomy on the Inside

We have already discussed some of the female internal organs, including the ovaries, uterus, cervix, and fallopian tubes. Your vagina and especially the G-spot have specific sexual functions that are often overlooked in health class.

The **vagina** is a muscular, tube-shaped cavity leading from the vulva to the **uterus**. It is usually around 4 to 5 inches in length and can expand to accommodate a penis or the passage of a baby. It can also contract and will hug or grasp a penis or tampon. The lining of the vagina is similar to the mucous membranes inside your mouth. Lubrication occurs on the vaginal lining, keeping the vagina moist and free of bacteria. Lubrication can be reduced by out-of-balance hormones. Some women notice that they are not as lubricated just after their period, childbirth, or during peri-menopause and post-menopause, whereas during ovulation and sexual arousal, lubrication may be increased.

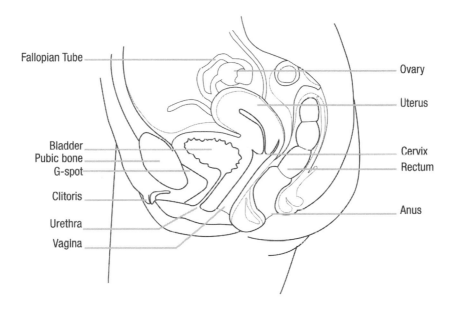

Just inside the vagina is a ridge of muscles that tighten around the penis during intercourse. Most women report that they have little feeling past the outer third of the vagina.

Beverly Whipple and John D. Perry identified the **G-spot** (Grafenberg spot after the German physician who first suggested the presence of the G-spot). The G-spot is about the size of a bean on the front wall of the vagina (belly button side), approximately in front of the urethra. The G-spot is sensitive in some women; when stimulated, it becomes engorged and will increase to about the size of a nickel. Some women have intense orgasms when the G-spot is stimulated during sexual play. Others have never found a G-spot. Most women have a much easier time achieving orgasm through clitoral stimulation.

The Big O

Orgasm is not the ultimate goal in a sexual experience. But it is a delightful, satisfying end to a time of intense pleasure either with a partner or by yourself. Women have told us that they do not have to have an orgasm to feel satisfied during lovemaking, although they sometimes find it necessary to fake an orgasm so their partner is content and can "come." Other women are not sure if they have ever had an orgasm.

Men and women experience orgasm differently. You will not hear a man say, "I don't think I have ever had an orgasm" because their climax is easy to see. Women may have pelvic floor orgasms, clitoral orgasms, or nipple-stimulated orgasms, to name a few, and these orgasms may be intense or mild. Most men are not aware that the vagina has very little sensation past the first third where the majority of nerves reside, so clitoral stimulation, along with other sexually arousing pleasures like kissing, touching, and petting are essential for women to become excited enough for vaginal penetration. Without enough foreplay, most women will not be ready to accept the man, and intercourse can be painful.

Beyond Sexual Anatomy

During the 1960s William H. Masters and Virginia E. Johnson (Masters and Johnson) brought sex out of the closet in their book *Human Sexual Response*. In their laboratory they were the first to observe and describe female sexual response, including orgasm. They found females responded in four phases: excitement, plateau, orgasm, and resolution.

In the excitement phase the vagina and clitoris begin to swell. Vaginal lubrication begins with secretions from the vaginal lining. Breathing rate also increases.

During the plateau phase the genitals become engorged with blood, causing the vaginal opening to narrow so it can grip the penis when inserted. A woman's nipples can become erect. The skin color of the labia deepens.

Orgasm phase is achieved when the clitoris is stimulated or enough pressure is applied to the cervix or surrounding vaginal wall to cause a build-up of tension or engorgement, eventually leading to a climax. Some women ejaculate from the urethra. Some women may think they are releasing a small amount of urine, but an analysis of the ejaculate revealed a chemical called acid phosphatase. Not all women ejaculate, nor is your pleasure diminished if you do not.

Resolution is a return to a non-aroused state. Some women feel alive and awake during this phase.

We must point out that no two individuals are the same. There is a complex interplay of factors involved in arousal and orgasm. For women especially, lovemaking is more pleasurable when foreplay and lots of stimulation are added to the mix. Both mental and physical stimulation are needed.

Loving Yourself

We mentioned earlier that orgasm does not have to happen every time you make love, but it is a nice conclusion. If you do not have a partner or you have not been able to have an orgasm with your partner, loving yourself is a sexually satisfying option for achieving orgasm. It is also a great way to teach your partner what you need to reach orgasm. The key to the best possible orgasm is to be honest and open with your partner about what you like and don't like and what you need to feel great, whether it be a certain type of touch, kissing, or caressing.

The "M word" has long been surrounded with taboos. Many illnesses have been attributed to masturbation—everything from hairy palms to blindness. Infants and children touch their genitals because it is pleasurable and makes them feel good. Depending on what you were told as a child by your parents to curb this behavior, you may think that masturbation is either a healthy, normal practice or a "dirty" one. Some people believe that masturbation should be censured because it stops people from seeking out another for sexual intimacy. Others believe if we promote masturbation, people will stop seeking out dangerous encounters that could lead to diseases like HIV, syphilis, or HPV infections. Whatever your opinion of masturbation, let us start off by saying masturbation is not only normal, it is healthy. Women and men equally enjoy masturbation.

According to Lou Paget in her book *The Big O, Orgasms: How to Have Them, Give Them, and Keep Them Coming*, almost 70 percent of women cannot reach orgasm through penetration. There is nothing wrong with you if you are in this group; this is quite normal. Manual stimulation of the clitoris is required by most women. Paget also says that, for most women, the reason for no or few orgasms with a partner boils down to two issues: one, she isn't being stimulated in a way that works for her; or two, she is not mentally present. As a result, it is often easier for a woman to be orgasmic on her own.

Self-Pleasure Steps

You have looked at the anatomical drawings of female genitals, and, we hope, you have gotten out a mirror and checked out your own so you know where all the parts are.

Put on some nice music, have a bath with your favorite aromatherapy products, light a candle, lock your bedroom door, put your lubricant on the bedside table, and relax. Don't forget to breathe. Breathing is one of the most important aspects of great orgasms.

Touch your genitals—they are a pleasure center like no other. Try stroking or massaging all the areas of your genitals to find out how it feels. Some women like to use two fingers together. They begin stroking or rubbing on the upper part of the hood of the clitoris. Apply pressure to the mons pubis, massage your nipples, and caress the inner areas of your thighs. Explore the inner third of your vagina. Contract your vaginal muscles, and release; contract, and release. Experiment with different pressures and movements. Breathe in and out in a rhythmic manner. Get in tune with how your genitals feel. Women are often disconnected from this area of their bodies. It is time to reconnect.

Fantasize. Dream up images that make you feel sexy. Remember: no negative self-talk. If all of a sudden you find you are chastising yourself for having these thoughts, remind yourself that you are a beautiful, healthy, sexy woman who deserves to have great orgasms. There are no "dirty" thoughts.

Self-stimulation is great if you are single or simply alone because it keeps your muscles working. Pelvic floor muscles get quite a workout during orgasm. The rhythmic contractions of orgasm give the walls of your vagina a workout too. Plus, orgasm can help those who have reduced lubrication by getting the secreting glands to keep working. Masturbation helps relieve sexual tension when you are without a partner. No boyfriend, no worries; masturbation to the rescue. For women who have partners with erectile problems, masturbation is a release and can take the pressure off his performance. And if you have yet to tell your partner how to satisfy you, then self-stimulation on your own is effective.

This experience is not about achieving orgasm. It is about getting to know what makes you feel great. If you reach orgasm, that's wonderful. Betty Dodson, a famous sexologist, has written an excellent book called *Sex for One*, designed to teach self-stimulation. Every woman should get this book as a graduation present to help her understand her body and feel good about her genitals. *Sex for One* is not about eliminating your partner from the equation; it is about getting to know yourself. If you are with a partner, this will only enhance your relationship and open the door to some hot lovemaking. Masturbation is fun and will put you in touch with your body and connect your body to your mind.

Vibrators and the History of "Hysteria"

Rachel P. Maines, author of the scholarly book *The Technology of Orgasm: Hysteria, the Vibrator, and Women's Sexual Satisfaction*, discusses how, during the late nineteenth and early twentieth centuries, a myriad of women's complaints associated with the "willful difficulties of the uterus" were medically treated with an assortment of vibrators designed to achieve orgasm. The medical profession of the time profitably treated a common condition of the day called "hysteria" with the medical intervention of vulva massage to relieve tension and bring the woman back to a "normal" state. Up until the 1920s, doctors did their duty to help "hysterical" women plagued by anxieties, fainting spells, and some conditions that are now classed as neuroses by inducing orgasm in their female patients. So many women required treatment (one doctor catalogued the possible symptoms in 76 pages, commenting that the list was "incomplete"), that expensive, large, mechanical vibrators were invented to take the pressure off manual manipulation and ensure more women could be treated faster. (This also ensured a healthy revenue stream for the physicians and fended off an attempt to have the treatment re-assigned to midwives.) Hysteria needing relief became an epidemic among middle- and upper-class women of the day, and many women's sexual needs were satisfied by their doctors. (Today's doctors would be prosecuted and lose their license to practice if they were found providing such a "service"!)

Near the end of the century, vibrators eventually became smaller and were sold as home appliances. Dr. Maines states that vibrators were the fifth household device to be electrified after, in order of importance, the sewing machine, fan, kettle, and toaster. The Sears and Roebuck catalogue sold vibrators for external use only as an aid to women's good health—to deliver rosy cheeks and youthful energy. Then vibrator advertising disappeared, and vibrators did not return to the public's attention until the sexual revolution of the late sixties and seventies. Today, the Sears catalogue carries vibrators as massage tools.

Vibrators can provide a different type of stimulation than what can be achieved with the human touch. Today, all kinds of women have vibrators: doctors, lawyers, mothers, and grandmothers. Vibrators are in more households than you can imagine. And no longer do you have to walk into a sex shop to buy your toys. They are now available online and at your local drugstore. Home sex toy parties similar to Tupperware parties are now commonplace.

Dr. Pettle and I like the Natural Contours line of vibrators (found at www.natural-contours.com). These vibrators are small, beautiful, not overwhelming, and they work. Or you can go to www.sharperimage.com and purchase a small massage vibrator. See the Appendix for information on the types we recommend. Your local pharmacy will sell a myriad of muscle massagers that are also very effective vibrators for self-stimulation. Do not buy the giant massager. It might be a bit too intense. You do not have to spend a lot of money; most vibrators are between $20 and $40. And you do not have to get too fancy with rabbit ears or 20 settings. Vibrators come in all shapes and sizes. Pick one you will feel comfortable using.

Vibrators can be for internal or external use, but most vibrators are for stimulating the outer areas. If you are new to using a vibrator, start by putting it on low speed. Many vibrators have a range of speeds, from low to intense. Start on low, and place the vibrator on the mons pubis. Move it around until you find an area that feels sensitive and responsive, and alternate speeds. Some women place the vibrator just above the hood of the clitoris. If you put it on your clitoris, it can be over-stimulating and then you may not be able to have an orgasm. Many women who try a vibrator for the first time are shocked that they can have an orgasm in minutes. According to new research, 98 percent of women who have never had an orgasm can achieve orgasm with the help of a vibrator.

A women is often worried that her husband will be offended or feel inferior if a vibrator is added to the sexual repertoire, or that the husband will worry that the woman will become addicted to the vibrator and not want her man any more? We can tell you that a vibrator will never replace warm, loving flesh and blood. Most men are totally turned on that their partner uses a vibrator.

Doctors have not withdrawn from the vibrator business altogether. You can have a vibrator prescribed by your doctor. The only FDA-approved device for women is the EROS clitoral therapy device, a small vacuum pump that applies suction to the clitoris. It is available by prescription only and costs about $350.00. Although insurance coverage for the product varies, according to manufacturer, UroMetrics, most insurers are covering the cost.

Lovely Lubricants

Lubrication occurs during arousal in most women. But for some, due to out-of-balance hormones, stress, performance anxiety, and/or prescription medications, lubrication just does not happen. If you are moaning from pain due to inadequate lubrication during sex or you cannot get excited because of lack of lubrication, then lubricants are a great solution.

Drugstores, health food stores, and websites sell vaginal lubricants. Some have stimulants in them like peppermint or menthol and are called warming lubricants. These are used to enhance sexual pleasure and orgasm. Other lubricants contain herbal extracts to aid dryness and soothe the vagina. Oil-based lubricants are not safe to use with condoms and can cause the vagina to harbor bacteria. Never use petroleum jelly. Look for water-based formulas. Always test the lubricant on your skin before applying it to your sensitive genitals. If any rash, redness, or irritation occurs, do not apply the lubricant to your genitalia.

On page 71 we discussed vaginal bioidentical estriol cream for hormone-related symptoms of vaginal dryness, vaginal atrophy, urinary incontinence, burning, and urinary frequency. Even with the use of vaginal estriol cream for these symptoms, you will also want to add a lubricant to enhance sexual inter-course. Vaginal dryness can also occur at different stages of the menstrual cycle (right after the period or just before), during pregnancy, when breastfeeding, or when using a condom.

Your lubricant should be:
- water-based
- latex friendly
- non-staining and non-toxic
- designed to be soothing and not disrupt normal vaginal Ph balance
- pleasant tasting or have no taste
- providing lots of lubrication that does not get sticky over time

Your lubricant should not:
- contain parabens, toxic preservatives, mineral oil, animal products, or petroleum ingredients

Begin using your lubricant during foreplay, spreading it liberally over the labia and clitoris and into the vagina. Apply it to your partner's penis too. You may need to add more during intercourse. Most women think a lube is for use only during intercourse, but a lubricant should be used throughout the day if you have vaginal dryness, in order to prevent infections, itching, burning, heat, and pain from the dryness. That is why it is important to pick a lubricant that has no odor and does not stain your panties.

Lubes We Like
LOVE, by Preferred Nutrition, contains no parabens or harmful preservatives. It has no taste, it has excellent lubrication, and the lubrication lasts during intercourse. It dries without being sticky or tacky. You can safely eat it as the ingredients are all water-based and natural.

- Oh My! comes in plain and many natural flavors.
- Emerita lubricant comes in a stimulant and plain variety.

Altoids Oral Pleasure

Who would have thought a peppermint could provide so much pleasure? The person who thought this up was very creative. Here is a tip to try with your partner. Have your partner suck on an Altoid, "the curiously strong peppermints" from England, while performing oral sex on your clitoris. This creates an amazing experience for the woman. Pure peppermint pleasure.

What have we learned?
- Some sexual concerns are related to hormones and health issues, and they should be addressed.
- A good sex life is an indicator of overall health.
- Exercise can help balance your sexy hormones.
- Masturbation is normal, and men and women enjoy it equally.
- Toys and lubes can spice up your sex life.
- You deserve to have it all—including great sex.

10

Program Yourself
for Pleasure

We all want to be loved and feel appreciated. Remember those feelings of anticipation, wondering what it would be like to kiss someone for the very first time? Or the sea of emotions you felt when you fell in love and made love for the first time? Emotions can turn hormones on or off. Sexy feelings are driven by emotions that turn on key hormones. Thought processes can and do make sexual experiences pleasurable. Or, conversely, emotions can disrupt how you feel about a situation.

Women have shared their deepest thoughts and feelings with Dr. Pettle and I in regards to their sex lives. Jokes are often made about wives and their indifference to sex, but from our experience, this indifference is a myth. Women are distressed when their desire for sexual intimacy is diminished (if not gone). Another myth is that a lack of interest in sex is a normal part of aging. According to the March 2003 issue of *Women's Health in Primary Care*, 50 percent of women between 66 and 71 still desire sex, and 29 percent of those over 78 are still active. So much for the "sex disappears with aging" theory.

Some women in menopause have told us they are done with sex and are happy never to have it again. We respect that decision. Other women miss sex terribly when their sex drive dies. Many more are desperate to get to the root of their sexual concerns. One woman told us that she was worried her husband would leave her if she did not figure out where her sex drive had gone. Other women, who have lost their partners due to death or divorce and have not found another lover, still want to have sexual enjoyment. Women have also told us they are terrified when their aging or heart-disease-affected male partner uses Viagra. They are afraid he might die on top of them, so fear has made these women avoid sex.

The fact remains that women's sexual complaints have largely been ignored in the research world. Doctors are not asking women about their sex lives during routine checkups. *The Lancet* reported in February 2007 that a patient's sexual health or lack of a sex life is not considered by most doctors as a sign of health or a symptom of disease—though it should be. Pain during every occasion of sex is more common than erectile dysfunction—it occurs in 40 percent of women younger than age 60. Yet research in this area is non-existent. Consumers are not being bombarded with advertisements for solutions for this extremely common female condition like they are about solutions for erectile dysfunction. Many of the same conditions that cause male sexual problems, including depression, disease, medications, stress, low thyroid, hormone dysfunction, and more, are the root causes of female sexual problems.

Is It All In Your Head?

A woman's sexual concerns are often dismissed as being "all in her head." Viagra research in women was abandoned in 2000 because researchers found it did not work on women the same way it worked on men. Researchers reported that a large part of female sex drive and function does start in the head. Yet this is a very important distinction because Dr. Pettle and I know that emotions and feelings can affect hormones; and hormones affect sex drive. For those of you who wish to have a healthy sex life, this chapter provides the tools to help modify how you think and feel about your sexuality so your emotions will not derail your pleasure.

Your psychological state can dramatically affect your sex drive, and a satisfying (or unsatisfying) sex life can dramatically affect your psychological state. When people improve their mental state by regaining a satisfying sex life, it has been found that this helps improve other health conditions, including immune function. Researchers at Wilkes University, Pennsylvania, stated that sex twice a week may even prevent the common cold. After studying the sex habits of undergraduate students, researchers concluded that students who had sex once or twice a week had one-third more immunoglobulin A (IgA) in their saliva. Elevated levels of IgA protect the body from colds, flu, and other infections. Surprisingly (or disappointingly for some undergrads), more sex is not better. Researchers found that those students who had sex more than three times a week had lower IgA levels than those who rarely had sex. Even with sex, moderation seems to be the key.

Hans Selye's classic book *The Stress of Life* educated the world on the connection between emotions and the body. Research has shown that positive emotions have positive effects on the body and, conversely, negative emotions can result in negative effects. Selye was not the first person to suggest that there might be some connection between physical illnesses and the mind. In 1796, William Falconer presented similar ideas in the book *The Influence of the Passions Upon Disorders of the Body*—"passions" meaning emotions. It was almost two centuries later that science again paid any attention to this theory. Candice Pert of Rutgers University has focused on hormones in the brain as the biochemical units of emotions. These hormone messengers link your nervous, immune, and endocrine systems, and they are profoundly affected by your emotions. Emotions, including anger, happiness, sadness, loneliness, shame, embarrassment, grief, guilt, fear, boredom, and particularly, love, all alter your sexy hormones.

Stress and emotions play such a large role in your sex life because they affect your hormones. Women who report decreased sexual sensations and satisfaction after hysterectomy are often told they are depressed and prescribed anti-depressant medications, which you have learned have negative side effects such as low sexual desire and reduced pleasure. The report in *The Lancet* suggested surgeons need to learn nerve-sparing surgical techniques for any type of pelvic surgery to protect a woman's sexual response, as we noted earlier. And yes, lack of desire may have to do with the psychological response to the removal of a woman's female organs, especially knowing the hormonal effect these organs have on emotions. Many female complaints related to hormones are dismissed as psychological or emotional even before evaluations are performed.

We mentioned earlier that the number of anti-depressant and anti-anxiety medication prescriptions written in North America for women is outrageously high. Most of this book has been about how physical factors can affect hormones and sexual health. Now we will look at the emotional side of hormones because emotions and stress do have a powerful effect on sexual health.

Stressors and Desire

Relationship problems (caused by poor communication, among other issues), and a stressful life can reduce your sex drive. And it is no surprise that a woman working full-time and raising children with a demanding partner may have no sex drive. Sex with that one special person you love is central to intimacy, your emotional wellbeing, and your quality of life. And, of course, you want to maintain all these things. So how does stress wreak havoc on your best intentions? For some women, the chicken and egg theory applies. Is it the stress in your life causing your lack of sexual desire, or is it the lack of sexual intimacy that is causing the stress in your life? Both are real possibilities, and we will provide some simple solutions for reducing stress.

The adrenal glands you read about earlier (see page 5) are central to how you feel and to your emotional response to stressors. Estrogens and testosterone are produced in your adrenal glands. These are your key sexy hormones. Cortisol, also secreted by your adrenals, disrupts these hormones, resulting in a lack of sexual desire, diminished pleasure, weak orgasms, and painful intercourse.

You also read earlier that the high levels of cortisol that are part of a prolonged stress response cause further sexy hormone disruption by filling receptor sites normally reserved for progesterone. And progesterone, among other functions, is an important hormone for helping you deal with stress. When your cortisol levels are chronically high, progesterone is not able to do its job of controlling estrogen. As a result, your estrogen levels go up, which then inhibits testosterone's effects and lowers your levels of thyroid hormone.

What happens as a result of this hormone mess? You would rather be taking out the trash than having sex. Keeping your cortisol levels in check by eliminating some of the things that create stress in your life is step one in enhancing your sex drive. Chronic stress elevates your cortisol, eventually burning out your adrenal glands and causing low cortisol (from depletion), which also affects sexual and overall health. (See pages 107, 163 for nutrients supporting adrenal health.)

High levels of cortisol don't just wreck your sex drive. One study looking at stress, cortisol, and vaginal infections found that women who suffer chronic stress have a higher incidence of vulvovaginal candida infections than those under less stress. Researchers looked at first morning salivary cortisol levels, which were abnormally low—a sign of adrenal exhaustion. These women had recurrent vulvovaginal candida infections compared to women with normal early morning cortisol. Remember: immune function is also suppressed in women under tremendous stress. Women with recurrent candida infections also do not feel like having sex for obvious reasons. If you are a woman with these infections, adopt our stress-reducing suggestions below.

These hormone-related reactions are definitely physiological. What does this have to do with your head? While your reaction to stress is physical, the initial "call to arms" comes from your brain and your emotions. In some cases, the alarm is legitimate and you need to make life changes that remove you from stressful situations. In other cases, you need to do some psychological work to change your response to unavoidable situations. You can change your response from a wash of stress hormones to a more measured, effective one that will help defuse the situation.

Negative Programming

Even though many of today's young women matured after the sexual revolution and its promotion of sexual freedom, some women still got messages when they were younger that sex is dirty or a sin. They carry that message with them during each sexual encounter. Women were taught that "good girls" don't enjoy sex or get pleasure from sex or have sex before marriage or like oral sex. You would think these outdated notions were no longer being taught, but we counsel many young women who are affected in bed by these negative thoughts. This guilt is a terrible, unnecessary emotion. Whenever you begin to feel guilt over your sexual desires, counteract it by telling yourself you are a beautiful, honest, caring person who deserves to have it all—including a great sex life.

Negative Body Esteem

If you do not feel good about yourself, it may be challenging to get undressed in front of someone else. We have had women tell us they will not have sex anymore because they do not like how their bodies look, even though their partners insist they are beautiful. If you are not having sex because you are unhappy with how you look, either turn the lights off before you get naked or start a program to get your body back in shape. As we noted in Chapter 8, sex burns calories so you can look at it as a form of weight loss.

When it comes to emotions and a healthy sex life, everything starts with communication. Touching, kissing, fondling, and cuddling also provide fabulous sexy hormone effects. Orgasm does not always have to be the goal. Intimacy is often confused with sexual intercourse. You do not have to have intercourse to be intimate, and intimacy is not sex. You can have a wonderful, loving, sexually intimate relationship without intercourse.

Poor Communication

Sex is one of the most important components of an intimate relationship, and most people never discuss it, other than the occasional short quip about not getting enough. You cannot expect your partner to give you miraculous pleasure if you have not communicated what you like. So many people think that their partner should somehow "just know" what to do in the bedroom. None of us received any training in how to pleasure another—if you cannot read your partner's mind, then assume he/she cannot read yours either. You had both better talk about what each of you like and do not like. Think about show-and-tell in kindergarten—this is a great approach.

You both have to feel safe to open up sexually. Safety for women means that their partners are not going to judge them or say hurtful things. (Men also fear being laughed at and ridiculed and will avoid communication because of this.) Safety for both partners also means knowing that they are protected from sexually transmitted diseases, including HPV and herpes. This is another topic that both partners must be honest about.

Too many women spend decades sacrificing their own pleasure, "faking it" because they are afraid to speak about their needs. Faking it tells your partner that everything is fine and sends the wrong message. The worst story we have heard was of a woman who had vaginal dryness and terrible pain during intercourse, which she had not told her doctor or partner about. She eventually had a tear in her vaginal wall during intercourse that hemorrhaged. She had to be rushed to hospital with a life-threatening problem, all because she too embarrassed to communicate. Fear of embarrassment is powerful and is an emotion that can keep you from experiencing it all. Never make decisions based on fear, unless it is about stepping off a bridge. We can guarantee that if you are not feeling satisfied, neither is your partner. Talk to each other—communication will build a better relationship.

Unresolved Anger

When we were discussing libido-enhancing nutrients we said, "You still have to like your partner." No nutrient, drug, or pill is going to help your sex life if you no longer like your partner. The number one reason couples fall out of "like" is because they resent their partners for something that was said or done that caused pain or anger. They still love them, but they do not like them anymore.

Do not let anger or resentment reside in your home. It spills into your bedroom, and a week without sex can turn into a month without sex and then a year. Couples tell us they have not been sexually intimate for a year or more because of an unresolved situation.

Above all, never use sex as a tool to get what you want. You can get into a rut and not know how to get out of it. If this is the case in your home, find an experienced counsellor to help you and your partner resolve your differences on neutral ground.

Performance Anxiety

Most men do not think women have performance anxiety, but they do. So many women have told us the same story about performance anxiety. When a woman starts to have hormone fluctuations, some develop vaginal dryness. Vaginal secretions are something that can be seen and felt and are often used as a barometer of sexual excitement or interest by partners. We compare the lack of vaginal secretions to the lack of an erection or a soft erection in men. Some women report anxiety because their partner may think they are not "turned on" even though they may well be. Some women have so much anxiety surrounding this, they avoid sex altogether. If your vaginal dryness is due to low estrogen, see Chapter 4 for more information on vaginal estriol. Using a good vaginal lubricant can take the stress out of vaginal dryness during intercourse. See pages 132, 209 for more information.

Mismatched Sex Drives

How do we define a normal sex drive? Your sex drive is normal if you are satisfied with it. The average married couple makes love once every 14 days. However it is very common for couples to have mismatched sex drives.

At the beginning of your relationship, you most likely could not get enough of each other. You had fantasies about the next encounter. You probably spent a lot of time getting ready for your partner with the right clothes, perfume, hygiene, and more. Sex cools off once you become overly familiar with your mate. But it does not have to be this way—go back to the dating days. Think erotic thoughts. Put as much energy into yourself as you did at the onset of your relationship and encourage your partner to do the same. Sparks will fly again. It takes work for partners to keep the passion in a relationship—it does not just happen. Boredom will shut down the hormones that create your interest in sex.

If you are a woman who is content with sex once a week and your partner wants sex twice a day, this will most likely create a problem in your relationship. You both actually have normal sex drives. If resentment and anger are surfacing around your mismatched sex drives, then negotiate a compromise over the amount of sex in your relationship.

Mismatched Sexual Preferences

Many men are confused about what their partners want because they remember when they were dating. At that time, their partner was more interested in variety and experimenting, including, for example, oral sex. After the couple got married, oral sex disappeared from the sexual menu. Some people are disgusted or turned off by some sex acts, including oral sex. For most women who have these feelings, the revulsion will never go away. Negative programming that "good girls" don't do these types of things is part of it. Sometimes, with open communication or work with a good therapist, this can be overcome. But honesty and communication is again very important; if you really hate something, you need to tell your partner.

One man told us that he always made sure his wife knew when he disliked a food she cooked because he did not want that food on his plate for 50 years. It is the same thing with sexual acts. If you really don't like what your partner is doing or wants you to do, just think: if you deceive your partner by faking pleasure or enthusiastic participation, you will be stuck doing it for the length of your relationship. You want the relationship to be a long and happy one. That should be enough to make you honest about your needs.

Take a Stress Test

Now let's look at ways you can de-stress, so your hormones are ready for more positive things in your day. Are you stressed? Take the test.

The following statements determine your happiness level, how you handle stress, and if you have negative thinking. Check off the situations that apply to you. Then total the points for the situations you checked off.

- ❏ I am worried about paying my bills this month.   1
- ❏ I look at myself in the mirror and think negative thoughts. 3
- ❏ I am not content with my body.   3
- ❏ I almost always fake orgasm.   2
- ❏ I am lonely.   3
- ❏ I dislike my job.   3
- ❏ I like my job but have too much work to do.   1
- ❏ I like my job, but my boss is too demanding.   2
- ❏ I am always trying to please everyone.   3
- ❏ I am exhausted but keep going.   3
- ❏ Sometimes my stomach feels like it has butterflies.   1
- ❏ I shop to make myself feel better.   1
- ❏ I have feelings of guilt or anger.   2
- ❏ I have feelings of inadequacy (not feeling good enough).   3
- ❏ I am afraid of failure.   2
- ❏ I have feelings of anxiety or low moods.   2
- ❏ I feel trapped or that I can't cope sometimes.   3
- ❏ I crave sugar.   1
- ❏ I am a single mother.   2
- ❏ I am a university student.   1
- ❏ I am in an unhappy marriage.   3

❑	I live with an alcoholic or drug abuser.	2
❑	I work shift work.	1
❑	I work too much and don't have enough play time.	1
❑	I get angry with myself.	2
❑	I hold resentment toward my partner.	3
❑	I cannot discuss my sexual desires with my partner.	2
❑	I do not eat regularly. (I wait more than four or five hours between meals.)	3
❑	I am sick more than three times a year.	1
❑	I lack sexual desire.	1
❑	I smoke.	3
❑	I drink alcohol more than twice a week.	3
❑	I drink too much caffeine.	2
❑	My family and friends are not supportive of the things I do.	2
❑	I am tired all the time.	3
❑	I have friends who take but never give.	2

How Did You Score?

■ If you scored 15 or less, you are handling stress but need to find more balance in your life.

■ If you scored from 16 to 30, you know you have to make some changes fast. You are at risk of adrenal exhaustion.

■ If you scored over 30, you are over the top and need to adopt strategies to reduce your risk of stress-related disease immediately.

In addition to the sex-drive-destroying stressors discussed above, you might be surprised at some of the stressors mentioned in the test. But these kinds of issues provide constant, low-grade stress that keeps your cortisol levels high and can lead to disruptions in your hormones.

Tackling the Stress in Your Life

The following tips can help you turn off the excess cortisol that is destroying your sex life.

Make More Time for Fun

Ask yourself what you are missing—time with friends, going for a walk, a swim at the pool, a sauna, reading a novel, playing games with the kids, kissing your spouse? Make a pact with yourself that once a week you will do one of the things that you miss. Then ask yourself what you hate doing—sitting in front of the television, doing laundry, cleaning, driving the kids to a dozen activities, dealing with your boss? Make a decision to change one thing a week. If you hate your boss, spend every spare moment looking for a new job. If you hate cleaning, hire a maid, even for one hour a week—or enlist the family to help. Teach the kids to do laundry (children as young as five can learn to sort clothes). Get Call Display so you can avoid people who make you tense or unhappy. Understand your life choices—do not do things that make you miserable. Fill your life with positives.

No More Negative Self-Talk

North American society is entrenched in a cult of "self-improvement." In order to drive the consumer economy, people must be constantly "reminded" that they need to buy goods and services that will improve their lives. Unfortunately, this means everyone is bombarded with negative thinking from a very young age. Beyond the fact that children hear the word "no" thousands of times by age three, all of us are constantly being asked to judge ourselves and find ways to "improve" things.

People often feel they are not good enough, that they are failures and hold associated feelings of guilt, shame, and fear. The idea comes from those who are trusted and loved the most—parents and teachers—and from nearly every piece of media encountered. These messages help each of us define who we think we are. Your self-regard is based on who you believe yourself to be and how you describe yourself. Retrain your thoughts, and believe you are fit, beautiful, and sexy. Say, "I am beautiful, sexy, and fit." Repeat it six times while looking at yourself in the mirror. Smile—it may feel strange, but do not stop.

Positive Affirmations

The first step in changing your negative self-concepts is to become present in the moment. It takes practice to become aware of only this moment. Find a quiet space where you will not be interrupted. Close the door. Sit in a comfortable chair, or lie on the bed. Be aware of your breathing, right down to the tips of your fingers and toes. Breathe in through your nose and out through your mouth. Breathe deep into your abdomen. Be aware of any sensations in your body. Follow this awareness by observing the thoughts in your mind. The process is to "just be," not to analyze or judge your feelings or thoughts. You will feel calm. Once you feel calm, you will be ready to introduce new ways of thinking, called patterning. It is important to create positive statements, called affirmations, that come from your heart. One affirmation that works well is, "I deserve to have it all, including a satisfying sex life." Here are some other positive affirmations:

"I am enjoying my sexy body."
"I love myself."
"I am making time for myself and my partner to share the day."
"I am being honest with my lover."
"I am a great person."

Affirmations are always in the present tense and are always positive. They teach you to stop thinking negatively. So if you find yourself thinking, "I don't have time for intimacy," change it to, "I will make time for intimacy."

What's Love Got to Do with It?

What is the point of all this positive self-talk? Deep, unconditional love is what most people seek. Loving yourself is the foundation for loving others. If you do not love yourself, you can not fully give of yourself to others. Nor can you graciously and joyously accept their love. (How many times have you brushed off a compliment because you did not agree with the speaker's positive assessment of you? Practice smiling and thanking them for the praise, even if it's about a sweater you've had for years.)

As someone who values herself, always choose what is good for you. It will be good for all those people you love too. Women must take care of themselves first. This means positive thoughts; excellent nutrition; time for exercise, de-stressing; and satisfying sex. And lots of love. Remember, a relationship with another person is not a prerequisite for being sexually satisfied. According to 2006 demographics, over 45 percent of North American women live without a partner. On page 205, we discuss ways to pleasure yourself.

Stress-Busting Tips

- Breathing is a powerful de-stressing tool. Several times a day, breathe in through your nose and fill your lungs with air until your abdomen rises. Then slowly exhale from your mouth until your lungs are empty. Repeat this technique five times whenever you do your deep breathing.
- Get eight hours of sleep every night, and try to sleep until 7:30 in the morning as often as possible.
- Say "no" when you have too much to humanly accomplish in one day. This will preserve healthy adrenal glands.
- Have the family share the household workload. Doing chores together can be fun, especially if maintain "family" standards rather than insisting everything be done "your way."
- Smile at everyone. It is impossible to be negative or unhappy with a smile on your face—just try it!
- Purge negative emotions by practising your chosen positive affirmations every day.
- Get help dealing with grief. The loss of a loved one, a divorce, or the loss of a job all merit grieving. Grieving is an ultimately healthy process you should accept and work through.
- *Carpe diem*—"seize the day"—and live it to the fullest. Don't worry so much about tomorrow.
- Believe in yourself. No more negative self-talk and continual self-doubt. Most of us are our own worst enemies. We focus on our weaknesses and minimize our strengths. Wake up each day, and tell yourself that you are a good and useful person.
- Notice the beauty around you. Smell the flowers, watch the sunset, and listen to the wind.
- Love your family and friends.
- Be good to yourself. Do the things you have always wanted to do. Learn to water ski, sing in a choir, write a book, tell stories to your grandchildren, walk, garden—whatever makes you happy.
- Seek your spiritual side. This does not have to be religious, although those with strong religious beliefs generally live at peace and feel protected. Most of us believe in something greater than ourselves, a spiritual power that offers solace and helps us find the quiet place within.

Rekindling the Mood

The Wonders of Pheromones

Women are aroused by certain aromas and turned off by others. Your nose is so sensitive that exposure to men's pheromones can affect your ovulation cycle, that is, your readiness and interest in sex. Yes, this has been researched. Pheromones are powerful cues. Underarm sweat has been shown to have a pheromone component—dehydroepiandrosterone (DHEA)—and it was discovered that when the underarm sweat of women in different menstrual phases was placed under the noses of female subjects, the length of these subjects' own cycles was synchronized over time. This explains why females living in close quarters (like mothers and daughters, sisters, or women living in college dormitories or working closely in offices every day) develop synchronized menstrual cycles.

Pheromones are hormone-like chemical signals that are detected between members of the same species even though the chemicals have no odor, feel, or taste. In cats, a male cat's incessant, desperate yowling is triggered by pheromones released from the female cat in heat. In humans, it is believed that pheromone signals are detected through an organ inside the nose called the Vomeronasal Organ (VNO). When the VNO detects pheromones, it sends a subconscious, sexual response signal to the brain. Research is ongoing in humans to find out exactly how pheromones work.

Current research has shown that when women smell an androgen-like compound, an area in their hypothalamus is activated. In contrast, when men smell an estrogen-like substance, a different portion of their hypothalamus is activated. Remember: the hypothalamus is the master controller of all of hormones. A double-blind, placebo-controlled study published in the *Journal of Sex Research* looked at how a sex-attractant pheromone from young, fertile women increased socio-sexual behavior in post-menopausal women. Researchers were evaluating if the pheromones increased these women's desire for sex over a six-week period. During the study, a significantly greater proportion of participants using the pheromone formula rather than the placebo reported an increase in frequency of petting, kissing, and affection. More pheromone users than placebo users experienced an increase in at least one of the four intimate socio-sexual behaviors. The results suggest that the pheromone formulation worn for a period of six weeks has sex-attractant effects for post-menopausal women. Just think what pheromones can do for your social life! Pheromones are available for sale in health food stores and on the Internet.

Are You Too Tired for Sex?

After a long day, many women are just too tired for sex (and to a lesser extent men are too). Seventy percent of North Americans report they have problems getting restful sleep, which compounds problems with sex drive and creates a cycle of fatigue. Yet sexual activity at bedtime acts as a natural sedative for many couples. Stressful jobs and daily anxiety about not having enough time to complete tasks push sex to the bottom of the to-do list. This is unfortunate because studies show that sexual intimacy produces hormones that reduce the negative effects of stress and aid sleep. Sex before sleep acts like a sleeping pill. For singles, self-induced orgasms work as a sedative as well. (See page 224 for more information.) Sex does not have to be a two-hour marathon. Quickies have the same effect on your body. Instead of carefully undressing at bedtime, disrobe and jump into the sack for some spontaneous passion without worrying about hanging up the rumpled clothes.

Create a Sexy Environment

You should not have to wait for a weekend getaway or an annual vacation to get yourself and your partner ready for sex. When there is no time to get away, you can still shift gears away from everyday events by creating an oasis in your home. A relaxing and inviting bedroom environment is very important. It is most often the last room in a house to get a makeover, but it should be the first.

Build your oasis by starting with a comfortable mattress, buy good sheets, a great duvet, and super fabulous pillows that make you want to spend more time under the covers. Replace harsh lighting with soft lights that have dimmers. Get a lock on your door, and advise other members of the household to always knock before entering when the door is closed. Most women find it hard to relax and enjoy sex if they are listening for children entering the bedroom.

A "family bed," where children sleep with their parents from birth until the child feels comfortable in a separate bed in another room, is the ultimate anti-sex pill. If you and your partner have made the decision to have a family bed, then you better have a back-up plan for your sex life.

Do not have a television in your bedroom—you will end up watching the news or sports at bedtime. Neither of these programs are fuel for erotica or cuddling—especially if his team misses the playoffs. News reports have been found to raise cortisol levels. This is a big no-no for testosterone levels.

Get in the habit of turning on your favorite soothing music as soon as you enter the bedroom. Even brushing your teeth will be more relaxing this way. If you and your partner go to bed at different times, break that habit and make bedtime a shared ritual, even if it is only a 10-minute ritual. Give each other a gentle massage in the places where muscle tension builds up before turning in for the night. Don't read or work in bed. Share bedtime with your partner.

And here is a hint for the guys—turn up the heat! Not that heat. *Room temperature* can mean the difference between wanting to get naked or wanting to wear fleece. Most men have a much lower tolerance for heat and like the environment cool, whereas women, until they hit menopause, are often seeking flannel in order to ward off the goose bumps.

Hormone recap:

- Hormones are messengers that control thousands of actions and reactions in the body, particularly your sexual health.
- Out-of-balance levels of hormones will have a powerful, negative effect on your health, your sex life, and your life in general.
- Out-of-balance levels of hormones can be brought back into balance with proper testing, appropriate lifestyle changes, nutrient support, and perhaps the use of bioidentical hormones.
- Foods have a powerful effect on hormones either by enhancing them or turning them off.
- Exercise is a fabulous way to enhance the hormones of desire while helping you achieve positive feelings about the way you look.
- Nutrients are essential for optimal hormone balance and can kick-start your sex drive.
- Loving yourself is the first step toward improving sexy hormones.
- Being good to yourself is an important booster of sexy hormones.

Appendix

Recommended Products and Services

Nutrient Support Products

Multivitamins with Minerals
A good multivitamin with minerals is the foundation of a hormone health program.
- In Canada, FemmEssentials (for women) is available from Preferred Nutrition Ltd. (See company information below for contact information.)
- In the U.S., MultiEssentials is available from Natural Factors Ltd. or at www.lornashop.com. (See company information below for contact information.)

Protein Powders
Protein powder is essential to maintain stable blood sugar and hormone balance. Taste is an important factor when choosing a brand; this product will be a snack or meal supplement for a good source of protein. We recommend:
- In Canada, BodySense ProteinEssentials powder, available in three delicious flavors including vanilla, chocolate cream, or tropical dream; or MenoFood with pomegranate; or Mood Food with L-theonine. Available from Preferred Nutrition Ltd.
- In the U.S., SlimStyles Meal Replacement Drink Mix with PGX in vanilla, chocolate, mango, strawberry, or peach. Available from Natural Factors Ltd.

Probiotics
Recommended to replenish friendly bacteria in the digestive tract, to aid digestion, elimination, and fat loss. Use Bifidobacterium BB536.
- In Canada, Bifidobacterium BB536 is available from Preferred Nutrition Ltd.
- In the U.S., Bifidobacterium BB536 is available from Natural Factors Ltd. and Jarrow Formulas Ltd.

Adrenal Support
Adrenal nutrients help reduce cortisol, the stress hormone. AdrenaSense contains ashwagandha, rhodiola, suma, Siberian ginseng, and schizandra berries.
- In Canada, AdrenaSense is available from Preferred Nutrition Ltd.
- In the U.S., AdrenaSense is available from Natural Factors Ltd.

BioSil
BioSil helps improve the look of skin, hair, and nails. Clinical studies confirm that BioSil offers superior absorption of silicon and increases collagen concentration in the skin.
- In Canada, BioSil is available from Preferred Nutrition Ltd.
- In the U.S., BioSil is available from Jarrow Formulas.

Estrogen Balancing
EstroSense is essential for those taking any type of hormone therapy, for protection from the production of dangerous metabolites. EstroSense can help those with fibroids, ovarian cysts, hormone imbalance, breast cancer, breast cysts, heavy periods, PCOS, acne, and cellulite.
- In Canada, EstroSense is available from Preferred Nutrition Ltd.
- In the U.S., EstroSense is available from Natural Factors.

MenoSense
MenoSense is an all-natural formula designed to provide support for symptoms associated with menopause, such as hot flashes and night sweats.
- In Canada, MenoSense is available from Preferred Nutrition Ltd.
- In the U.S., MenoSense is available from Natural Factors.

SexEssentials
SexEssentials is a combination of L-arginine, eurycoma longifolia, Vitamin B5, choline, gingko biloba, tribulus terrestris.
- In Canada, SexEssentials is available in local health food stores.

- U.S. customers can purchase Sex Essentials online at www.shoplorna.com.

Thyroid Support

We recommend ThyroSense, to be taken along with thyroid medication or for those who have the symptoms of low thyroid but cannot get medication. ThyroSense includes L-tyrosine, ashwagandha, guggals, pantothenic acid, copper, manganese, and potassium iodide.
- In Canada, ThyroSense is available from Preferred Nutrition Ltd.
- In the U.S., ThyroSense is available from Natural Factors Ltd. or online at www.shoplorna.com.

Progesterone Cream in U.S.

In the U.S. progesterone creams are sold over the counter in health food stores and pharmacies and also through compounding pharmacies.

Life-Flo Health Products

- Progesta-care is progesterone in a metered pump providing 20 mg of USP progesterone.
- Available at all health food stores in the U.S. Visit www.life-flo.com for more information.

Lubricants

Our favorite personal lubricant is called LOVE from Preferred Nutrition Ltd. in Canada or at www.shoplorna.com. It is paraben-free and has no taste; it is silky smooth and does not stain sheets or panties.

We also like:

O'My personal lubricants from
O'My Products Inc.
188 Pemberton Avenue, North Vancouver, BC V7P 2R5
www.omyonline.com
Telephone: 604-990-9700

Emerita is another parabens-free personal lubricant.
Emerita
621 SW Alder Street, Suite 900, Portland, Oregon 97205 USA
Telephone: 503-226-1010 or 1 800-648-8211
www.emerita.com

Vibrators or Massagers

Natural Contours Vibrators and Kegel exerciser
The Energie Kegel exerciser is the one we recommend and the Liberte vibrator is a good one to start with as it is ergonomically comfortable
To order discreetly online, go to www.natural-contours.com

Sharper Image AcuVibe Rechargeable Personal Massager is a two-speed model or the Little-vibe is a single-speed smaller version. We like both.
To order discreetly online, go to www.sharperimage.com, and go to the personal care massage button.

Most pharmacies now carry personal massage devices. After looking online at these websites, a similar one may be available at your local store.

Company Contact Information

Preferred Nutrition Ltd.
153 Perth Street, Acton, Ontario L7J 1C9
Telephone: 519-853-1118 • Toll-free: 1 888-826-9625
www.pno.com

Natural Factors Nutritional Products Inc.
1111 - 80th Street SW, Suite 100, Everett, Washington 98203 USA
Telephone: 425-513-8800 • Toll-free: 1 800-322-8704
www.naturalfactors.com

Life-Flo Health Care Products Inc.
11202 N. 24th Avenue, Phoenix, Arizona 85029 USA
Telephone: 602-995-8715 • Toll-free: 1 888-999-7440
www.life-flo.com

Jarrow Formulas
1824 S. Robertson Blvd., Los Angeles, CA 90035 USA
Telephone: 310-204-6936 • Toll-Free 1 800-726-0886
www.jarrow.com

Services

Hormone Saliva Testing

IN CANADA

Rocky Mountain Analytical Laboratories
Unit A, 253147 Bearspaw Road NW, Calgary, Alberta Canada T3L 2P5
Telephone: 403-241-4513
info@rmalab.com

IN THE U.S.

ZRT Laboratory
8605 SW Creekside Place, Beaverton, OR 97008
Telephone: 503-466-2445 • Toll Free: 1-866-600-1636
Hormone Hotline: 503-466-9166
info@zrtlab.com

Compounding Pharmacies

IN CANADA

York Downs Pharmacy
3910 Bathurst Street, Toronto, Ontario, Canada M3H 5Z3
Telephone: 416-633-2244 • Toll Free: 1 800-564-5020
info@yorkdownsrx.com

IN THE U.S.

The International Academy of Compounding Pharmacists
Use the Compounding Pharmacy Locator at www.iacprx.org
Go to the "find a compounding pharmacist" button
Toll Free: 1-800-927-4227

References

Aardal E, et al. Cortisol in saliva-reference ranges and relation to cortisol in serum. *Eur J Clin Chem Clin Biochem.* 1995;33:927–932.

Aardal-Eriksson E, et al. Salivary cortisol–an alternative to serum cortisol determinations in dynamic function tests. *Clin Chem Lab Med.* 1998;36:215–222.

Adashi EY. The climacteric ovary as a functional gonadotropin-driven androgen-producing gland. *Fertil Steril.* 1994;62:20–27.

Adlercreutz H. Phyto-oestrogens and cancer. *Lancet Oncol.* 2002;3:364373.

Agarwal VR, et al. (CYP19) gene in breast adipose tissues of cancer-free and breast cancer patients. *J Clin Endocrinol Metab.* 1996;81:3843–3849.

Aleander GM, et al. Sex steroids, sexual behavior, and selection attention for erotic stimuli in women using oral contraceptives. *Psychoneuroendocrinology.* 1993;18:91–102.

Allen WM. Physiology of the corpus luteum, V: the preparation and some chemical properties of progestin, a hormone of the corpus luteum which produces progestational proliferation. *American Journal of Physiology.* 1930;92:174–188.

Allen WM. Progesterone: how did the name originate? *Southern Medical Journal.* 1970;63:1151–1155.

Allen WM, et al. Normal growth and implantation of embryos after very early ablation of the ovaries, under the influence of extracts of the corpus luteum. *American Journal of Physiology.* 1929;88:340–346.

Allolio B, et al. Diurnal salivary cortisol patterns during pregnancy and after delivery: relationship to plasma corticotrophin-releasing hormone. *Clin Endocrinol.* 1990;33:279–289.

Amann W. Improvement of acne vulgaris following therapy with Agnus castus. *Ther Ggw.* 1967;106:124–126.

American Herbal Products Association. *Use of Marker Compounds in Manufacturing and Labeling Botanically Derived Dietary Supplements.* Silver Spring, MD: American Herbal Products Association; 2001.

Anderson TJ, et al. Oral contraceptive use influences resting breast proliferation. *Human Pathology.* 1989;20:1139–1144.

Anderson WA, et al. Similarities and differences in the ultrastructure of two hormone-dependent and one independent human breast carcinoma grown in athymic nude mice: comparison with the rat DMBA-induced tumor and normal secretory mammocytes. *Journal of Submicroscopic Cytology.* 1984;16:673–690.

Andersson S, et al. Expression cloning and regulation of steroid 5-reductase, an enzyme essential for male sexual differentiation. *Journal of Biological Chemistry.* 1989;264: 16249–16255.

Andersson T, et al. Progesterone metabolism in the microsomal fraction of the testis, head kidney, and trunk kidney from the rainbow trout. *General and Comparative Endocrinology.* 1990;79:130–135.

Andriole GL, et al. Effect of the dual 5-reductase inhibitor dutasteride on markers of tumor regression in prostate cancer. *The Journal of Urology.* 2004;172:915–919.

Ang HH, et al. Aphrodisiac evaluation in non-copulator male rats after chronic administration of Eurycoma longifolia Jack. *Fundamental and Clinical Pharmacology.* 2001;15(4):265–268.

Ang HH, et al. Effect of Eurycoma longifolia Jack on orientation activities in middle-aged male rats. *Fundamental and Clinical Pharmacology.* 2002;16:479–483.

Ang HH, et al. Effects of Eurycoma longifolia Jack (Tongkat Ali) on the initiation of sexual performance of inexperienced castrated male rats. *Experimental Animal.* 2000;49(1):35–38.

Ang HH, et al. Enhancement of sexual motivation in sexually naïve male mice by Eurycoma longifolia. *International Journal of Pharmacognosy.* 1997;35(2):144–146.

Ang HH, et al. Euyrcolactones A-C, novel quassinoids from Eurycoma longifolia. *Tetrahedron Letters.* 2000;41:6849–6853.

Ang HH, et al. Eurycoma longifolia Jack and orientation activities in sexually experienced male rats. *Biological and Pharmaceutical Bulletin.* 1998;21(2):153–155.

Ang HH, et al. In vitro antimalarial activity of quassinoids from Eurycoma longifolia against Malaysian chloroquine-resistant plasmodium falciparum isolates. *Planta Medica.* 1995;61(2):177–178.

Ang HH, et al. Quassinoids from Eurycoma longifolia. *Phytochemistry.* 2002;59(8):833–837.

Anisimov VN. The role of pineal gland in breast cancer development. *Crit Rev Oncol Hematol.* 2003 Jun;46(3):221–234.

Araghiniknam M, et al. Antioxidant activity of dioscorea and dehydroepiandrosterone (DHEA) in older humans. *Life Sci.* 1996;11:147–57.

Arici A, et al. Progesterone metabolism in human endometrial stromal and gland cells in culture. *Steroids.* 1999;64:530–534.

Atherden LM. Progesterone metabolism; investigation of the products of metabolism with human liver in vitro. *Biochemical Journal.* 1959;71:411–415.

Auborn KJ, et al. The interaction between HPV infection and estrogen metabolism in cervical carcinogenesis. *Int J Cancer.* 1991 Dec 2;49(6):867–869.

Aviram M, et al. Pomegranate juice consumption for 3 years by patients with carotid artery stenosis reduces common carotid intima-media thickness, blood pressure and LDL oxidation. *Clin Nutr.* 2004;23(3):423–433.

Aviram M, et al. Pomeganate juice consumption inhibits serum angiotensin coverting enzyme activity and reduces systolic blood pressure. *Atherosclerosis.* 2001; 158(1):195–198.

Aviram M, et al. Pomegranate juice consumption reduces oxidative stress, atherogenic modifications to LDL, and platelet aggregation: studies in humans and in atherosclerotic apolipoprotein E-deficient mice. *Am J Clin Nutr.* 2000;71(5):1062–1076.

Bailey GS, et al. Enhancement of carcinogenesis by the natural anticarcinogen indole-3-carbinol. *J Natl Canc Inst.* 1987 May;78(5):931–934.

Balthazart J, et al. Changes in progesterone metabolism in the chicken hypothalamus during induced egg laying stop and molting. *General and Comparative Endocrinology.* 1988;72:282–295.

Bancroft J, et al. Oral contraceptives, androgens, and the sexuality of young women, II: the role of androgens. *Arch Sex Behav.* 1991;20:121–135.

Bao TT, et al. A comparison of the pharmacological actions of seven constituents isolated from Fructus schisandrae [in Chinese; English abstract]. *Acta Pharm Sin.* 1980 Jan;93(1):41–47.

Barcelo S, et al. CYP2E1-mediated mechanism of anti-genotoxicity of the broccoli constituent sulforaphane. *Carcinogenesis.* 1996;17:277–282.

Barentsen R, et al. Continuous low dose estradiol released from a vaginal ring versus estriol vaginal cream for urogenital atrophy. *Eur J Obstet Gynecol Reprod Biol.* 1997 Jan;71(1):73–80.

Barrou Z, et al. Overnight dexamethasone suppression test; comparison of plasma and salivary cortisol measurement for the screening of Cushing's syndrome. *Eur J Endocrin.* 1996;134:93–96.

Beck C, et al. Acute, non-genomic actions of the gonadal and neural steroid, 3-hydroxy-4-pregnen-20-one (3HP), in FSH release, studied in perifused rat anterior pituitary cells. *Endocrine.* 1997;6:221–229.

Beckham N. Phyto-oestrogens and compounds that affect oestrogen metabolism. *Aust J Med Herbalism.* 1995;7(1):11–16.

Bedin M, et al. Deficiency in placental sulfatase. Clinical and biochemical study of 3 cases. [French]. *Nouv Presse Med.* 1976 Sep 18;5(30):1889–1892.

Beecher CWW. Cancer prevention properties of varieties of Brassica oleracea: a review. *Amer J Clin Nutr.* 1994;59 (suppl):1166S–1170S.

Beling CG, et al. Progesterone metabolism in cultured amniotic fluid cells. *International Journal of Gynaecology and Obstetrics.* 1978;15:317–321.

Belkien LD, et al. Estradiol in saliva for monitoring follicular stimulation in an in vitro fertilization program. *Fertil Steril.* 1985;44:322.

Ben-Ze'ev A. The cytoskeleton in cancer cells. *Biochimica et Biophysica Acta.* 1985;780: 197–212.

Berglund H, et al. Brain response to putative pheromones in lesbian women. *Proc Natl Acad Sci USA.* 2006 May 23;103(21):8269–8274.

Berliner DL, et al. The extra-hepatic metabolism of progesterone in rats. *Journal of Biological Chemistry.* 1956;221:449–459.

Bershadsky AD, et al. The state of actin assembly regulates actin and vinculin expression by a feedback loop. *Journal of Cell Science.* 1995;108:1183–1193.

Bertics SJ, et al. Distribution and ovarian control of progestin-metabolizing enzymes in various rat hypothalamic regions. *Journal of Steroid Biochemistry.* 1987;26:321–328.

Birrell SN, et al. Androgens induce divergent proliferative responses in human breast cancer cell lines. *Journal of Steroid Biochemistry and Molecular Biology.* 1995;52:459–467.

Block G, et al. Fruit, vegetables, and cancer prevention: a review of the epidemiological evidence. *Nutr Cancer.* 1992;12:1–29.

Blumenthal M, et al. *The Complete German Commission E Monographs: Therapeutic Guide to Herbal Medicines.* Austin, TX: American Botanical Council; 1998.

Blumenthal M, et al. *Herbal Medicine: Expanded Commission E Monographs.* Austin, TX: American Botanical Council; 2000.

Boccuzzi G, et al. Growth inhibition of DMBA-induced rat mammary carcinomas by the antiandrogen flutamide. *Journal of Cancer Research and Clinical Oncology.* 1995;121: 150–154.

Bone K. Vitex agnus-castus: scientific studies and clinical applications. *Eur J Herbal Med.* 1994;1:12–15.

Bolaji II, et al. Assessment of bioavailability of oral micronized progesterone using a salivary progesterone enzymeimmunoassay. *Gynecol Endocrinol.* 1993;7:101–110.

Bolaji II. Sero-salivary progesterone correlation. *Int J Gynaecol Obstet.* 1994;45:125–131.

Bolton JL, et al. Role of quinoids in estrogen carcinogenesis. *Chem Res Toxicol.* 1998;11(10):1113–1127.

Booth A, et al. Testosterone and child and adolescent adjustment: the moderating role of parent-child relationships. 2000 October. Unpublished manuscript.

Boswell KJ, et al. Estradiol increases consumption of a chocolate cake mix in female rats. *Pharmacol Biochem Behav.* 2006 May;84(1):84–93.

Bottiglione F, et al. Transvaginal estriol administration in postmenopausal women: a double blind comparative study of two different doses. *Maturitas.* 1995 Nov;22(3):227–232.

Bradlow HL, et al. Multifunctional aspects of the action of indole-3-carbinol as an antitumor agent. *Ann NY Acad Sci.* 1999;889:204–213.

Bradlow HL, et al. Steroids as procarcinogenic agents. *Ann NY Acad Sci.* 2004;1028:216–232.

Bradlow HL, et al. 2-hydroxyestrone: the 'good' estrogen. *J Endocrinol.* 1996;150 Suppl:S259–265.

Bramson HD, et al. Unique preclinical characteristics of GG745, a potent dual inhibitor of 5AR. *Journal of Pharmacology and Experimental Therapeutics.* 1997;282:1496–1502.

Braunsberg H, et al. Action of a progesterone on human breast cancer cells: mechanism of growth stimulation and inhibition. *European Journal of Cancer and Clinical Oncology.* 1987;23:563–572.

Bravo L. Polyphenols: chemistry, dietary sources, metabolism, and nutritional significance. *Nutr Rev.* 1998;56:317–333.

Brehkman I. *Man and Biologically Active Substances: the Effects of Drugs, Diet and Pollution on Health.* New York, NY: Pergamon Press, 1980.

Brown CT, et al. Dutasteride: a new 5-reductase inhibitor for men with lower urinary tract symptoms secondary to benign prostate hyperplasia. *International Journal of Clinical Practice.* 2003;57:705–709.

Bryson MJ, et al. Metabolism of progesterone in human myometrium. *Endocrinology.* 1969;84:1071–1075.

Bryson MJ, et al. Metabolism of progesterone in human proliferative endometrium. *Endocrinology.* 1967;81:729–734.

Bulun SE, et al. The human CYP19 (uromatase P450) gene: update on physiologic roles and genomic organization of promoters. *J Steroid Biochem Mol Biol.* 2003;86:219–224.

Butenandt A, et al. Über das Hormon des Corpus luteum. *Zeitschrift für Physiologische Chemie.* 1934;227:84–98.

Campbell BC, et al. Menstrual variation in salivary testosterone among regularly cycling women. *Horm Res.* 1992;37:132–136.

Campbell DR, et al. Flavonoid inhibition of aromatase enzyme activity in human preadipocytes. *J Steroid Biochem Mol Biol.* 1993;46:381–388.

Canadian Consensus Conference on Menopause. *J Obstet Gynecol.* 2006;28:Special Edition Update.

Canosa LF, et al. Pregnenolone and progesterone metabolism by the testes of Bufo arenarum. *Journal of Comparative Physiology.* 1998;168:491–496.

Cappelletti V, et al. Effect of progestin treatment on estradiol- and growth factor-stimulated breast cancer cell lines. *Anticancer Research.* 1995;15:2551–2556.

Carreau S, et al. Aromatase expression and role of estrogens in male gonad: a review. *Reprod Biol Endrocrinol.* 2003;1:35.

Casper F, et al. Local treatment of urogenital atrophy with an estradiol-releasing vaginal ring: a comparative and a placebo-controlled multicenter study. Vaginal Ring Study Group. *Int Urogynecol J Pelvic Floor Dysfunct.* 1999;10(3):171–176.

Castro M, et al. Out-patient screening for Cushing's Syndrome: the sensitivity of the combination of circadian rhythm and overnight dexamethasone suppression salivary cortisol tests. *J Clin Endocrinol Metab.* 1999;84:878–882.

Chan KL, et al. *Chemical prospecting in Malayan Forest.* "Antipyretic activity of quassinoids from Eurycoma longifolia Jack." Subang Jaya, Malaysia: Pelanduk Publications; 1995:219–224.

Chan KL, et al. Plants as sources of antimalarial drugs. Part 3. Eurycoma longifolia. *Planta Medica.* 1986;52:105–107.
Chan KL, et al. A quassinoid glycoside from the roots of Eurycoma longifolia. *Phytochemistry.* 1989;28(10):2857–2859.

Chan KL, et al. 6alpha-hydroxyeurycomalactone, a quassinoid from Eurycoma longifolia. *Phytochemistry.* 1992;31(12):4295–4298.

Chan KL, et al. 13alpha,18-dihydroeurycomanol, a quassinoids from Eurycoma longifolia. *Phytochemistry.* 1991;30(9): 3138–3141.

Chang HM, et al. *Pharmacology and Applications of Chinese Materia Medica.* Toh Tuk Link, Singapore: World Scientific; 1986.

Chang L, et al. Mammalian MAP kinase signalling cascades. *Nature.* 2001;410:37–40.

Chatani F, et al. Stimulatory effect of luteinizing hormone on the development and maintenance of 5-reduced steroid-producing testicular interstitial cell tumors in Fischer 344 rats. *Anticancer Research.* 1990;10:337–342.

Cherry N, et al. Relation between hormone replacement therapy and ischaemic heart disease in women: prospective observational study. *BMJ.* 2003;326(7386):426.

Cheung AP. Acute effects of estradiol and progesterone on insulin, lipids and lipoproteins in postmenopausal women: a pilot study. *Maturitas.* 2000 Apr 28;35(1):45–50.

Chiu PY, et al. Hepatoprotective mechanism of schisandrin B: role of mitochondrial glutathione antioxidant status and heat shock proteins. *Free Radic Biol Med.* 2003 Aug 15;35(4):368–380.

Chiu PY, et al. In vivo antioxidant action of a lignan-enriched extract of Schisandra fruit and an anthraquinone-containing extract of Polygonum root in comparison with schisandrin B and emodin. *Planta Med.* 2002 Nov;68(11):951–956.

Chiu PY, et al. Schisandrin B protects myocardial ischemia-reperfusion injury partly by inducing Hsp25 and Hsp70 expression in rats. *Mol Cell Biochem.* 2004 Nov;266(1–2):139–144.

Chiu PY, et al. Time-dependent enhancement in mitochondrial glutathione status and ATP generation capacity by schisandrin B treatment decreases the susceptibility of rat hearts to ischemia-reperfusion injury. *Biofactors.* 2003;19(1–2):43–51.

Choe JK, et al. Progesterone and estradiol in the saliva and plasma during the menstrual cycle. *Am J Obstet Gynecol.* 1983;147:557–562.

Choo CY, et al. High performance liquid chromatography analysis of canthinone alkaloids from Eurycoma longifolia. *Planta Medica.* 2002;68:382–384.

Christiansen K, et al. Androgen levels and components of aggressive behaviour in men. *Horm Behav.* 1987;21:170–180.

Christiansen K, et al. Sex hormones and cognitive functioning in men. *Neuropsychobiol.* 1987;18:27–36.

Chronobiology: its role in clinical medicine, general biology, and agriculture. *Prog Clin Biol Res.* 1990;341A:105–117.

Chung FL, et al. Chemoprevention of colonic aberrant crypt foci in Fischer rats by major isothiocyanates in watercress and broccoli. *Proceedings of the American Association for Cancer Research.* 2000;41:660.

Chung F, et al. Dose–response effects of *Lepidium meyenii* (Maca) aqueous extract on testicular function and weight of different organs in adult rats. *Journal of Ethnopharmacology.* 2005 Apr 8;98(1–2):143–147.

Clapper ML, et al. Preclinical and clinical evaluation of broccoli supplements as inducers of glutathione S-transferase activity. *Clin Cancer Res.* 1997;3:25–30.

Clark CL, et al. Progestin regulation of cellular proliferation. *Endocrine Reviews.* 1990;11: 266–302.

Clark RV, et al. Marked suppression of dihydrotestosterone in men with benign prostatic hyperplasia by dutasteride, a dual 5-reductase inhibitor. *Journal of Clinical Endocrinology and Metabolism.* 2004;89:2179–2184.

Clarke R, et al. Hormonal carcinogenesis in breast cancer: cellular and molecular studies of malignant progression. *Breast Cancer Research and Treatment.* 1994;31:237–248.

Clements AD, et al. The relationship between salivary cortisol concentrations in frozen versus mailed samples. *Psychoneuroendocrinol.* 1998;23:613–616.

Clevenger CV, et al. Prolactin as an autocrine/paracrine factor in breast tissue. *Journal of Mammary Gland Biology and Neoplasia.* 1997; 2:59–68.

Clur A. Di-iodothyronine as part of the oestradiol and catechol oestrogen receptor—the role of iodine, thyroid hormones and melatonin in the aetiology of breast cancer. *Med Hypotheses.* 1988 Dec;27(4):303–311.

Cohen SM, et al. Cell proliferation in carcinogenesis. *Science.* 1990;249:1007–1011.

Collins JA, et al. Progesterone metabolism in adenocarcinoma of the endometrium. *American Journal of Obstetrics and Gynecology.* 1974;120:779–784.

Cooper A, et al. Systemic absorption of progesterone from progest cream in postmenopausal women. *Lancet.* 1998;351:1255–1256 [letter] and *Lancet* 1998;352:905–906 [comments].

Croxtall JD, et al. Glucocorticoids act within minutes to inhibit recruitment of signalling factors to activated EGF receptors through a receptor-dependent, transcription- independent mechanism. *British Journal of Pharmacology.* 2000;130:289–298.

Dabbs JM, et al. Reliability of salivary testosterone measurements: a multicenter evaluation. *Clin Chem.* 1995;41:1581–1584.

Dabbs JM. Salivary testosterone measurements: collecting, storing and mailing saliva samples. *Phys Behav.* 1991;49:815–817.

Dabbs JM. Salivary testosterone measurements: reliability across hours, days and weeks. *Phys Behav.*1990;48:83–86.

Das R, et al. Prolactin as a mitogen in mammary cells. *Journal of Mammary Gland Biology and Neoplasia.* 1997;2:29–39.

Dauchy RT, et al. Dim light during darkness stimulates tumor progression by enhancing tumor fatty acid uptake and metabolism. *Cancer Letters.* 1999;144:131–136.

Davidson MH, et al. Safety and endocrine effects of 3-acetyl-7-oxo DHEA (7-keto DHEA). *FASEB J.* 1998;12:A4429.

Davies RH, et al. Salivary testosterone levels and major depressive illness in men. *Br J Psychiatry.* 1992 Nov;161:629–632.

Davis DL, et al. Rethinking breast cancer risk and the environment: the case for the precautionary principle. *Environ Health Perspect.* 1998;106(9):523–529.

Davis EP, et al. The start of a new school year: individual differences in salivary cortisol response in relation to child temperament. *Dev Psychobiol.* 1999;35:188–196.

de la Llosa-Hermier MP, et al. Inhibitory effect of ovine and human placental lactogens on progesterone catabolism in luteinized rat ovaries in vitro. *Placenta.* 1983;4:479–487.

Delfs TM, et al. 24-Hour profiles of salivary progesterone. *Fertil Steril.* 1994;62:960–966.

Dennerstein L, et al. Are changes in sexual functioning during midlife due to aging or menopause? *Fertil Steril.* 2001 Sep;76(3):456–460.

Dennerstein L, et al. The menopause and sexual functioning: a review of the population-based studies. *Annu Rev Sex Res.* 2003;14:64–82.

Dentali S. Hormones and yams: what's the connection? *The American Herb Assoc.* 1994;10:4–5.

Desgres J, et al. Progesterone metabolism in newborn rat heart cell cultures. *Advances in Myocardiology.* 1980;1:339–344.

Dhanvantari S, et al. Suppression of follicle-stimulating hormone by the gonadal-and neurosteroid, 3-hydroxy-4-pregnen-20-one involves actions at the level of the gonadotrope membrane/calcium channel. *Endocrinology.* 1994;134:371–376.

Di Monaco M, et al. Dihydrotestosterone affects the growth of hormone-unresponsive breast cancer cells: an indirect action. *Anticancer Research.* 1995;15:2581–2584.

Dinsdale CJ, et al. Glycerol alters cytoskeleton and cell adhesion while inhibiting cell proliferation. *Cell Biology International Reports.* 1992;16:591–602.

Dittmar FW, et al. Premenstrual syndrome: treatment with a phytopharmaceutical. *TW Gynakol.* 1992; 5: 60–68.

Dollbaum CM. Lab analyses of salivary DHEA and progesterone following ingestion of yam-containing products. *Townsend Letter for Doctors and Patients.* 1995 Oct;104.

Dorfman RI. In vivo metabolism of neutral steroid hormones. *Journal of Clinical Endocrinology and Metabolism.* 1954;14:318–325.

Duclos M, et al. Corticotroph axis sensitivity after exercise in endurance-trained athletes. *Clin Endocrin.* 1998;48:493–501.

Eechaute W, et al. Steroid metabolism and steroid receptors in dimethylbenz(a)anthracene-induced rat mammary tumors. *Cancer Research.* 1983;43:4260–4265.

Ehrstrom SM, et al. Signs of chronic stress in women with recurrent candida vulvovaginitis. *Am J Obstet Gynecol.* 2005 Oct;193(4):1376–1381.

Emanuele MA, et al. Alcohol and the male reproductive system. *Alcohol Res Health.* 2001;25(4):282–287.

Endogenous Hormones and Breast Cancer Collaborative Group. Endogenous sex hormones and breast cancer in postmenopausal women: reanalysis of nine prospective studies. *J Natl Cancer Inst.* 2002 Apr 17;94(8):606–616.

Erlund I, et al. Plasma concentrations of the flavonoids hesperetin, naringenin and quercetin in human subjects following their habitual diets, and diets high or low in fruit and vegetables. *Eur J Clin Nutr.* 2002;56:891–898.

Fahey JW, et al. Antioxidant functions of sulforaphane: a potent inducer of Phase II detoxication enzymes. *Food Chem Toxicol.* 1999;37:973–979.

Fahey JW, et al. Broccoli sprouts: an exceptionally rich source of inducers of enzymes that protect against chemical carcinogens. *Proc Natl Acad Sci.* 1997;94:10367–10372.

Fahey JW, et al. Sulforaphane inhibits extracellular, intracellular, and antibiotic-resistant strains of Helicobacter pylori and prevents benzo[a]pyrene-induced stomach tumors. *PNAS.* 2002 May 28;99(11):7610–7615.

Fennessey PV, et al. Progesterone metabolism in T47Dco human breast cancer cells–I, 5-pregnan-3ß,6-diol-20-one is the secreted product. *Journal of Steroid Biochemistry.* 1986;25(5A):641–648.

Ferguson MM, et al. Progesterone metabolism in the murine submandibular salivary gland. *Journal of Dental Research.* 1983;62:1031–1032.

Fettes I. Migraine in the menopause. *Neurology.* 1999;53(4 Suppl 1):S29–33. Review.

Filaire E, et al. Dehydroepiandrosterone (DHEA) rather than testosterone shows saliva androgen responses to exercise in elite female handball players. *Int J Sports Med.* 2000;21:17–20.

Filaire E, et al. Saliva cortisol, physical exercise and training: influences of swimming and handball on cortisol concentrations in women. *Eur J Appl Physiol.* 1996;74:274–278.

Finn MM, et al. The frequency of salivary progesterone sampling and the diagnosis of luteal phase insufficiency. *Gynecol Endocrinol.* 1992;6:127–134.

Fotherby K. Bioavailability of orally administered sex steroids used in oral contraception and hormone replacement therapy. *Contraception.* 1996;54:59–69.

Fournier A, et al. Breast cancer risk in relation to different types of hormone replacement therapy in the E3N-EPIC cohort. *Int J Cancer.* 2005;114:448–454.

Fowke JH, et al. Brassica vegetable consumption shifts estrogen metabolism in healthy postmenopausal women. *Cancer Epidemiol Biomarkers Prev.* 2000;9(8):773–779.

Friebely J, et al. Pheromonal influences on sociosexual behavior in postmenopausal women. *J Sex Res.* 2004 Nov;41(4):372–380.

Frost P, et al. Metabolism of progesterone-4-^{14}C in vitro in human skin and vaginal mucosa. *Biochemistry.* 1969;8:948–952.

Gaby A. Multilevel yam scam. *Townsend Letter for Doctors and Patients.* 1996 Jan:96–97.

Galan MV, et al. Oral broccoli sprouts for the treatment of *Helicobacter pylori* infection: a preliminary report. *Dig Dis Sci.* 2004 Aug;49(7–8):1088–1090.

Gamet-Payrastre L, et al. Sulforaphane, a naturally occurring isothiocyanate, induces cell cycle arrest and apoptosis in HT29 human colon cancer cells. *Cancer Research.* 2000;60:1426–1433.

Garritano S, et al. Estrogen-like activity of seafood related to environmental chemical contaminants. *Environ Health.* 2006 Mar 30;5:9.

Gibson EL, et al. Increased salivary cortisol reliably induced by a protein-rich midday meal. *Psychosom Med.* 1999;61:214–224.

Gilles PA, et al. Effect of 20-dihydroprogesterone, progesterone, and their 5-reduced metabolites on serum gonadotropin levels and hypothalamic LHRH content. *Biology of Reproduction.* 1981;24:1088 1097.

Gingras S, et al. Induction of 3ß-hydroxysteroid dehydrogenase/^{5}-^{4} isomerase type 1 gene transcription in human breast cancer cell lines and in normal mammary epithelial cells by interleukin-4 and interleukin-13. *Molecular Endocrinology.* 1999;13:66–81.

Girgert R, et al. Tracking the elusive antiestrogenic effect of melatonin: a new methodological approach. *Neuroendocrinol Lett.* 2003 Dec;24(6):440–444.

Glasier MA, et al. Progesterone metabolism by guinea pig intrauterine tissues. *Journal of Steroid Biochemistry and Molecular Biology.* 1994;51:199–207.

Going JJ, et al. Proliferative and secretory activity in human breast during natural and artificial menstrual cycles. *American Journal of Pathology.* 1988;130:193–204.

Gonzales GF, et al. Effect of Lepidium meyenii (Maca), a root with aphrodisiac and fertility-enhancing properties, on serum reproductive hormone levels in adult healthy men. *J Endocrinol.* 2003 Jan;176(1):163–168.

Gonzales GF, et al. Effect of Lepidium meyenii (MACA) on sexual desire and its absent relationship with serum testosterone levels in adult healthy men. *Andrologia.* 2002 Dec;34(6):367–372.

Gordon GG, et al. Effect of alcohol (ethanol) administration on sex-hormone metabolism in normal men. *N Engl J Med.* 1976 Oct 7;295(15):793–797.

Graham S, et al. Diet in the epidemiology of cancer of the colon and rectum. *J Nat Cancer Inst.* 1978;61(3):709–714.

Granberg S, et al. Endometrial sonographic and histologic findings in women with and without hormonal replacement therapy suffering from postmenopausal bleeding. *Maturitas.* 1997;27(1):35–40.

Granger DA, et al. Neuroendocrine reactivity, internalizing behavior problems, and control-related cognitions in clinic-referred children and adolescents. *J Abn Psychology.* 1994;103:267–276.

Granger DA, et al. Reciprocal influences among adrenocortical activation, psychosocial processes, and the behavioral adjustment of clinic-referred children. *Child Dev.* 1996;67:3250–3262.

Granger DA, et al. Salivary testosterone determination in studies of child health and development. *Horm Behav.* 1999;35:18–27.

Grin W, et al. A significant correlation between melatonin deficiency and endometrial cancer. *Gynecol Obstet Invest.* 1998;45(1):62–65.

Groshong SD, et al. Biphasic regulation of breast cancer cell growth by progesterone:

role of the cyclin-dependent kinase inhibitors, p21 and p27 Kip1. *Molecular Endocrinology.* 1997;11:1593–1607.

Grube B, et al. St. John's Wort extract: efficacy for menopausal symptoms of psychological origin. *Adv Ther.* 1999 Jul-Aug;16(4):177–86.

Gruenwald J, et al. *PDR for Herbal Medicines.* Montvale, NJ: Medical Economics Company; 1998.

Guerra MC, et al. Comparison between Chinese medical herb Pueraria lobata crude extract and its main isoflavone puerarin antioxidant properties and effects on rat liver CYP-cataly-sed drug metabolism. *Life Sci.* 2000;67(24):2997–3006.

Gupta M, et al. Estrogenic and antiestrogenic activities of 16 alpha- and 2-hydroxy metabolites of 17 beta-estradiol in MCF-7 and T47D human breast cancer cells. *J Steroid Biochem Mol Biol.* 1998;67(5–6):413–419.

Hackenberg R, et al. Androgen sensitivity of the new human breast cancer cell line MFM-223. *Cancer Research.* 1991;51:5722–5727.

Haggans CJ, et al. Effect of flaxseed consumption on urinary estrogen metabolites in postmenopausal women. *Nutr Cancer.* 1999;33(2):188–195.

Halaska, M. et al. [Treatment of cyclical mastodynia using an extract of Vitex agnus castus: results of a double-blind comparison with a placebo] [In Czech]. *Ceska Gynekol.* 1998;63(5):388–392.

Hammond GL, et al. Serum distribution of the major metabolites of norgestimate in relation to its pharmacological properties. *Contraception.* 2003;67:93–99.

Hanahan D, et al. The hallmarks of cancer. *Cell.* 2000;100: 57–70.

Hancke JL, et al. Schisandra chinensis (Turcz.) Baill. *Fitoterapia.* 1999;70:451–471

Hanukoglu I, et al. Progesterone metabolism in the pineal, brain stem, thalamus and corpus callosum of the female rat. *Brain Research.* 1977;125:313–324.

Harada N, et al. Tissue-specific expression of the human aromatase cytochrome P-450 gene by alternative use of multiple exons 1 and promoters, and switching of tissue-specific exons 1 in carcinogenesis. *Proc Natl Acad Sci USA.* 1993;90:11312–11316.

Hargrove JT, et al. An alternative method of hormone replacement therapy using the natural sex steroids. *Infert Repro Med Clin N Am.* 1995;6:653–74.

Hargrove JT, et al. Menopausal hormone replacement therapy with continuous daily oral micronized estradiol and progesterone. *Obstet Gynecol.* 1989;73:606–12.

Harris B, et al. Maternity blues and major endocrine changes: cardiff puerperal mood and hormone study II. *BMJ.* 1994 Apr;308:949–953.

Havas S, et al. 5-A-Day for Better Health: a new research initiative. *J Am Diet Assoc.* 1994; 94:32–36.

Head KA. Estriol: safety and efficacy. *Altern Med Rev.* 1998 Apr;3(2):101–13. Review.

Hecht SS. Chemoprevention of cancer by isothiocyanates, modifiers of carcinogen metabolism. *J Nutr.* 1999;129:768S–774S.

Heim C, et al. Abuse-related posttraumatic stress disorder and alterations of the hypothalamic-pituitary-adrenal axis in women with chronic pelvic pain. *Psychosom Med.* 1998;60:309–318.

Heine RP, et al. Accuracy of salivary estriol testing compared to traditional risk factor assessment in predicting preterm birth. *Am J Obstet Gynecol.* 1999;180:S214–218.

Helige C, et al. Interrelation of motility, cytoskeletal organization and gap junctional communication with invasiveness of melanocyte cells in vitro. *Invasion and Metastasis.* 1997;17:26–41.

Henriksson L, et al. A comparative multicenter study of the effects of continuous low-dose estradiol released from a new vaginal ring versus estriol vaginal pessaries in postmenopausal women with symptoms and signs of urogenital atrophy. *Am J Obstet Gynecol.* 1994 Sep;171(3):624–632.

Henwood SM, et al. An escalating dose oral gavage study of 3beta-acetoxyandrost-5-ene-7, 17-dione (7-oxo-DHEA-acetate) in rhesus monkeys. *Biochem Biophys Res Commun.* 1999;254:124–126.

Henzl MR. Norgestimate: from the laboratory to three clinical indications. *Journal of Reproductive Medicine.* 2001;46:647–661.

Herbert J, et al. Adrenal secretion during major depression in 8- to 16-year-olds, 1. Altered diurnal rhythms in salivary cortisol and dehydroepiandrosterone (DHEA) at presentation. *Psychol Med.* 1996;26: 245–256.

Hermann AC, et al. Over-the-counter progesterone cream produces significant drug exposure compared to a food and drug administration-approved oral progesterone product. *J Clin Pharmacol.* 2005;45:614–619.

Hernandez D, et al. Evaluation of the antiulcer and antisecretory activity of extracts of Aralia elata root and Schisandra chinensis fruit in the rat. *J Ethnopharmacol.* 1988 May-Jun;23(1):109–114.

Hickey RJ, et al. Essential hormones as carcinogenic hazards. *J Occup Med.* 1979 Apr;21(4):265–268. Review.

Hobkirk R, et al. The effect of chorion-uterine interaction upon free progesterone metabolism during advanced gestation in the guinea pig. *Journal of Steroid Biochemistry and Molecular Biology.* 1997;62:185–193.

Holme TC. Cancer cell structure: actin changes in tumour cells—possible mechanisms for malignant tumour formation. *European Journal of Surgery and Oncology.* 1990;16 161–169.

Holth LT, et al. Chromatin, nuclear matrix and the cytoskeleton: role of cell structure in neoplastic transformation. *International Journal of Oncology.* 1998;13:827–837.

Horwitz KB, et al. MCF-7; a human breast cancer cell line with estrogen, androgen, progesterone, and glucocorticoid receptors. *Steroids.* 1975;26:785–795.

Horwitz KB, et al. Progesterone metabolism in T47Dco human breast cancer cells–II, Intracellular metabolic path of progesterone and synthetic progestins. *Journal of Steroid Biochemistry.* 1986;25:911–916.

Horwitz KB, et al. Progestin action and progesterone receptor structure in human breast cancer: a review. *Recent Progress in Hormone Research.* 1985;41:249–316.

Huang Z, et al. 16 alpha-hydroxylation of estrone by human cytochrome P4503A4/5. *Carcinogenesis.* 1998;19(5):867–872.

Humphries MJ, et al. The structure of cell adhesion molecules. *Trends in Cell Biology.* 1998;8:78–83.

Ibrahim AR, et al. Aromatase inhibition by flavonoids. *J Steroid Biochem Mol Biol.* 1990;37:257–260.

Ichikawa H, et al. Role of component herbs in antioxidant activity of shengmai san—a traditional Chinese medicine formula preventing cerebral oxidative damage in rat. *Am J Chin Med.* 2003;31(4):509–521.

Iczkowski KA, et al. The dual 5-reductase inhibitor dutasteride induces atrophic changes and decreases relative cancer volume in human prostate. *Urology.* 2005;65:76–82.

Ip SP, et al. Differential effect of schisandrin B and dimethyl diphenyl bicarboxylate (DDB) on hepatic mitochondrial glutathione redox status in carbon tetrachloride intoxicated mice. *Mol Cell Biochem.* 2000 Feb;205(1–2):111–114.

Ip SP, et al. Effect of schisandrin B on hepatic glutathione antioxidant system in mice: Protection against carbon tetrachloride toxicity. *Planta Med.* 1995;6:398–401.

Ip SP, et al. Schisandrin B protects against carbon tetrachloride toxicity by enhancing the mitochondrial glutathione redox status in mouse liver. *Free Radic Biol Med.* 1996;21(5):709–712.

Ip SP, et al. Schisandrin B protects against menadione-induced hepatotoxicity by enhancing DT-diaphorase activity. *Mol Cell Biochem.* 2000 May;208(1–2):151–155.

Itokawa H, et al. Cytotoxic quassinoids and tirucallane-type triterpene from the woods of Eurycoma longifolia. *Chemical and Pharmaceutical Bulletin.* 1992;40:1053–1055.

Itokawa H, et al. Eurylene, a new squalene-type triterpene from Eurycoma longifolia. *Tetrahedron Letters.* 1991;32(15):1803–1804.

Itokawa H, et al. A new squalene-type triterpene from the woods of Eurycoma longifolia. *Chemistry Letters.* 1991;2221–2222.

Itokawa H, et al. Novel quassinoids from Eurycoma longifolia. *Chemical and Pharmaceutical Bulletin.* 1993;41(2):403–405.

Jabara AG. Effects of progesterone on 9,10-dimethyl-1,2-benzanthracene-induced mammary tumours in Sprague-Dawley rats. *British Journal of Cancer.* 1967;21:418–429.

Jeong HJ, et al. Inhibition of aromatase activity by flavonoids. *Arch Pharm Res.* 1999 Jun;22(3):309–312.

Ji Q, et al. Selective loss of AKR1C1 and AKR1C2 in breast cancer and their potential effect on progesterone signaling. *Cancer Research.* 2004;64:7610–7617.

Ji Q, et al. Selective reduction of AKR1C2 in prostate cancer and its role in DHT metabolism. *The Prostate.* 2003;54:275–289.

Jiwajinda S, et al. In vitro anti-tumor promoting and anti-parasitic activities of the quassinoids from Eurycoma longifolia, a medicinal plant in Southeast Asia. *Journal of Ethnopharmacology.* 2002;82:55–58.

Jiwajinda S, et al. Quassinoids from Eurycoma longifolia as plant growth inhibitors. *Phytochemistry.* 2001;58:959–962.

Johansson A, et al. Adrenal steroid dysregulation in dystrophia myotonica. *J Int Med.* 1999;245:345–351.

Judd HL, et al. Endocrine function of the postmenopausal ovary: concentration of androgens and estrogens in ovarian and peripheral vein blood. *J Clin Endocrinol Meta.* 1974;39:1020–1024.

Kabat GC, et al. Urinary estrogen metabolites and breast cancer: a case-control study. *Cancer Epidemiol Biomarkers Prev.* 1997;6(7):505–509.

Kall MA, et al. Effects of dietary broccoli on human drug metabolising activity. *Cancer Letters.* 1997;114:169–170.

Kanchanapoom T, et al. Canthin-6-one and beta-carboline alkaloids from Eurycoma harmandiana. *Phytochemistry.* 2001;56:383–386.

Kandouz M, et al. Proapoptotic effects of antiestrogens, progestins and androgen in breast cancer cells. *Journal of Steroid Biochemistry and Molecular Biology.* 1999;69:463–471.

Kao YC, et al. Molecular basis of the inhibition of human aromatase (estrogen synthetase) by flavone and isoflavone phytoestrogens: A site-directed mutagenesis study. *Environ Health Perspect.* 1998 Feb;106(2):85–92.

Karnat A, et al. Mechanisms in tissue-specific regulation of estrogen biosynthesis in humans. *Trends Endocrinol Metab.* 2002; 13:122–128.

Kavaliers M, et al. Analgesic effects of the progesterone metabolite, 3-hydroxy-5-pregnan-20-one, and possible modes of action in mice. *Brain Research.* 1987;415:393–398.

Kawaii S, et al. Differentiation-promoting activity of pomegranate (Punica granatum) fruit extracts in HL-60 human promyelocytic leukemia cells. *J Med Food.* 2004;7(1):13–18.

Kellis JT Jr, et al. Inhibition of human estrogen synthetase (aromatase) by flavones. *Science.* 1984 Sep 7;225(4666):1032–1034.

Kenny FS, et al. Effect of dietary GLA+/-tamoxifen on the growth, ER expression and fatty acid profile of ER positive human breast cancer xenografts. *Int J Cancer.* 2001 May 1;92(3):342–347.

Kenny FS, et al. Gamma linolenic acid with tamoxifen as primary therapy in breast cancer. *Int J Cancer.* 2000 Mar 1;85(5):643–648.

Keshamouni VG, et al. Mechanism of 17-ß-Estradiol-induced Erk1/2 activation in breast cancer cells. *Journal of Biological Chemistry.* 2002;277:22558–22565.

Key TJ, et.al. Endogenous Hormones Breast Cancer Collaborative Group. Body mass index, serum sex hormones, and breast cancer risk in postmenopausal women. *J Natl Cancer Inst.* 2003 Aug 20;95(16):1218–1226.

Khan-Dawood FS, et al. Salivary and plasma bound and "free" testosterone in men and women. *Am J Obstet Gynecol.* 1984;148:441–445.

Kicovic PM, et al. The treatment of postmenopausal vaginal atrophy with Ovestin vaginal cream or suppositories: clinical, endocrinological and safety aspects. *Maturitas.* 1980 Dec;2(4):275–282.

Kiess W, et al. Salivary cortisol levels throughout childhood and adolescence: relation with age, pubertal stage and weight. *Pediatr Res.* 1995;37:502–506.

Kim ND, et al. Chemopreventive and adjuvant therapeutic potential of pomegranate (Punica granatum) for human breast cancer. *Breast Cancer Res Treat.* 2002 Feb;71(3):203–217.

Kim SR, et al. Dibenzocyclooctadiene lignans from Schisandra chinensis protect primary cultures of rat cortical cells from glutamate-induced toxicity. *J Neurosci Res.* 2004 May 1;76(3):397–405.

King RJB. Estrogen and progestin effects in human breast carcinogenesis. *Breast Cancer Research and Treatment.* 1993;27:3–15.

Kitts DD. Studies on the estrogenic activity of a coffee extract. *J Toxicol Environ Health.* 1987;20(1–2):37–49.

Klassen AD, et al. Sexual experience and drinking among women in a U.S. national survey. *Arch Sex Behav.* 1986 Oct;15(5):363–392.

Ko KM, et al. Schisandrin B modulates the ischemia-reperfusion induced changes in non-enzymatic antioxidant levels in isolated-perfused rat hearts. *Mol Cell Biochem.* 2001 Apr;220(1–2):141–147.

Ko KM, et al. Schisandrin B protects against tert-butylhydroperoxide induced cerebral toxicity by enhancing glutathione antioxidant status in mouse brain. *Mol Cell Biochem.* 2002 Sep;238(1–2):181–186.

Kohlmeier L, et al. Cruciferous vegetable consumption and colorectal cancer risk: meta-analysis of the epidemiological evidence. *FASEB Journal.* 1997;11(3):A369.

Kohno H, et al. Pomegranate seed oil rich in conjugated linolenic acid suppresses chemically induced colon carcinogenesis in rats. *Cancer Sci.* 2004;95(6):481–486.

Korneyev A, et al. Regional and interspecies differences in brain progesterone metabolism. *Journal of Neurochemistry.* 1993;61:2041–2047.

Kudielka BM, et al. Psychological and endocrine responses to psychosocial stress and dexamethasone/corticotropin-releasing hormone in healthy postmenopausal women and young controls: the impact of age and a two-week estradiol treatment. *Neuroendocrinol.* 1999;70:422–430.

Kuhl H. Comparative pharmacology of newer progestogens. *Drugs.* 1996;51:188–215.

Kuhl H. Pharmacology of estrogens and progestogens: influence of different routes of administration. *Climacteric.* 2005;8 (Suppl 1):3–63.

Kuntz S, et al. Comparative analysis of the effects of flavonoids on proliferation, cytotoxicity, and apoptosis in human colon cancer cell lines. *Eur J Nutr.* 1999;38:133–142.

Kuppusamy UR, et al. Effects of flavonoids on cyclic AMP phosphodiesterase and lipid mobilization in rat adipocytes. *Biochem Pharmacol.* 1992;44:1307–1315.

Kuwata M, et al. Progesterone metabolism in vitro by testes from germ cell-free mice of different ages. *Biochimica et Biophysica Acta.* 1976;486:127–135.

Lac G, et al. Dexamethasone in resting and exercising men. II. Effects on adrenocortical hormones. *J Appl Physiol.* 1999 Jul;87(1):183–188.

Lac G, et al. Steroid assays in saliva: a method to detect plasmatic contaminations. *Arch Int Physiol Biochim Biophys.* 1993;101:257–262.

Lachelin GC, et al. A comparison of saliva, plasma unconjugated and plasma total oestriol levels throughout normal pregnancy. *Brit J Obstet Gyn.* 1984;91:1203–1209.

Lacy LR, et al. Progesterone metabolism by the ovary of the pregnant rat: discrepancies in the catabolic regulation model. *Endocrinology.* 1976;99:929–934.

Laduron PM. Criteria for receptor sites in binding studies. *Biochemical Pharmacology.* 1984;33:833–839.

Laine M, et al. Progesterone metabolism by major salivary glands of rat-I, Submandibular and sublingual glands. *Journal of Steroid Biochemistry.* 1990;35:723–728.

Laine MA, et al. Progesterone metabolism in human saliva in vitro. *Journal of Steroid Biochemistry and Molecular Biology.* 1999;70:109–113.

Lanari C, et al. Induction of mammary adenocarcinomas by medroxyprogesterone acetate in BALB/c female mice. *Cancer Letters.* 1986;33:215–223.

Lapointe J, et al. Role of the cyclin-dependent kinase inhibitor p27(Kip1) in androgen-induced inhibition of CAMA-1 breast cancer cell proliferation. *Endocrinology.* 2001;142: 4331–4338.

Lardy H, et al. An acute oral gavage study of 3beta-acetoxyandrost- 5-ene-7,17-dione (7-oxo-DHEA-acetate) in rats. *Biochem Biophys Res Commun.* 1999;254:120–123.

Lardy H, et al. Ergosteroids. II: Biologically active metabolites and synthetic derivatives of dehydroepiandrosterone. *Steroids.* 1998;63:158–165.

Lauritzen CH, et al. Treatment of premenstrual tension syndrome with Vitex agnus castus: controlled, doubleblind study versus pyridoxine. *Phytomed.* 1997; 4: 183–189.

Le Bail JC, et al. Effects of phytoestrogens on aromatase, 3beta and 17beta-hydroxysteroid dehydrogenase activities and human breast cancer cells. *Life Sci.* 2000;66: 1281–1291.

Lechner W, et al. Correlation of oestriol levels in saliva, plasma and urine of pregnant women. *Acta Endocrinol.* 1985;109:266–268.

Lemon HM. Pathophysiologic considerations in the treatment of menopausal patients with oestrogens; the role of oestriol in the prevention of mammary carcinoma. *Acta Endoocrinol.* 1980;Suppl 233:17–27.

Leonetti HB, et al. Transdermal progesterone cream as an alternative progestin in hormone therapy. *Altern Ther Health Med.* 2005;11:36–38.

Leonetti HB, et al. Transdermal progesterone cream for vasomotor symptoms and postmenopausal bone loss. *Obstet Gynecol.* 1999; 94:225–228.

Levine H, et al. Comparison of the pharmacokinetics of crinone 8% administered vaginally versus Prometrium administered orally in postmenopausal women(3). *Fertil Steril.* 2000 Mar;73(3):516–521.

Lewis MJ, et al. Expression of progesterone metabolizing enzyme genes (AKR1C1, AKR1C2, AKR1C3, SRD5A1, SRD5A2) is altered in human breast carcinoma. *BMC Cancer.* 2004;4(27):1–12. Available at: http://www.biomedcentral.com. Accessed 2007.

Li X-Y. Bioactivity of neolignans from Fructus schisandrae. *Mem Inst Oswaldo Cruz.* 1991;86:31–37.

Lichtenstein P, et al. Environmental and heritable factors in the causation of cancer—analyses of cohorts of twins from Sweden, Denmark, and Finland. *N Engl J Med.* 2000;343(2):78–85.

Limbird LE. *Cell Surface Receptors: A Short Course on Theory and Methods.* 2nd ed. "Identification of receptors using direct radioligand techniques." Norwell, MA: Klewer Academic Publishers; 1996.

Lippert C, et al. The effect of endogenous estradiol metabolites on the proliferation of human breast cancer cells. *Life Sci.* 2003 Jan 10;72(8):877–883.

Lipson SF, et al. Development of protocols for the application of salivary steroid analyses to field conditions. *Am J Human Biol.* 1989;1:249–255.

Lipson SF, et al. Normative study of age variation in salivary progesterone profiles. *J Biosoc Sci.* 1992;24:233–244.

Little B, et al. The conversion of progesterone to delta 4 pregnene-20 alpha-ol, 3-one by human placenta in vitro. *Acta Endocrinologica (Copenh)*. 1959;30:530–538.

Liu G-T. Pharmacological actions and clinical use of Fructus schisandrae. *Chin Med J*. 1989;102:740–749.

Liu H, et al. Indolo[3,2-b]carbazole: a dietary-derived factor that exhibits both antiestrogenic and estrogenic activity. *J Natl Cancer Inst*. 1994;86:1758–1765.

Liu KT. Studies on fructus schisandrae chinensis. Plenary lecture, World Health Organization (WHO). Seminar on the Use of Medicinal Plants in Health Care, Sept 1977. Tokyo, Japan. In: WHO Regional Office for the Western Pacific, Final Report, November 1977, Manila, 101–121.

Lloyd RV. Studies on the progesterone receptor content and steroid metabolism in normal and pathological human breast tissues. *Journal of Clinical Endocrinology and Metabolism*. 1979;48:585–593.

Lo MS, et al. Clinical applications of salivary cortisol measurements. *Sing Med J*. 1992;33:170.

Lomaestro B, et al. Glutathione in health and disease: pharmacotherapeutic issues. *Ann Pharmacother*. 1995;29:1263–1273.

Lorrain J, et al. Sleep in menopause: differential effects of two forms of hormone replacement therapy. *Menopause*. 2001 Jan-Feb;8(1):10–16.

Lu Y, et al. Salivary estradiol and progesterone levels in conception and nonconception cycles in women: evaluation of a new assay for salivary estradiol. *Fertil Steril*. 1999; 71:863–868.

Lu YC, et al. Direct radioimmunoassay of progesterone in saliva. *J Immunoassay*. 1997;18:149–163.

Luna EJ, et al. Cytoskeleton-plasma membrane interactions. *Science*. 1992;258:955–964.

Luo S, et al. Inhibitory effect of the novel anti-estrogen EM-800 and medroxyprogesterone acetate on estrone-stimulated growth of dimethylbenz[a]anthracene-induced mammary carcinoma in rats. *International Journal of Cancer*. 1997;73:580–586.

McCann SE, et al. Dietary lignan intakes and risk of breast cancer by tumor estrogen receptor status. *Breast Cancer Res Treat*. 2006 Oct;99(3):309–311.

McGregor JA, et al. Diurnal variation in saliva estriol level during pregnancy: a pilot study. *Am J Obstet Gynecol*. 1999;180:S223–225.

McGregor JA, et al. Salivary estriol as risk assessment for preterm labor: a prospective trial. *Am J Obstet Gynecol*. 1995;173:1337–1342.

McGuire WL. Prognostic factors for recurrence and survival in human breast cancer. *Breast Cancer Res Treat*. 1987;10:5–9.

McGuire WL, et al. A role for progesterone in breast cancer. *Ann NY Acad Sci.* 1977;286:90–100.

Macario AJ. Heat-shock proteins and molecular chaperones: implications for pathogenesis, diagnostics, and therapeutics. *Int J Clin Lab Res.* 1995;25(2):59–70.

Mady EA, et al. Sex steroid hormones in serum and tissue of benign and malignant breast tumor patients. *Dis Markers.* 2000;16(3–4):151–157.

Maheo K, et al. Inhibition of cytochromes P-450 and induction of glutathione S-transferases by sulforaphane in primary human and rat hepatocytes. *Cancer Res.* 1997;57:3649–3652.

Majewska MD, et al. Steroid hormone metabolites are barbiturate-like modulators of the GABA receptor. *Science.* 1986;232:1004–1007.

Malaysian Monograph Committee. Radix eurycomae eurycoma root. Malaysian Monograph Committee: Kuala Lumpur. *Malaysian Herbal Monograph.* 1999;(1):29–32.

Manach C, et al. Polyphenols: food sources and bioavailability. *Am J Clin Nutr.* 2004;79:727–747.

Manjer J, et al. Postmenopausal breast cancer risk in relation to sex steroid hormones, prolactin and SHBG (Sweden). *Cancer Causes Control.* 2003 Sep;14(7):599–607.

Marrone BL. Ovarian steroidogenesis in vitro during the first month posthatching in the domestic chick: gonadotropin responsiveness and [^{3}H]progesterone metabolism. *General and Comparative Endocrinology.* 1986;62:62–69.

Marrone BL, et al. Progesterone metabolism by the hypothalamus, pituitary, and uterus of the rat during pregnancy. *Endocrinology.* 1981;109:41–45.

Marrone BL, et al. Progesterone metabolism by the hypothalamus, pituitary, and uterus of the aged rat. *Endocrinology.* 1982;111:162–167.

Martel FL, et al. Salivary cortisol levels in socially phobic adolescent girls. *Depression Anxiety.* 1999;10:25–27.

Martini L, et al. Androgen and progesterone metabolism in the central and peripheral nervous system. *Journal of Steroid Biochemistry and Molecular Biology.* 1993;47:195–205.

Maskarinec G, et al. Alcohol and dietary fibre intakes affect circulating sex hormones among premenopausal women. *Public Health Nutr.* 2006 Oct;9(7):875–881.

Matsumoto K, et al. Progesterone metabolism in vitro by rabbit testes at different stages of development. *Endocrinology.* 1976;99:1269–1272.

Matsunaga M, et al. Identification of 3ß,5ß-tetrahydroprogesterone, a progesterone metabolite, and its stimulatory action on preoptic neurons in the avian brain. *Brain Research.* 2004;1007:160–.

Matthews KA, et al. Influence of hormone therapy on the cardiovascular responses to stress of postmenopausal women. *Biol Psychol.* 2005 Apr;69(1):39–56.

Mauvais-Jarvis P, et al. In vivo studies on progesterone metabolism by human skin. *Journal of Clinical Endocrinology and Metabolism*. 1969;29:1580–1585.

Meilahn EN, et al. Do urinary oestrogen metabolites predict breast cancer? Guernsey III cohort follow-up. *Br J Cancer*. 1998;78(9):1250–1255.

Melcangi RC, et al. Progesterone 5-reduction in neuronal and in different types of glial cell cultures: type 1 and 2 astrocytes and oligodendrocytes. *Brain Research*. 1994;639:202–206.

Menendez JA, et al. Effect of gamma-linolenic acid on the transcriptional activity of the Her-2/neu (erbB-2) oncogene. *J Natl Cancer Inst*. 2005 Nov 2;97(21):1611–1615.

Menendez JA, et al. Inhibition of fatty acid synthase-dependent neoplastic lipogenesis as the mechanism of gamma-linolenic acid-induced toxicity to tumor cells: an extension to Nwankwo's hypothesis. *Med Hypotheses*. 2005;64(2):337–341.

Menendez JA, et al. Omega-6 polyunsaturated fatty acid gamma-linolenic acid (18:3n-6) enhances docetaxel (Taxotere) cytotoxicity in human breast carcinoma cells: relationship to lipid peroxidation and HER-2/neu expression. *Oncol Rep*. 2004 Jun;11(6):1241–1252.

Menendez JA, et al. Synergistic interaction between vinorelbine and gamma-linolenic acid in breast cancer cells. *Breast Cancer Res Treat*. 2002 Apr;72(3):203–319.

Metcalf MG, et al. Indices of ovulation: comparison of plasma and salivary levels of progesterone with urinary pregnanediol. *J Endocr*. 1984;100:75–80.

Meulenberg PM, et al. Salivary progesterone excellently reflects free and total progesterone in plasma during pregnancy. *Clin Chem*. 1989;35:168–172.

Michnovicz JJ, et al. Changes in levels of urinary estrogen metabolites after oral indole-3- carbinol treatment in humans. *J Natl Cancer Inst*. 1997;89(10):718–723.

Milewicz A, et al. Vitex agnus castus extract in the treatment of luteal phase defects due to hyperprolactinemia: results of a randomized placebo-controlled, double-blind study. *Arzneim-Forsch Drug Res*. 1993;43:752–756.

Milewich L, et al. Initiation of human parturition, VI: identification and quantification of progesterone metabolites produced by the components of human fetal membranes. *Journal of Clinical Endocrinology and Metabolism*. 1977;45:400–411.

Miller WR. Pathways of hormone metabolism in normal and non-neoplastic breast tissue. *Ann NY Acad Sci*. 1990;586:53–59.

Minjarez D, et al. Regulation of uterine 5-reductase type 1 in mice. *Biology of Reproduction*. 2001;65:1378–1382.

Mitsunaga K, et al. Canthin-6-one alkaloids from Eurycoma longifolia. *Phytochemistry*. 1994;35(3):799–802.

Mol JA, et al. New insights in the molecular mechanism of progestin-induced proliferation of mammary epithelium: induction of the local biosynthesis of growth hormone (GH) in the mammary gland of dogs, cats and humans. *Journal of Steroid Biochemistry and Molecular Biology.* 1996;57:67–71.

Montplaisir J, et al. Effect of oral micronized progesterone on androgen levels in women with polycystic ovary syndrome. *Fertil Steril.* 2002 Jun;77(6):1125–1127.

Moon YS, et al. Effects of prostaglandins E2 and F2 alpha on progesterone metabolism by rat granulosa cells. *Biochemical and Biophysical Research Communications.* 1986;135:764–769.

Moon YS, et al. Time-dependent effects of follicle-stimulating hormone on progesterone metabolism by cultured rat granulosa cells. *Biochemical and Biophysical Research Communications.* 1987;144:67–73.

Morales A, et al. Is yohimbine effective in the treatment of organic impotence? Results of a controlled trial. *J Urol.* 1988 Apr;139(4): 849–852.

Moran DJ, et al. Lack of normal increase in saliva estriol/progesterone ratio in women with labor induced at 42 weeks' gestation. *Am J Obstet Gynecol.* 1992;167:1563–1564.

Morgenthaler J, et al. *The Smart Guide to Better Sex.* Petaluma, CA: Smart Publications; 1999.

Mori M, et al. In vitro metabolism of progesterone in the mammary tumour and the normal mammary gland of GRS/A strain of mice and dependency of some steroid-metabolizing enzyme activities upon ovarian function. *European Journal of Cancer.* 1980;16:185–193.

Mori M, et al. Steroid metabolism in the normal mammary gland and in the dimethylbenz-thracene-induced mammary tumour of rats. *Endocrinology.* 1978;102:1387–1397.

Mori-Okamoto J, et al. Pomegranate extract improves a depressive state and bone properties in menopausal syndrome model ovariectomized mice. *J Ethnopharmacol.* 2004;92(1):93–101.

Morita H, et al. Biphenylneolignans from wood of Eurycoma longifolia. *Phytochemistry.* 1992;31(11):3993–3995.

Morita H, et al. Highly oxygenated quassinoids from Eurycoma longifolia. *Phytochemistry.* 1993;33(3):691–696.

Morita H, et al. New quassinoids from the roots of Eurycoma longifolia. *Chemistry Letters.* 1990;749–752.

Morita H, et al. Squalene-derivatives from Eurycoma longifolia. *Phytochemistry.* 1993;34(3):765–771.

Moss HB, et al. Salivary cortisol responses and the risk for substance abuse in prepubertal boys. *Biol Psych.* 1995;38:547–555.

Mousavi Y, et al. Enterolactone and estradiol inhibit each other's proliferative effect on MCF-7 breast cancer cells in culture. *J Steroid Biochem Mol Biol.*

1992;41(3–8):615–619.

Murray M, et al. *Encyclopedia of Natural Medicine*. 2nd ed. Rocklin, CA: Prima Publishing; 1999.

Musgrove EA, et al. Cell cycle control by steroid hormones. *Seminars in Cancer Biology*. 1994;5:381–389.

Muti P, et al. Estrogen metabolism and risk of breast cancer: a prospective study of the 2:16 alpha-hydroxyestrone ratio in premenopausal and postmenopausal women. *Epidemiology*. 2000;11(6):635–640.

Nahoul K, et al. Comparison of saliva and plasma 17-hydroxyprogesterone time-course response to hCG administration in normal men. *J Steroid Biochem*. 1987;26:251–257.

Nahoul K, et al. Saliva testosterone time-course response to hCG in adult normal men, comparison with plasma levels. *J Steroid Biochem*. 1986;24:1011–1015.

Nakajima T, et al. Expression of 20-hydroxysteroid dehydrogenase mRNA in human endometrium and decidua. *Endocrine Journal*. 2003;50:105–111.

National Research Council. *Diet and Health: Implications for Reducing Chronic Disease Risk*. Washington, DC: National Academy Press; 1989.

Navarro MA, et al. Salivary excretory pattern of testosterone in substitutive therapy with testosterone enanthate. *Fertil Steril*. 1994;61:125–128.

Navarro MA, et al. Salivary testosterone in postmenopausal women with rheumatoid arthritis. *J Rheumatol*. 1998;25:1059–1062.

Nestle M. Broccoli sprouts as inducers of carcinogen-detoxifying enzyme systems: clinical, dietary, and policy implications. *Proc Natl Acad Sci*. 1997;94:11149–11151.

Nestle M. Broccoli sprouts in cancer prevention. *Nutr Rev*. 1998;56:127–130.

Nijhoff WA, et al. Effects of consumption of Brussels sprouts on plasma and urinary glutathione S-transferase class-alpha and -pi in humans. *Carcinogenesis*. 1995;16:955–957.

Nimrod A. Studies on the synergistic effect of androgen on the stimulation of progestin secretion by FSH in cultured rat granulosa cells: progesterone metabolism and the effect of androgens. *Molecular and Cellular Endocrinology*. 1977;8:189–199.

Ohno S, et al. Effects of flavonoid phytochemicals on cortisol production and on activities of steroidogenic enzymes in human adrenocortical H295R cells. *J Steroid Biochem Mol Biol*. 2002;80:355–363.

Onland-Moret NC, et al. Urinary endogenous sex hormone levels and the risk of postmenopausal breast cancer. *Br J Cancer*. 2003 May 6;88(9):1394–1399.

O'Leary P, et al. Salivary, but not serum or urinary levels of progesterone are elevated after topical application of progesterone cream to pre and postmenopausal women. *Clin Endocrinol*. 2000;53:615–620.

Oravec S, et al. Disorders of thyroid function and fertility disorders. *Ceska Gynekol.* 2000 Jan;65(1):53–57.

O'Rourke MT, et al. Salivary estradiol levels decrease with age in healthy, regularly-cycling women. *End J.* 1993;1:487–494.

Ortmann J, et al. Testosterone and 5-dihydrotestosterone inhibit in vitro growth of human breast cancer cell lines. *Gynecological Endocrinology.* 2002;16:113–120.

Osborne MP. Chemoprevention of breast cancer. *Surg Clin North Am.* 1999;79(5):1207–1221.

Ottosson UB, et al. Subfractions of high-density lipoprotein cholesterol during estrogen replacement therapy: a comparison between progestogens and natural progesterone. *Am J Obstet Gynecol.* 1985;151:746–750.

Pan SY, et al. Schisandrin B protects against tacrine- and bis(7)-tacrine-induced hepatotoxicity and enhances cognitive function in mice. *Planta Med.* 2002 Mar;68(3):217–220.

Panda S, et al. Changes in thyroid hormone concentrations after administration of ashwagandha root extract to adult male mice. *J Pharm Pharmacol.* 1998 Sep;50(9):1065–1068.

Panda S, et al. Guggulu (Commiphora mukul) induces triiodothyronine production: possible involvement of lipid peroxidation. *Life Sci.* 1999;65(12):PL137–141.

Panda S, et al. Guggulu (Commiphora mukul) potentially ameliorates hypothyroidism in female mice. *Phytother Res.* 2005 Jan;19(1):78–80.

Pao T-T, et al. Protective action of Schizandrin B on hepatic injury in mice. *Chin Med J.* 1977;3:173–180.

Patte-Mensah C, et al. Substance P inhibits progesterone conversion to neuroactive metabolites in spinal sensory circuit: a potential component of nociception. *PNAS.* 2005;102:9044–9049.

Pawlak KJ, et al. Membrane 5-pregnane-3,20-dione (5P) receptors in MCF-7 and MCF-10A breast cancer cells are up-regulated by estradiol and 5P and down-regulated by the progesterone metabolites, 3-dihydroprogesterone and 20-dihydroprogesterone, with associated changes in cell proliferation and detachment. *Journal of Steroid Biochemistry and Molecular Biology.* 2005;97:278–288.

Pawlak KJ, et al. Regulation of estrogen receptor (ER) levels in MCF-7 cells by progesterone metabolites. Paper presented at: The Endocrine Society 87th Annual Meeting; June 4–7, 2005; San Diego CA.

Pearson D, et al. *The Life Extension Companion.* New York, NY: Warner Books; 1984.

Pearson G, et al. Mitogen-activated protein (MAP) kinase pathways: regulation and physiological functions. *Endocrine Reviews.* 2001;22:153–183.

Pelissero C, et al. Effects of flavonoids on aromatase activity, an in vitro study. *J Steroid Biochem Mol Biol.* 1996 Feb;57(3–4):215–223.

Perlman D, et al. Metabolism of progestereone and testosterone by mammalian cells growing in suspension culture. *Canadian Journal of Biochemistry and Physiology.* 1960;38:393–395.

Petsos P, et al. Comparison of blood spot, salivary and serum progesterone assays in the normal menstrual cycle. *Clin Endocrin.* 1986;24:31 38.

Phillips A, et al. Comparative effect of estriol and equine conjugated estrogens on the uterus and the vagina. *Maturitas.* 1984 Mar;5(3):147–152.

Pignataro L, et al. Biosynthesis of progesterone derived neurosteroids by developing avian CNS: in vitro effects on the GABAA receptor complex. *International Journal of Developmental Neuroscience.* 1998;16:433–441.

Pike MC, et al. Estrogens, progestogens, normal breast cell proliferation, and breast cancer risk. *Epidemiologic Reviews.* 1993;15:17–35.

Pizzorno Joseph, et al. *Textbook of Natural Medicine.* 2nd ed. Oxford, UK: Churchill Livingstone; 1999.

Plu-Bureau G, et al. Percutaneous progesterone use and risk of breast cancer: results from a French cohort study of premenopausal women with benign breast disease. *Cancer Detect Prev.* 1999;23:290–296.

Plumb GW, et al. Are whole extracts and purified glucosinolates from cruciferous vegetables antioxidants? *Free Radic Res.* 1996;25:75–86.

Pollow K, et al. Progesterone metabolism in normal human endometrium during the menstrual cycle and in endometrial carcinoma. *Journal of Clinical Endocrinology and Metabolism.* 1975;41:729–737.

Pomata PE, et al. In vivo evidences of early neurosteroid synthesis in the developing rat central nervous system and placenta. *Developmental Brain Research.* 2000;120:83–86.

Potten CS, et al. The effect of age and menstrual cycle upon proliferative activity of the normal human breast. *British Journal of Cancer.* 1988;58:163–170.

Poulin R, et al. Androgens inhibit basal and estrogen-induced cell proliferation in the ZR-75-1 human breast cancer cell line. *Breast Cancer Research and Treatment.* 1988;12:213–225.

Pruessner JC, et al. Burnout, perceived stress, and cortisol responses to awakening. *Psychosom Med.* 1999;61:197–204.

Purves-Tyson TD, et al. Rapid actions of estradiol on cyclic AMP response-element binding protein phosphorylation in dorsal root ganglion neurons. *Neuroscience.* 2004;129: 629–637.

Quissell D. Steroid hormone analysis in human saliva. *Ann N Y Acad Sci.* 1993;694:143–145.

Raff H, et al. Late-night salivary cortisol as a screening test for Cushing's Syndrome. *J Clin Endocrinol Metab.* 1998;83:2681–2686.

Raz A. Adhesive properties of metastasizing tumor cells. *Ciba Foundation Symposia.* 1988;141:109–122.

Read GF. Status report on measurement of salivary estrogens and androgens. *Ann NY Acad Sci.* 1993; 694:146–160.

Read GF, et al. Changes in male salivary testosterone concentrations with age. *Int J Androl.* 1981;4:623–627.

Read GF, et al. Salivary cortisol and dehydroepiandrosterone sulphate levels in postmenopausal women with primary breast cancer. *Eur J Cancer Clin Oncol.* 1983;19:477–483.

Read GF, et al. Steroid analysis in saliva for the assessment of endocrine function. *Ann NY Acad Sci.* 1993;595:260–274.

Redmond AF, et al. Uterine progesterone metabolism during early pseudopregnancy in the rat. *Biology of Reproduction.* 1986;35:949–955.

Reed GA, et al. A phase I study of indole-3-carbinol in women: tolerability and effects. *Cancer Epidemiol Biomarkers Prev.* 2005 Aug;14(8):1953–1960.

Rhodes ME, et al. Inhibiting progesterone metabolism in the hippocampus of rats in behavioral estrus decreases anxiolytic behaviors and enhances exploratory and antinociceptive behaviors. *Cognitive, Affective and Behavioral Neuroscience.* 2001;1:287–296.

Riad-Fahmy D, et al. Salivary steroid assays for assessing variation in endocrine activity. *J Steroid Biochem.* 1983;19:265–272.

Robb-Nicholson C. By the way, doctor. I'm 53 and have been taking HRT with Estradiol and Prometrium daily for about a year. Should I also take a soy vitamin supplement? I took one before starting HRT because I thought it was supposed to prevent breast cancer. But I want to be on as little estrogen as possible. Will soy along with estrogen increase my risk of breast tumors? *Harv Womens Health Watch.* 2000 Feb;7(6):8.

Rosmond R, et al. The hypothalamic-pituitary-adrenal axis activity as a predictor or cardiovascular disease, type 2 diabetes and stroke. *J Int Med.* 2000;247:188–197.

Rosser A. The day of the yam. *Nurs Times.* 1985 May 1-7;81(18):47.

Ruiz-Luna AC, et al. Lepidium meyenii (Maca) increases litter size in normal adult female mice. *Reprod Biol Endocrinol.* 2005 May 3;3:16.

Ruutiainen K, et al. Salivary testosterone in hirsutism: correlations with serum testosterone and the degree of hair growth. *J Clin Endocrinol Metab.* 1987;64:1015–1020.

Saarinen N, et al. No evidence for the in vivo activity of aromatase-inhibiting flavonoids. *J Steroid Biochem. Mol. Biol.* 2001;78:231–239.

Saarinen NM, et al. Flaxseed attenuates the tumor growth stimulating effect of soy protein in ovariectomized athymic mice with MCF-7 human breast cancer xenografts. *Int J Cancer.* 2006 Aug 15;119(4):925–931.

Sadano H, et al. Differential expression of vinculin between weakly and highly metastatic B16-melanoma cell lines. *Japanese Journal of Cancer Research.* 1992;83:625–630.

Sanderson J'I, et al. Induction and inhibition of aromatase (CYP19) activity by various classes of pesticides in H295R human adrenocortical carcinoma cells. *Toxicol Appl Pharmacol.* 2002;182:44–54.

Santen RJ, et al. Endocrine treatment of breast cancer in women. *Endocrine Reviews.* 1990;11:221–265.

Santen RJ, et al. The role of mitogen-activated protein (MAP) kinase in breast cancer. *Journal of Steroid Biochemistry and Molecular Biology.* 2002;80:239–256.

Sannikka E, et al. Testosterone concentrations in human seminal plasma and saliva and its correlation with non-protein-bound and total testosterone levels in serum. *Int J Andrology.* 1983;6:319–330.

Savard K, et al. Biosynthesis of androgens from progesterone by human testicular tissue *in vitro. Journal of Clinical Endocrinology and Metabolism.* 1956;16:1629–1630.

Scheer FA, et al. Light affects morning salivary cortisol in humans. *J Clin Endocrinol.* 1999;84:3395–3398.

Schernhammer ES, et al. Night-shift work and risk of colorectal cancer in the nurses' health study. *J Natl Cancer Inst.* 2003 Jun 4;95(11):825–828.

Schliwa M, et al. A tumor promoter induces rapid and coordinated reorganization of actin and vinculin in cultured cells. *Journal of Cell Biology.* 1984;99:1045–1059.

Schmidbauer CP. Vaginal estriol administration in treatment of postmenopausal urinary incontinence. *Urologe A.* 1992 Nov;31(6):384–389.

Schramm W, et al. Determination of free progesterone in an ultrafiltrate of saliva collected in situ. *Clin Chem.* 1990;36:1488–1493.

Schramm W, et al. Testosterone concentration is increased in whole saliva but not in ultrafiltrate after toothbrushing. *Clin Chem.* 1993;39:519–521.

Schroeder MD, et al. Prolactin modulates cell cycle regulators in mammary tumor epithelial cells. *Molecular Endocrinology.* 2002;16:45–57.

Schwartz EB, et al. Assessing salivary cortisol in studies of child development. *Child Dev.* 1998;69:1503–1513.

Schurmeyer T, et al. Effect of ketoconazole and other imidazole fungicides on testosterone biosynthesis. *Acta Endocrinol (Copenh).* 1984;105:275–280.

Seamark RF, et al. Progesterone metabolism in ovine blood: the formation of 3-hydroxypregn 4 en 20 one and other substances. *Steroids.* 1970;15:589–604.

Segaloff A. Steroids and carcinogenesis. *Journal of Steroid Biochemistry.* 1975;6:171–175.

Selye H. Correlations between the chemical structure and the pharmacological actions of the steroids. *Endocrinology.* 1942;30:437–453.

Sheldrick EL, et al. Placental production of 5ß-pregnane-3,20-diol in goats. *Journal of Endocrinology.* 1981;90:151–158.

Sherwin BB, et al. The role of androgen in the maintenance of sexual functioning in oophorectomized women. *Psychosom Med.* 1987;49:397–409.

Shirtcliff EA, et al. Assessing estradiol in biobehavioral studies using saliva and blood spots: simple radioimmunoassay protocols, reliability, and comparative validity. *Horm Behav.* 2000;38:137–147.

Shirtcliff EA, et al. Use of salivary biomarkers in biobehavioral research: cotton-based sample collection methods can interfere with salivary immunoassay results. *Psychoneuroendocrinol.* 2001;26:165–173.

Shyamala G, et al. Cellular expression of estrogen and progesterone receptors in mammary glands: regulation by hormones, development and aging. *Journal of Steroid Biochemistry and Molecular Biology.* 2002;80:137–148.

Sikora R, et al. Ginkgo biloba extract in the therapy of erectile dysfunction. *J Urol.* 1989; 141:188A.

Siliutz G, et al. Agnus castus extracts inhibit prolactin secretion of rat pituitary cells. *Horm Metab Res.* 1993;25:253–255.

Simoncini T, et al. Genomic and non-genomic effects of estrogens on endothelial cells. *Steroids.* 2004;69:537–542.

Sitruk-Ware R. Pharmacological profile of progestins. *Maturitas.* 2004;47:277–283.

Slaunwhite WR, Jr, et al. Progesterone as a precursor of testicular androgens. *Journal of Biological Chemistry.* 1956;220:341–352.

Slotta KH, et al. Reindarstellung der Hormone aus dem Corpus-Luteum. *Berichte der Deutschen Chemischen Gesellschaft.* 1934;67:1270–1273.

Soto AM, et al. Control of cell proliferation: evidence for negative control on estrogen-sensitive T47D human breast cancer cells. *Cancer Research.* 1986;46:2271–2275.

Soule HD, et al. Isolation and characterization of a spontaneously immortalized human breast epithelial cell line, MCF-10. *Cancer Research.* 1990;50:6075–6086.

Sporn MB. The war on cancer. *Lancet.* 1996;347:1377–1381.

Stanczyk FZ, et al. Percutaneous administration of progesterone: blood levels and endometrial protection. *Menopause.* 2005;12:232–237.

Stegner HE, et al. Steroid metabolism in an androblastoma (Sertoli-Leydig cell tumor): a histopathological and biochemical study. *International Journal of Gynecological Pathology.* 1984;2:410–425.

Steinmetz K, et al. Vegetables, fruit, and cancer prevention: a review. *J Am Diet Assoc.* 1996;96:1027–1039.

Stephenson PU, et al. Modulation of cytochrome P4501A1 activity by ascorbigen in murine hepatoma cells. *Biochem Pharmacol.* 1999;58(7):1145–1153.

Steptoe A, et al. Job strain and anger expression predict early morning elevation in salivary cortisol. *Psychosom Med.* 2000;62:286–292.

Stones A, et al. The effect of stress on salivary cortisol in panic disorder patients. *J Affect Disorders.* 1999;52:197–201.

Stuerenburg HJ, et al. Effect of age on synthesis of the GABAergic steroids 5—pregnane-3,20-dione and 5—pregnane-3—ol-20-one in rat cortex in vitro. *Journal of Neural Transmission.* 1997;104:249–257.

Sugino N, et al. Progesterone inhibits 20-hydroxysteroid dehydrogenase expression in the rat corpus luteum through the glucocorticoid receptor. *Endocrinology.* 1997;138:4497–4500.

Sumiala S, et al. Salivary progesterone concentrations after tubal sterilization. *Obstet Gynecol.* 1996;88:792–796.

Suzuki H, et al. Decrease in gamma-actin expression, disruption of actin microfilaments and alterations in cell adhesion systems associated with acquisition of metastatic capacity in human salivary gland adenocarcinoma cell clones. *International Journal of Oncology.* 1998;12:1079–1084.

Suzuki T, et al. 5-Reductases in human breast carcinoma: possible modulator of in situ androgenic actions. *Journal of Clinical Endocrinology and Metabolism.* 2001;86:2250–2257.

Sweat ML, et al. The synthesis and metabolism of progesterone in the human and bovine ovary. *Biochimica et Biophysica Acta.* 1960;40:289–296.

Swinkels LM, et al. Concentrations of total and free dehydroepiandrosterone in plasma and dehydroepiandrosterone in saliva of normal and hirsute women under basal conditions and during administration of dexamethasone/synthetic corticotropin. *Clin Chem.* 1990;16:2042–2046.

Tada H, et al. New antiulcer quassinoids from Eurycoma longifolia. *European Journal of Medical Chemistry.* 1991;26:345–349.

Talalay P, et al. Chemoprotection against cancer by isothiocyanates and glucosinolates. *Biochem Soc Trans.* 1996;24:806–810.

Tan S, et al. HPLC analysis of plasma 9-methoxycanthin-6-one from Eurycoma longifolia and its application in a bioavailability/pharmacokinetic study. *Planta Medica.* 2002;68:355–358.

Tang MH, et al. Hepatoprotective action of schisandrin B against carbon tetrachloride toxicity was mediated by both enhancement of mitochondrial glutathione status and induction of heat shock proteins in mice. *Biofactors.* 2003;19(1–2):33–42.

Telang NT, et al. Inhibition of proliferation and modulation of estradiol metabolism: novel mechanisms for breast cancer prevention by the phytochemical indole-3-

carbinol. *Proc Soc Exp Biol Med.* 1997;216(2):246–252.

Thijssen JH, et al. Determination of dexamethasone in saliva. *Clin Chem.* 1996;42:1238–1242.

Thompson CB. Apoptosis in the pathogenesis and treatment of disease. *Science.* 1995;267:1456–1462.

Thompson LU, et al. Dietary flaxseed alters tumor biological markers in postmenopausal breast cancer. *Clin Cancer Res.* 2005 May 15;11(10):3828–3835.

Tilbe KS, et al. Sertoli cell capacity to metabolize progesterone: variation with age and the effect of follicle-stimulating hormone. *Endocrinology.* 198;108:597–604.

Toi M, et al. Preliminary studies on the anti-angiogenic potential of pomegranate fractions in vitro and in vivo. *Angiogenesis.* 2003;6(2):121–128.

Tripathi YB, et al. Thyroid stimulating action of Z-guggulsterone obtained from Commiphora mukul. *Planta Med.* 1984 Feb;50(1):78–80.

Tschop M, et al. A time-resolved fluorescence immunoassay for the measurement of testosterone in saliva: monitoring of testosterone replacement therapy with testosterone buciclate. *Clin Chem Lab Med.* 1998;36:223–230.

Tschudin S, et al. [Treatment of cyclical mastalgia with a solution containing a Vitex agnus castus extract: results of a placebo-controlled double-blind study. *Breast J.* 1999;8:175–181]. *Forsch Komplementarmed Klass Naturheilkd.* 2000;7(3):162–164.

Tulppala M, et al. Luteal phase defect in habitual abortion: progesterone in saliva. *Fertil Steril.* 1991;56:41–44.

Tunn S, et al. Simultaneous measurement of cortisol in serum and saliva after different forms of cortisol administration. Clin Chem. 1992;38:1491–1494.

Turgeon C, et al. Regulation of sex steroid formation by interleukin-4 and interleukin-6 in breast cancer cells. *Journal of Steroid Biochemistry and Molecular Biology.* 1998;6:151–162.

Turner S, et al. A double blind clinical trial on a herbal remedy for premenstrual syndrome: a case study. *Complimentary Therapies in Medicine.* 1993;1:73–77.

Uebelhack R, et al. Black cohosh and St. John's wort for climacteric complaints: a randomized trial. *Obstet Gynecol.* 2006 Feb;107(2 Pt 1):247–255.

Ukena K, et al. Developmental changes in progesterone biosynthesis and metabolism in the quail brain. *Brain Research.* 2001;898:190–194.

Ulrich LG. Accumulated knowledge of Kliogest safety aspects. *Br J Obstet Gynaecol.* 1996 May;103 Suppl 13:99–102; discussion 102–103. Review.

U.S. Department of Agriculture/U.S. Department of Health and Human Services. *Nutrition and Your Health: Dietary Guidelines for Americans.* 4th ed; 1995.

U.S. Food and Drug Administration. Report: Limited FDA Survey of Compounded Drug Products. Available at: http://www.fda.gov/cder/pharmcomp/survey.htm. Accessed 2007.

Valentova K, et al. The in vitro biological activity of Lepidium meyenii extracts. *Cell Biol Toxicol.* 2006 Mar;22(2):91 99.

Vanderbilt JN, et al. Intercellular receptor concentration limits gluco-corticoid-dependent enhancer activity. *Molecular Biology.* 1987;1:68–74.

Vedhara K, et al. Acute stress, memory, attention and cortisol. *Psychoneuroendocrinol.* 2000;25:535–549.

Verhoeven DT, et al. Epidemiological studies on brassica vegetables and cancer risk. *Cancer Epidemiol Biomarkers Prev.* 1996;5:733–748.

Verhoeven DT, et al. A review of mechanisms underlying anticarcinogenicity by brassica vegetables. *Chem Biol Interact.* 1997;103:79–129.

Vincent A, et al. Soy isoflavones: are they useful in menopause? *Mayo Clin Proc.* 2000;75(11):1174–1184.

Vining RF,et al. Hormones in saliva: mode of entry and consequent implications for clinical interpretation. *Clin Chem.* 1983;29:1752–1756.

Vining RF, et al. The measurement of hormones in saliva: possibilities and pitfalls. *J Steroid Biochem.* 1987;27(1–3):81–94.

Viscoli CM, et al. A clinical trial of estrogen-replacement therapy after ischemic stroke. *N Engl J Med.* 2002;346(12):942–943.

Vittek J, et al. Direct radioimmunoassay (RIA) of salivary testosterone: correlation with free and total serum testosterone. *Life Sciences.* 1985;37:711–716.

Volicer L, et al. Some pharmacological effects of Schisandra chinensis. *Arch Int Pharmacodyn Ther.* 1966;163:249–262.

Vooijs GP, et al. Review of the endometrial safety during intravaginal treatment with estriol. *Eur J Obstet Gynecol Reprod Biol.* 1995 Sep;62(1):101–106. Review.

Voss HF. Saliva as a fluid for measurement of estradiol levels. *Am J Obstet Gynecol.* 1999;180:S226–231.

Vuorento T, et al. Daily measurements of salivary progesterone reveal a high rate of anovulation in healthy students. *Scand J Clin Lab Invest.* 1989;49:395–401.

Waddell BJ, et al. Distribution and metabolism of topically applied progesterone in a rat model. *J Steroid Biochem Mol Biol.* 2002;80:449–455.

Walker RF, et al. Chronobiology in laboratory medicine: principles and clinical applications illustrated from measurements of neutral steroids in saliva. *Prog Clin Biol Res.* 1990;341A:105–117.

Wang DY, et al. Salivary oestradiol and progesterone levels in premenopausal women with breast cancer. *Eur J Cancer Clin Oncol.* 1986 Apr;22(4):427–433.

Wang DY, et al. Salivary progesterone: relation to total and non-protein-bound blood levels. *J Steroid Biochem.* 1985;23:975–979.

Wang L, et al. The inhibitory effect of flaxseed on the growth and metastasis of estrogen receptor negative human breast cancer xenograftsis attributed to both its lignan and oil components. *Int J Cancer.* 2005 Sep 20;116(5):793–798.

Wantanabe M, et al. Forskolin up-regulates aromatase (CYP19) activity and gene transcripts in the human adrenocortical carcinoma cell line H295R. *J Endocrinol.* 2004;180:125–133.

Watson CS, et al. Rapid actions of estrogens in GH3/B6 pituitary tumor cells via a plasma membrane version of estrogen receptor-. *Steroids.* 1999;64:5–13.

Webb P, et al. The limits of the cellular capacity to mediate an estrogen response. *Molecular Endocrinology.* 1992;6:157–167.

Webster K, et al. Oestrogen and progesterone increase the levels of apoptosis induced by the human papillomavirus type 16 E2 and E7 proteins. *J Gen Virol.* 2001 Jan;82(Pt 1):201–213.

Weeks C, et al. Preclinical toxicology evaluation of 3-acetyl-7-oxo-dehydroepiandrosterone (7-keto DHEA). *FASEB J.* 1998;12:A4428.

Wehling M. Specific, nongenomic actions of steroid hormones. *Annual Review of Physiology.* 1997;59:365–395.

Weiderpass E, et al. Low-potency oestrogen and risk of endometrial cancer: a case-control study. *Lancet.* 1999;353:1824–1828.

Weiler PJ, et al. Plasma membrane receptors for the cancer-regulating progesterone metabolites, 5-pregnane-3,20-dione and 3-hydroxy-4-pregnen-20-one in MCF-7 breast cancer cells. *Biochemical and Biophysical Research Communications.* 2000;272:731–737.

Wellen JJ, et al. Testosterone and androstenedione in the saliva of patients with Klinefelter's Syndrome. *Clin Endocrinol.* 1983;18:51–59.

Welsh CW. 1982. *Hormonal Regulation of Mammary Tumors.* "Hormones and murine mammary tumorigenesis: an historical view." Montreal, Canada: Eden Press; 1-29.

Wiebe JP. Isolated Sertoli cells from immature rats produce 20-hydroxy-pregn-4-en-3-one from progesterone and 5-pregnane-3ß,20-diol from pregnenolone. *Biochemical and Biophysical Research Communications.* 1978;84:1003–1008.

Wiebe JP. Nongenomic actions of steroids on gonadotropin release. *Recent Progress in Hormone Research.* 1997;52:71–101.

Wiebe JP. Role of progesterone metabolites in mammary cancer. *Journal of Dairy Research.* 2005;72:51–57.

Wiebe JP, et al. Activity and expression of progesterone metabolizing 5-reductase, 20-hydroxysteroid oxidoreductase and 3(ß)-hydroxysteroid oxidoreductases in tumorigenic (MCF-7, MDA-MB-231, T-47D) and nontumorigenic (MCF-10A) human breast cancer cells. *BMC Cancer.* 2003;3:(9) 1–15. Available at: http://www.biomedcentral.com/1471-2407/3/9. Accessed June 2007.

Wiebe JP, et al. Analgesic effects of the putative FSH- suppressing gonadal steroid, 3-

hydroxy-4-pregnen-20-one: possible modes of action. *Brain Research.* 1988; 461:150–157.

Wiebe JP, et al. An analysis of the metabolites of progesterone produced by isolated Sertoli cells at the onset of gametogenesis. *Steroids.* 1980;35:561–577.

Wiebe JP, et al. *De novo* synthesis of steroids (from acetate) by isolated rat Sertoli cells. *Biochemical and Biophysical Research Communications.* 1979;89:1107–1113.

Wiebe JP, et al. Dutasteride affects progesterone metabolizing enzyme activity/expression in human breast cell lines resulting in suppression of cell proliferation and detachment. *Journal of Steroid Biochemistry and Molecular Biology.* 2006;100:129–140.

Wiebe JP, et al. The endogenous progesterone metabolite, 5-pregnene-3,20-dione, decreases cell-substrate attachment, adhesion plaques, vinculin expression, and polymerized F-actin in MCF-7 breast cancer cells. *Endocrine.* 2001;16:7–14.

Wiebe JP, et al. Metabolism of progesterone by avian granulosa cells in culture. *Journal of Steroid Biochemistry and Molecular Biology.* 1990;37:113–120.

Wiebe JP, et al. Modification of steroidogenesis in rat adrenocortical cells transformed by Kirsten Murine Sarcoma virus. *Cancer Research.* 1987;47:1325–1332.

Wiebe JP, et al. The progesterone metabolites, 5-dihydroprogesterone (5P) and 3-hydroxy-4-pregnen-20-one (3HP), have opposing effects on cell substrate adhesion, amount of polymerized actin and adhesion plaque-associated vinculin in MCF-7, MCF-10A, MDA-MB-231 and T47D breast cell lines. Paper presented at: The Endocrine Society 86th Annual Meeting; June 16–19, 2004; New Orleans, LA.

Wiebe JP, et al. A radio-immunoassay for the regulatory allylic steroid, 3-hydroxy-4-pregnen-20-one (3HP). *Journal of Steroid Biochemistry and Molecular Biology.* 1991;38:505–512.

Wiebe JP, et al. The role of progesterone metabolites in breast cancer: potential for new diagnostics and therapeutics. *Journal of Steroid Biochemistry and Molecular Biology.* 2005;93:201–208.

Wiebe JP, et al. Synthesis, metabolism and levels of the neuroactive steroid, 3-hydroxy-4-pregnen-20-one (3HP), in rat pituitaries. *Brain Research.* 1997;764:158–166.

Wiebe JP, et al. Suppression in gonadotropes of gonado-tropin-releasing hormone-stimulated follicle-stimulating hormone release by the gonadal- and neurosteroid, 3-hydroxy-4-pregnen-20-one involves cytosolic calcium. *Endocrinology.* 1994b;134:377–382.

Wiebe JP, et al. Synthesis of the allylic regulatory steroid, 3-hydroxy-4-pregnen-20-one, by rat granulosa cells and its regulation by gonadotropins. *Biology of Reproduction.* 1994a;50:956–964.

Wiebe JP, et al. The 4-pregnene and 5-pregnane progesterone metabolites formed in non-tumorous and tumorous breast tissue have opposite effects on breast cell proliferation and adhesion. *Cancer Research.* 2000;60:936–943.

Wiest WG. The metabolism of progesterone to delta4-pregnen-20-ol-3-one in eviscerated female rats. *Journal of Biological Chemistry.* 1956;221:461–467.

Wilkins JA, et al. High-affinity interaction of vinculin with actin filaments. *Cell.* 1982;28:83–90.

Wong GY, et al. Dose-ranging study of indole-3-carbinol for breast cancer prevention. *J Cell Biochem Suppl.* 1997;29:111–116.

Wong YF, et al. Salivary estradiol and progesterone during the normal ovulatory menstrual cycle in Chines women. *Eur J Obstet Gynecol Reprod Biol.* 1990;34:129–135.

Wood PH, et al. Selective suppression of FSH secretion in anterior pituitary cells in culture by the gonadal steroid, 3-hydroxy-4-pregnen-20-one (3HP). *Endocrinology.* 1989;125:41–48.

Worthman CM, et al. Sensitive salivary estradiol assay for monitoring ovarian function. *Clin Chem.* 1990;36:1769–1773.

Wren B, et al. Effect of sequential transdermal progesterone cream on endometrium, bleeding pattern, and plasma progesterone and salivary progesterone levels in postmenopausal women. *Cliamcteric.* 2000;3:155–160.

Wright J, et al. *Maximize Your Vitality & Potency For Men Over 40.* "Reported Effects of Low Testosterone." Petaluma, CA: Smart Publications; 1999.

Wu J, et al. The hypolipidemic natural product guggulsterone acts as an antagonist of the bile acid receptor. *Mol Endocrinol.* 2002 Jul;16(7):1590–1597.

Wu WH, et al. Estrogenic effect of yam ingestion in healthy postmenopausal women. *J Am Coll Nutr.* 2005 Aug;24(4):235–243.

Xu M, et al. Post-initiation effects of chlorophyllin and indole-3-carbinol in rats given 1,2-dimethylhydrazine or 2-amino-3-methyl-imidazo[4,5-f]quinoline. *Carcinogenesis.* 2001;22:309–314.

Xu X, et al. Effects of soy isoflavones on estrogen and phytoestrogen metabolism in premenopausal women. *Cancer Epidemiol Biomarkers Prev.* 1998;7(12):1101–1118.

Xu X, et al. Soy consumption alters endogenous estrogen metabolism in postmenopausal women. *Cancer Epidemiol Biomarkers Prev.* 2000;9(8):781–786.

Xue JY, et al. Antioxidant activity of two dibenzocyclooctene lignans on the aged and ischemic brain in rats. *Free Radic Biol Med.* 1992;12(2):127–135.

Yager JD. Endogenous estrogens as carcinogens through metabolic activation. *J Natl Cancer Inst Monogr.* 2000;27: 67–73.

Yang TS, et al. Efficacy and safety of estriol replacement therapy for climacteric women. *Zhonghua Yi Xue Za Zhi (Taipei).* 1995 May;55(5):386–391.

Yim TK, et al. Schisandrin B protects against myocardial ischemia-reperfusion injury by enhancing myocardial glutathione antioxidant status. *Mol Cell Biochem.* 1999 Jun;196(1 2):151 156.

Young MC, et al. Androstenedione rhythms in saliva in congenital adrenal hyperplasia. *Arch Dis Child.* 1988;63:624–628.

Yu H, et al. Plasma sex steroid hormones and breast cancer risk in Chinese women. *Int J Cancer.* 2003 May 20;105(1):92–97.

Zainah A. [master's thesis]. Penang, Malaysia: Universiti Sains Malaysia, School of Pharmceutical Sciences; 2003.

Zand RS, et al. Steroid hormone activity of flavonoids and related compounds. *Breast Cancer Res Treat.* 2000;62:35–49.

Zava DT, et al. Estrogen and progestin bioactivity of foods, herbs, and spices. *Proc Soc Exp Biol Med.* 1998 Mar;217(3):369–378.

Zeleniuch-Jacquotte A, et al. Postmenopausal levels of oestrogen, androgen, and SHBG and breast cancer: long-term results of a prospective study. *Br J Cancer.* 2004 Jan 12;90(1):153–159.

Zhai S, et al. Comparative Inhibition of Human Cytochromes P450 1A1 and 1A2 by flavonoids. *Drug Metab Dispos.* 1998 Oct;26(10):989–992.

Zhang G, et al. Opposing effects of the progesterone metabolites, 5-pregnane-3,20-dione (5P) and 3-hydroxy-4-pregnen-20-one (3HP) on apoptosis in MCF-7 and T-47D breast cancer cells. Abstract #P3-652, p 705. The Endocrine Society 87th Annual Meeting; June 4–7, 2005; San Diego, CA.

Zhang J, et al. Progesterone metabolism in human fibroblasts is independent of P-glycoprotein levels and Niemann-Pick type C disease. *Journal of Steroid Biochemistry and Molecular Biology.* 1999;70:123–131.

Zhang JG, et al. Mitochondrial electron transport inhibitors cause lipid peroxidation-dependent and -independent cell death: protective role of antioxidants. *Arch Biochem Biophys.* 2001;393:87–96.

Zhang Y, et al. Effect of ethanol extract of Lepidium meyenii Walp. on osteoporosis in ovariectomized rat. J Ethnopharmacol. 2006 Apr 21;105(1–2):274–279.

Zhang Y, et al. A major inducer of anticarcinogenic protective enzymes from broccoli: isolation and elucidation of structure. *Proc Natl Acad Sci.* 1992;89:2399–2403.

Zhang Y, et al. Anticarcinogenic activities of sulforaphane and structurally related synthetic norbornyl isothiocyanates. *Proceedings of the National Academy of Sciences USA.* 1994;91:3147–3150.

Zhong L, et al. Prolactin-mediated inhibition of 20-hydroxysteroid dehydrogenase gene expression and the tyrosine kinase system. *Biochemical and Biophysical Research Communications.* 1997;235:587–592.

Zmigrod A, et al. Reductive pathways of progesterone metabolism in the rat ovary. *Acta Endocrinologica (Copenh).* 1972;69:141–152.

Index

low thyroid and, 38
progesterone and, 36
St. John's wort for, 135–36
testosterone for, 75
D-glucarate, 85–86, 171
DHA (docosahexaenoic acid), 156
DHEA (dehydroepiandrosterone),
17, 23, 25, 27, 37, 40, 76
DHEAS (dehydroepiandrosterone-
sulfate), 25, 44
DHT blood test, 44
diabetes, 15, 37, 40, 44
diet,
for boosting sexy hormones,
164–78
for maintaining hormonal
balance, 147–63
dioscorea. See wild yam
docosahexaenoic acid, 156
doctors, biodentical-friendly, 78
dong quai, 129
drugs, 61, 137.
See also names of individual drugs
dysglycemia, 50
dysmenorrhea (painful
menstruation), 38, 127, 129
dyspareunia (painful intercourse),
37, 38, 40, 72, 212

E

echium oil,
for endometriosis, 98
for FBD, 103
GLA and, 92, 93,155–56
for heavy menstruation, 96
for ovarian cysts, 102
for PCOS, 102
for uterine fibroids, 96
EFAs, 154
Eleutherococcus senticosus, 108–109
endometrial cancer, 56, 72, 119

endometriosis,
biodentical hormones for, 98
CA-125 blood test, 53
estrogens and, 37
fat cells and, 14
immune system and, 99
laparascopy for, 98
low thyroid and, 38
non-drug treatments for, 98
in peri-menopause, 40
progesterone and, 36
symptoms, 97–98
xenoestrogens and, xx
Energie Kegel, 200
essential fatty acids (EFAs), 154
Estrace, 61, 77
Estraderm, 61, 77
estradiol (E2), xx–xxi, 20, 32, 42–43,
175
Estradot, 77
Estratab, 61
Estring, 61, 77
estriol (E3), 20, 21, 33, 65–67,
71–72, 77, 124
Estrogel, 77
estrogen dominance, xvii, 175–76
estrogen-dominant conditions, xx,
37, 94–95, 104. See also names of
individual conditions
Estrogen HRT patch, 145
estrogenic foods, 176–77
estrogens,
alcohol and, 176
androstenedione and, 22
aromatase and, 22
biodentical, 70–72
breast cancer and, 23
cortisol and, 7
cycle in women, 81–83
dietary regulators of, 168, 170
environmental.
See xenoestrogens

vitamin D, 8, 114–15
vitamin K, 96, 97
Vitex (chaste tree berry), 83,
    91–92, 96, 98, 102, 129–30

W

weight-bearing exercise, 182,
    183–84
weight loss, 38, 121
weights, 183–84
WHI research study, 57–58, 69,
    78
wild yam, 61, 72–73, 169
Wiler / PCCA Canada, 79
Withania somnifera. See
    ashwagandha
withdrawal from synthetic
    hormones, 144–46
Women's Health Initiative
    (WHI), 57–58, 69, 78

X

xenoestrogens, xix–xxii,
    xxvii–xxviii
xylitol, 151

Y

yam, wild, 61, 72–73, 169
York Downs Pharmacy, 79

Z

zinc deficiency, 166
Zoloft, 122, 137
ZRT Laboratory, 46

About the Authors

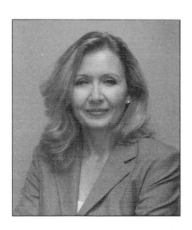

Lorna R. Vanderhaeghe, M.S. is Canada's leading women's natural health expert. Lorna has a Masters in Health Studies in nutrition and a degree in biochemistry. She is the author of eight books and thousands of articles. Lorna believes in empowering people with health knowledge so they may achieve optimal wellness. Lorna has an award winning website www.healthyimmunity.com and a monthly health e-letter. She is also the host of the internet talk show *Ask Lorna*.

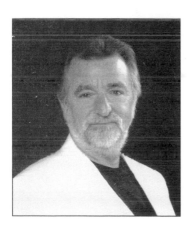

Alvin Pettle, M.D. is a pioneer Canadian Gynecologist who practices integrative medicine. He graduated from the University of Toronto Medical School in 1969 and received his fellowship in Obstetrics and Gynecology in 1974. Dr. Pettle is viewed as an authoritative figure in integrative medicine and therapies for women. He is a preeminent specialist in natural hormone replacement therapy. Dr. Pettle has an informative website at www.drpettle.com